# Food for Thought

Nutrition and the Aging Brain

**Richard A. Dienstbier**

Professor Emeritus, Psychology Department,
University of Nebraska

**Cognitive Science and Psychology**

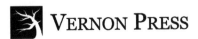
VERNON PRESS

www.vernonpress.com

*In the Americas:*
Vernon Press
1000 N West Street, Suite 1200
Wilmington, Delaware, 19801
United States

*In the rest of the world:*
Vernon Press
C/Sancti Espiritu 17,
Malaga, 29006
Spain

Cognitive Science and Psychology

Library of Congress Control Number: 2022939068

ISBN: 978-1-64889-556-2

Also available: 978-1-64889-470-1 [Hardback]; 978-1-64889-501-2 [PDF, E-Book]

Cover design by Vernon Press. The cover image is from a photo by the author of a market in Guatemala.

# Table of contents

# Introduction

Perhaps because aging and I are becoming inseparable companions, I am increasingly interested in anything that might slow or even prevent the cognitive decline that often accompanies the aging brain. In a previous book, I analyzed how activities such as systematic exercise, cognitive stimulation, and even affectionate and social activities could lead to cognitive sharpening and psychological resilience. I realized subsequently that the impact of nutrition on delaying cognitive decline was at least as important as those activities. Hence this book.

With cognitive decline in mind, consider that while much of modern nutrition research assesses impacts on lifespan, the newer term "healthspan" describes our years of living with good health. Nutritionists interested in healthspan usually emphasize cardiovascular health, diabetes, cancer, obesity, or similar indicators of physical health. Lifespan and healthspan are not always correlated; indeed, some nutritive interventions that extend the one can limit the other (e.g., Wilson et al., 2021). But the focus of this book is on nutrition's impacts on the aging brain, on our possibly-declining cognitive abilities, and on our changing emotional dispositions. Perhaps we need a different term for that—one that more accurately describes mental preservation. Just free-associating, perhaps "cogspan" or even "smartspan" could indicate our later years of lucidity. Unfortunately and obviously, neither of those terms has any real pizzazz, so I withdraw them from official consideration. But pizzazz or not, I am fond of "smartspan" and I hope mine is long and steady.

Of course, my concerns with aging and cognition are not unique. As we approach our "best by" date, most of us hope that our life pattern reflects healthy elderly years with all our mental faculties intact, at least until we are overtaken by our genetic limitations. The pattern of a healthy and lucid elderly life followed by death that arrives without dragging her feet is the "squaring of the curve." Thus the "squaring" is not a gradual decline, but rather a late-but-quick one.

Assessing impacts on brain health from nutrition leads to unique recommendations because nutrition that does not extend life or save us from cardiovascular disasters should not necessarily be dismissed; it may add to the curve squaring of mental health and cognitive capacities. Consider, for example, recent observations that multi-vitamin supplements have not been proven to extend life and may therefore be "a waste of money." However, as noted extensively below, vitamin supplements may still contribute to brain health, cognitive preservation, and other aspects of mental health, especially for those of us with some nutritive deficiencies. And as for "wasting money," even multivitamin formulations for older people like me cost only US $.10; they are affordable. Actually, the stand taken by many nutritionists against supplements is justified by their recognition that many essential nutrients can only be obtained from food—not from supplements, and they recognize that many of us substitute supplements to allay concerns about poor dietary choices.

Another reason for emphasizing brain health and preserving cognition is that some nutrients may have different impacts on brain health than they do on other aspects of physical health. For example, there is some evidence that moderate doses of alcohol enhance cardiovascular health, but those same moderate levels have sometimes been found to be harmful for brain and/or cognition, or sometimes beneficial (yes!) depending on the important factors discussed in Chapter 14.

Other nutrients like tryptophan that have positive effects on neurochemical balances and thus moods and energy may have no known positive impacts on longevity (Canfield & Bradshaw, 2019).

**Consistency.** The history of research on nutrition seems filled with inconsistent findings—sometimes outright contradictions. Those of us lucky enough to have progressed to "old" or even all the way to "elderly" have experienced the whip-lash of research informing us that previously good nutrients were actually bad for us, and vice versa. To mention just a few examples, assessments of eggs have gone from bad to good—especially good for brains, whereas some margarine, that used to save us from "awful" butter, has progressed largely from good to bad; transfats that used to be added to everything delicious are now considered almost deadly, and sugar-filled drinks keep getting worse and worse. Some of the artificial sweeteners that otherwise could "save" us from the sugar have proven to be awful for us. Whole milk may not be so bad after all, and some cheeses are absolutely great for us (perhaps only slightly exaggerated for personal reasons). Long-term coffee consumption has emerged from probably bad to quite good, and thankfully even chocolate turns out to be increasingly wonderful.

Keep in mind that inconsistencies in nutrition research are not unique. Rather than dismissing nutrition research because of its occasional inconsistencies, we should examine the research with caution and the reservations discussed in Chapter 3, and even then perhaps view at least some of the inconsistencies as signs of scientific progress.

**Smart supplements.** An overarching issue of inconsistent nutrition research is whether *any* diet or supplement has substantial benefits for preserving brain and cognition, and for delaying dementia. It was only in 2015 that the lead journal of the Association for Psychological Science called nutritional mental health an "emerging" field (Kaplan et al., 2015, p. 964). Yet even well before 2015, research on major dietary approaches such as the Mediterranean diet showed that smart nutrition choices do indeed support brain maintenance and development, enhance cognition, buttress our better moods, and even delay dementia.

But what about specific nutrients, and supplements? In the editor's introduction to a special section on nutrition and mental health in the journal *Clinical Psychological Science*, Kazdin (2016, p. 1080) noted that there are "controlled clinical trials showing that psychiatric symptoms and disorders respond to micronutrient interventions." However, summaries of the larger body of research on specific nutrients and supplements are mixed. Those inconsistencies often bother people who try to be conscientious about their nutrition, and the sometimes-bogus information from some purveyors of supplements does not help.

According to the US Government Accountability Office report from 2017, many advertisements that describe the benefits of various supplements are simply untrue, and some are even illegal. Specifically focusing on cognition, a *Consumer Reports* article recently asked "Do memory supplements really work?" and answered with quotations from authorities that "dietary supplements cannot cure, mitigate, treat, or prevent Alzheimer's dementia, or any disease" (Calderone, 2018, p. 2).

A major purpose of this book is to address that issue, mostly by examining research published in the last decade or so. But before we go there, reconsider the phrase that "dietary supplements cannot cure, mitigate, treat, or prevent Alzheimer's dementia, or any disease." I shall show that modern research justifies denying that phrase. As written, it is simply wrong. But beyond questioning its accuracy as written, note also that "*or delay*" was *not* included. Perhaps we should not reject a supplement that has solid research support for *delaying* cognitive decline or *delaying* dementias such as Alzheimer's, or one that delays or *mitigates* depression. After all, a delay could extend a decade or two. Nor should we write off the potential for major benefits to brain, cognition, or mental health from some supplements merely because of occasional bogus and fraudulent claims.

We should remain especially aware of the potential needs for "essential nutrients." Essential nutrients are nutrients that we require from our food because we humans cannot synthesize them in our bodies in sufficient quantities. There seem to be 40 to 50 of them—around 15 each of vitamins and minerals, some amino acids, and a few essential fatty acids. In ideal conditions, we would be able to derive those nutrients from the foods we consume, but that may not always be the case. Supplements may be required, or at least very beneficial, and those supplements may be important for maintaining balances of nutrients that are not technically essential. For example, with exposure to sufficient sunlight, our bodies can usually synthesize enough vitamin D, but when winter arrives in Northern lands, we benefit from an occasional salmon, or, failing that, even from a drugstore supplement. Naturally, our concern with important nutrients goes beyond those that are technically called essential.

**Expertise.** It would be appropriate for readers to question my authority for saying such things. The answer, like nutrition itself, is complicated. Because I am not a nutritionist I recognize that my occasionally questioning real nutritionists must seem a bit audacious. My interests as a psychologist are in how neurochemistry and various neural and brain processes affect our cognitive capacities and our resilience. As mentioned above, my previous book, titled *"Building resistance to stress and aging: The toughness model"* was about how activities such as physical exercise, some social activities, cognitive challenges, etc. enhance neurochemistry and neural structures (i.e., toughen us), and then how those physiological modifications lead to enhanced cognition and to psychological resilience. But for those activities to enhance neurochemistry and neural structures the right nutritive elements must be available in sufficient amounts. And they do make a difference.

To continue being audacious, I believe that a case can be made for a book such as this being produced by a non-nutritionist. Without pre-conceived notions about the effectiveness of any of the nutrients or supplements described within, I have dived into the modern research; and the reference section of well over 300 research papers is heavy with reviews, sometimes with meta-analyses—reviews and analyses mostly by real nutritionists to whom I owe a great debt.

**What lies ahead.** First, note that this is not designed to be a "self help" book. Rather it is a book about nutrition science, and neuroscience, cognitive science, and to a lesser extent about the science of stress tolerance, depression, and anxiety. Although I make some dietary recommendations that leak into some of the chapters and are summarized in Chapter 20, my primary goal is to provide the scientific information to allow readers to make their own nutrition choices.

In fact, if you need more information to feel confident about your choices, doing further scholarship on your own is really not that difficult. Simply access "Google Scholar" and then enter your own keywords such as "lutein cognition review" and limit the search to (say) papers published after 2010. The article abstracts you obtain from such searches may be readable and all that you really need. However, if you need the entire paper, clicking an icon for "PDF" or something similar may quickly download your paper. If you have access to an academic library, the Interlibrary Loan office can get the paper for you. If worst comes to it, you can almost always pay for a copy.

The structure of the book is that the first three chapters provide a foundation for understanding impacts on brain, cognition, and resilience. Chapter 1 very lightly sketches relevant brain structure and neurochemistry. Chapter 2 discusses in only slightly more detail how aging and stress affect neurochemistry, brain structure, cognitive capacities, and resilience. Chapter 3 introduces basic nutrition research issues—the good, the bad, and the ugly. The brain scientists among you may wish to skim or even skip the first two or even three of those chapters. Chapters 4 through 17 consolidate the credible modern research on impacts of nutrition on brain and cognitive capacities. Chapter 18 describes nutrition that affects psychological resilience, interpreted there as stress tolerance, and resistance to both anxiety and depression.

Chapter 19 describes how activities that toughen us can interact with nutrition that has similar effects. Although toughening activities include the wide array listed above, Chapter 19 will be limited to the interplay of nutrition with physical exercise and cognitive challenge. After all, I must stop somewhere. Chapter 20 offers afterthoughts and briefly summarizes the highlights of nutrition impacts on brain and cognition.

The Glossary is meant to be an informative and substantial part of the book, designed to relieve any pain I may have inflicted with scanty explanations in the text. Please use it.

**Thanks and acknowledgements.** My wife Karen has been most patient. Being cooped up together during the pandemic has led to interesting interactions. Often she has come upon me talking to my computer screen, obviously confused, but trying desperately to figure it all out. At such times I have not been the great communicator she may have wished. My thanks for putting up with all of it.

Most sincerely, I thank the thousand or so scholars who prepared the research papers and reviews that I have devoured to obtain a reasonable level of understanding of this most interesting topic.

Chapter 1

# Basic brain processes and genetics

To understand how aging and stress can degrade brain and cognition, and how nutrition and some toughening activities have beneficial impacts, in this brief chapter, I discuss relevant neural structures and neurochemistry and then process some words about basic genetic functions. This chapter is only modestly technical, and therefore like the rest of the book, with minimal consternation it should be accessible to non-scientists. If some terms seem unfamiliar, remember that the occasionally-useful Glossary is provided, but on the other hand, scientists who are good with brains may wish to skim this chapter.

## Neurons, glia, and structures of concern

**Neurons.** It is the activity of our neurons that results in the mental processes that we cherish—at least we cherish them when the neurons are behaving. Unfortunately, aging and stress both negatively affect their functioning, but as noted in other chapters, our neurons are supported and enhanced by appropriate nutrition and various toughening activities. Please glance at Figure 1.1. There is little information besides the figure and its caption that needs to be covered at this time.

**Glia.** The glia are the cells of the brain that perform many supporting roles for the neurons. Although the glia cells were thought previously to vastly outnumber the neurons, modern evidence suggests equal numbers of neurons and glia, with close to 100 billion of each. There are several types of glia, but the astrocytes and microglia are most relevant for us because they perform immune functions in the brain and clean waste products and the distorted proteins that otherwise can accumulate and degrade neural functions. Those immune functions and cleaning tasks defend us against dementia, and as described later, one of the paths for nutrition to enhance cognition is by boosting the effectiveness of the microglia and astrocytes.

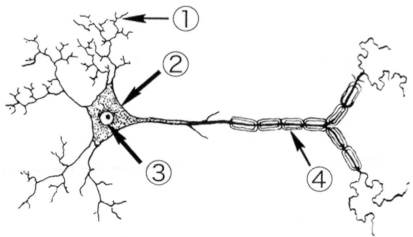

**Figure 1.1. A Basic Neuron**

The basic structures of a neuron, rendered with great artistic license. The parts represented are (1) the dendrites covered by spines with synapses, (2) the neural cell body, (3) the cell nucleus, and (4) the axon covered with a myelin sheath. The neural impulse travels from left to right, ultimately activating synapses at the ends of the axons. The image is modified from Wickimedia Commons; it was published initially by Pearson Scott Foresman and is available at http://commons.wikimedia.org/wiki/File:Neuron_%28PSF%29.png.

**The gray cortex and white matter.** The brain's cortex is the remarkably thin outer covering consisting of neural cell bodies and the dendrites that are the branches that receive impulses. Although only up to a half centimeter thick, because of being folded in various ways the volume of the gray cortex of the human brain is over half the total brain's volume. In other mammals, the ratio of cortex to total brain is much smaller. That large cortical volume is handy in us humans because the cortex is where our higher-order mental processing takes place. In fact, given our great human cortex, one would have thought we humans might have avoided our wars, been better at protecting the environment, and at choosing less-narcissistic politicians. But as emphasized by the psychologists taken with the notion of emotional intelligence, a big cortex isn't everything.

The axons of the neurons that connect far-flung neural networks are coated by myelin—the white fatty substance supplied by the glia cells called oligodendrocytes; myelin is shown in Figure 1.1. Myelin acts metaphorically like an insulator on an electrical wire, allowing neural impulses to travel quickly. Large tracts of such white myelin-coated axons in the brain are called (no real surprise here) "white matter." The corpus callosum shown in Figure

1.2 is such a tract of white matter, consisting of 200 million well-myelinated axons that provide the connection between the two hemispheres.

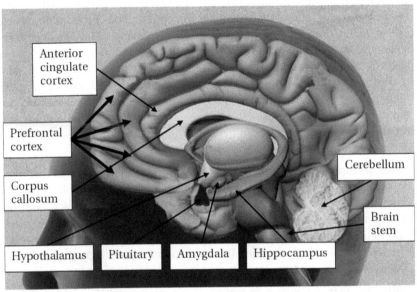

**Figure 1.2. A labeled brain**
Although this gentleman's brain was sliced between the two hemispheres, the hippocampi emerge from mid-brain outward toward the sides of the brain into the temporal lobes. The two easily-excited amygdalae are located near the temporal-lobe ends of the hippocampi. The image has been modified from one provided by the USA's National Institute on Aging/National Institutes of Health and is available at http://www.nia.nih.gov/alzheimers/scientific-images#brain.

**Hippocampi.** The brain structures mentioned the most throughout the book are the hippocampi. (The singular is hippocampus.) The hippocampi assemble episodic memories. Episodic memories are memories of the events of our lives—not how to play chess or speak French—but rather where, how, and what it was like to learn chess or French. The components of such memories include emotional feelings, and elements that may be visual, auditory, tactile, olfactory (smell), etc. Those different types of elements are stored in different brain areas—the visual components in brain structures that process vision, and so on. When later recalled, our hippocampi reactivate the same scattered brain areas that stored the components and reassemble those components into a (hopefully) coherent memory (Danker & Anderson, 2010). Episodic memories are gradually lost when people experience profound cognitive decline and/or dementia. Because they are the stories of our lives, their loss is usually tragic.

**Prefrontal cortex.** The frontal lobes consist of most of the front half of the adult human's brain. The front section of those frontal lobes—essentially the part above our eyes—is the prefrontal cortex. We cannot take our prefrontal cortex for granted because it is where we do much of the mental heavy lifting needed for our conscious cognitive functions. The prefrontal cortex's executive functions include reasoning, problem-solving, planning, organizing goals, and building the plans for reaching our goals, etc. The prefrontal cortex also contributes to working memory (i.e., conscious mental processing), and it contributes to regulating our emotional responses, and to focusing and maintaining attention. Because many of those cognitive activities do not typically function automatically, they require our conscious attention and often require widespread neural networks working together diligently for our occasional novel solutions.

Like the hippocampi the prefrontal cortex is the kind of busy area that must be modified as we develop new memories and skills; thus, it is plastic, implying that it is susceptible to structural modifications. In fact, both the hippocampi and the prefrontal cortex shrink with chronic stress, aging, and with deficient nutrition, but they can increase in volume with combinations of relief from stress, brain-friendly nutrients, and the toughening activities described in Chapter 19.

**Mitochondria.** I sketch information about mitochondria only briefly here because the mitochondria star in their own Chapter 15. Our mitochondria are the energy-generating organelles found in huge quantities in all of our cells—not just in the brain. Actually, thousands can be packed (carefully) into a single cell. By producing all our energy, in many ways, our mitochondria regulate our lives. But unfortunately, a byproduct of their exertions is an especially reactive type of oxygen molecule technically termed "reactive oxygen species." Those reactive oxygen molecules cause mutations and other forms of damage to the mitochondria themselves and to the cells that host them. The genetic damage accelerates with stress and accumulates with age.

The organs most susceptible to the damage from reactive oxygen species are the heart and the brain, because both are huge energy consumers. Even when we are merely day-dreaming, the brain uses 20-25% of all the energy that our body produces. Thus a huge proportion of that dangerously reactive oxygen is produced in the brain where it can molest neurons and glia. Fortunately, however, that damage can be limited by antioxidants that are supplied by our food or even from supplements.

## Neurochemistry

**Neurotransmitters.** All mental activity depends upon communication between neurons, but the neurons that try to signal each other do not make physical contact; instead, they are separated by a gap—a synapse. When a signal is sent from a sending neuron to a receiving neuron, neurotransmitter molecules are released from the axon ends of the sending neuron into the synapse between the neurons. When receptors on the dendrites (i.e., the receiving ends) of the receiving neuron detect enough of those neurotransmitter molecules, the receiving neuron transmits the signal onward. At least that is what happens when things go well (and if the receiving neurons are not texting someone). Unfortunately, both stress and aging deplete levels of available neurotransmitters, degrading communication between neurons.

I do not want to overload details here concerning the specialized roles for different neurotransmitters like dopamine, serotonin, acetylcholine and GABA; some relevant information will come later. For the moment, note that the different neurotransmitters have different functions, and whether due to aging, stress, inadequate nutrition, or other factors, shortages of neurotransmitters have noticeable impacts. Good nutrition helps, but the neurotransmitters are sufficiently different from each other so that (to some extent) they are nurtured by different nutrients.

**Neurotropins.** The blessed neurotropins comprise another important class of neurochemicals with a variety of essential functions. One crucial function is to transcribe the genes responsible for neural maintenance and growth. One of our most beloved neurotropins is brain-derived neurotropic factor, usually written throughout simply as BDNF. You will see it written in that form and mentioned often in various chapters.

Neural activity, physical exercise, and certain nutrients can all lead to the transcription of the genes that produce BDNF. Those BDNF molecules transcribe other genes that (indirectly) produce various proteins. Those modifications may result in other neurochemicals being produced, or new synapses created, or even new neurons created from the neural stem cells that have been waiting patiently our entire lifetimes. Over time and with repeated neural activity, the brain structures affected may increase in volume— increases sufficient to be detectable by brain scans (e.g., magnetic-resonance imaging—MRIs—or other scanning methods).

**The blood-brain barrier.** More than in other parts of our body, the capillaries in our brains benefit from the cells of their inner lining—the endothelial cells—being tightly packed together like rock fans in a mosh pit. Thus some potentially-harmful substances (and some potentially helpful ones too), usually in the form or large and rambunctious molecules, cannot pass through the walls of the brain's capillaries to enter the brain's cerebro-spinal fluid. As examples of substances kept out of the brain, the hormone adrenaline, some antibiotics, and (important for our later considerations) some nutrients cannot cross the blood-brain barrier.

## Genes and epigenetics

**Transcribing genes.** We humans have only 23,000 genes. Each consists of a segment of DNA. Although their initial design role is the one we usually celebrate, our genes do far more than provide instructions for our initial design. They are also involved in the day-to-day changes in the functioning and the structure of our bodies—even our adult bodies. Thus they play a major role in our aging and our responses to stressors. Genetic activation occurs when molecules called transcription factors transcribe or activate a gene. Following genetic transcription, through several intermediate steps, the transcribed gene produces the specific protein that is its responsibility. With that newly created protein, physical structures are maintained, or modified, or even newly created. Those processes are happening in our brains and bodies right now. For example, those processes modify the structure of the neurons that are busy with new learning.

**Genetic mutations.** As mentioned above, stress results in the need for our mitochondria to produce more energy; unfortunately, as a byproduct of that enhanced energy production the mitochondria also produce higher levels of mutation-causing reactive oxygen species. A downside of aging is that it also accelerates the rate of mutations. Naturally, genetic functions are affected by those mutations. Recent research has shown that the rate of mutations accelerates during or soon after puberty, and that people who have faster rates of mutations have shorter lifespans (Cawthon et al., 2020). That is not a happy observation, but protection from acquiring those mutations is provided by nutrients that are rich in antioxidants.

**Telomeres.** Besides the protection our genes receive from good nutrition, our telomeres also defend our genes from acquiring mutations. Telomeres are complexes of proteins and DNA that cap the ends of our chromosomes. Unfortunately, those protective telomeres shrink steadily as we age, and they shrink even faster with stress. However, there are ways to minimize that shrinkage and thus potentially to slow the rate of our mutations, sustain health, and then even possibly prolong life. Being regularly engaged with the toughening activities of physical exercise, cognitive challenge, meditation, and even nurturing activities reduces telomere shrinkage. And most relevant to our concerns here, some dietary elements like coffee (but not caffeine) can slow the age-induced decline of our telomeres; more about that later. (See

Jacobs et al., 2010, Shalev et al., 2013, and Epel, 2009, for more on telomeres and see Dienstbier, 2015, for more on toughening activities.)

**Epigenetics.** The 23,000 genes that actively determine our human characteristics and our individual bodies, brains, and personalities are sometimes thought to be *way* too few to design and build all that on their own. But they do. If each of those individual genes had a single transcription factor that resulted in a single protein being produced, the complex system of structures and chemicals that is "us" could not exist. But life is not that simple. Each transcription factor may activate a handful of different genes, and each gene may be transcribed by a handful of transcription factors. Add to that complexity that those activities interact with environmental factors. Then events external to our bodies change our internal environments (e.g., enhancing some neurochemicals) that have impacts on immediate genetic transcription or more long-term epigenetic processes.

The modern science of epigenetics helps us to understand those processes, including how aging or stress can make some genes less (and others more) susceptible to transcription. A gene becomes less responsive to transcription factors when a methyl-group molecule becomes attached to that gene. That clinging methyl molecule may inhibit that gene temporarily, or for months, years, or even for a lifetime. For example, abuse and neglect of children can methylate (suddenly, it's a verb) the genes that produce the spectacular neurotropin BDNF. The reduced responsivity of the methylated (and then an adjective) *BDNF* genes can last a lifetime, so that BDNF levels are inadequate, and the brain's development and maintenance never reaches its full potential (Roth et al., 2009). (Modern gene-reading methods have identified 20 million methylation sites in the human genome; Fitzgerald et al., 2021.)

But epigenetic modifications can enhance gene function too. The long-term sensitivity of specific genes can be enhanced when an acetyl-group molecule makes the gene more responsive to a transcription factor. To illustrate, consider the opposite of abuse and neglect. Great nurturing can lead to the acetylation of the genes that create receptors for the hormones oxytocin and estrogen. Having more receptors for both oxytocin and estrogen disposes a person to be more responsive to those hormones, leading to becoming both affectionate and nurturing; those impacts too can last for years, or even for a lifetime (Champagne, 2010).

Methylation and acetylation patterns change in response to experiences such as stressors or new learning—experiences that may be unique to each of us and that should therefore impact our epigenetic patterns in unique ways. For example, identical twins, especially when living apart, have patterns of methylation and acetylation that grow increasingly different from each other (Fraga et al., 2005).

Most important for our interests here, the availability or shortage of nutrition at any age can affect epigenetic processes, but young individuals are especially affected by the adequacy of nutrition. Because of their impacts on fetuses, various supplements that affect epigenetic processes can be very important for pregnant women to consume, whereas other nutrients, like caffeine, can be detrimental to fetal brain development.

Aging also affects epigenetic processes. With aging, it is not that overall levels of methylation or acetylation increase but rather that the pattern of those epigenetic modifications changes in a predictable manner as we age. In Chapters 19 and 20, I confront the intriguing question of how we might reverse our age-related pattern of methylation and acetylation with diet and with toughening activities.

Chapter 2

# Aging and stress impact brain, cognition, and resilience

Aging and stress have somewhat similar negative impacts on brain and cognition. As with Chapter 1, none of the material presented here is technically difficult, although some readers may be disturbed by the details of how stress and aging pummel our brains and cognitive capacities. However, that sometimes-depressing information about negative impacts from aging and stress eventually gives way to subsequent chapters that describe first *how much* nutrition can sustain and enhance brain and cognition, and *how* nutrition achieves that magic.

## Aging

The young should be aware that aging is not a gift presented exclusively to the elderly. Age- and stress-induced modifications to our human brains may be hardly noticed in our early years, but those modifications really do begin early and may be noticed only in later years when the brain becomes more vulnerable. To illustrate that progression, note that throughout adulthood the brain as a whole shrinks at the rate of 2% per decade, and the vitally-important prefrontal cortex and hippocampi shrink at least twice that fast. But in later adulthood, some estimates for hippocampal shrinkage put that decline at 10% per decade. As frequently reported by the elderly, aging is not for sissies. Modern thought is that the central underlying cause of aging is DNA damage, although DNA methylation also plays a role (Schumacher et al., 2021). But some nutrients slow or even reverse those degrading processes, and thus may mimic the fountain of youth. In subsequent chapters, we shall see.

## Stress and challenge

Stress is available to us irrespective of age. Stress has many definitions, but I define it simply as an internal response to stressors. The stress response itself usually has the cognitive components of worry and rumination, some negative emotional responses, and physiological arousal in brain and body, with high arousal, especially in the early stages of an extended stress response. The stressors that cause stress are often threats of bad outcomes that may happen, or our recognition that the vultures have already landed—that harm or loss has happened. Because we humans are very social creatures, major stressors are often social, such as conditions that portend embarrassment, threats to our status or to our relationships, or the aftermath of damaged relationships. Stress responses often follow appraisals that a poor outcome is unpredictable or uncontrollable (Dickerson & Kemeny, 2004; Chida & Hamer, 2008).

Recall from Chapter 1 that because the hippocampi busily process information into memories, the hippocampi are the most plastic or modifiable structures of our brain. Unfortunately, one of the aspects of that plasticity is that they shrink in substantial ways with stress as well as with aging. But after shrinking with stress, the hippocampi recover some lost volume with successful therapies, and with activities that toughen the brain. They can also grow measurably with brain-friendly nutrition. Thus researchers who assess impacts of nutrition on the brain often assess changes in the hippocampi, providing us with many occasions to marvel at their plasticity.

**Challenge.** To further refine my definition of stress, consider the contrasting concept of challenge. Even if coping with challenges requires energy and effort, challenges usually feel manageable, evoke expectations of positive outcomes, and elicit positive emotions. Unlike stressors, challenges are not usually about social relationships. Some writers consider challenges to be a form of stressor, and challenge to be a form of stress. I do not follow that path, but writers who do sometimes use terms like "eustress" for "good stress." There is no absolutely right or wrong way to settle these issues of definition. However, as described below, the arousal that is a component of a stress response is different from the arousal of challenge, and of course, the emotional and cognitive responses are different too. Because of those differences, a life filled with challenges tends to be healthy for brain and body, building both physiological toughness and psychological resilience. By comparison, a life filled with stress is often a short life, and a life more likely to include poor mental and physical health. (Physiological toughness and psychological resilience are defined and explained in Chapter 19, or, with lots of time on your hands, see Dienstbier, 2015 for my book-length presentation of those issues, or consider Dienstbier & PytlikZillig, 2021 for a lighter chapter-length summary.)

### Aging and stress together

In the previous chapter, I noted that heroic neurotropins like BDNF can stimulate the building of brain tissue. Unfortunately, with our aging and with accumulating stress, it becomes increasingly difficult to transcribe the genes that release BDNF and other benevolent neurotropins. Then, with neurotropin levels in short supply, even general maintenance functions in the brain are neglected and various brain structures atrophy—especially the prefrontal cortex and the hippocampi (Erickson et al., 2010).

But three observations are especially important here: First, note that cortical deterioration and even the accumulation of the Alzheimer's-related proteins described below do not occur in noticeable ways in all aging brains. Second, perhaps in league with Pollyanna, Harrington et al. (2021) noted that if elderly people with usually-undetected neurodegenerative diseases are eliminated from participant samples (by neuroimaging or detecting cerebrospinal fluid biomarkers), that the remaining elderly show far less-than-expected cognitive decline as they age. The third is that half of the people who have already developed measurable Alzheimer's-related *physiological* pathology still experience no noticeable dementia. Dhana et al. (2021) note, for example, that subjects with *asymptomatic* Alzheimer's dementia (i.e., have observable brain pathology without cognitive evidence of dementia) represent approximately 50% of individuals older than 75 years of age.

When neural deterioration does occur, our poor brain enters an unfortunate downward spiral where declining neural tissue cannot easily produce the neurotropins that would stem further decline. The brain must now contend with the pruning back of dendrites, fewer synapses, and even the death of some neurons. Happily, in addition to those impacts being minimal in some aging brains, some nutrients can come to the rescue by enhancing the availability of neurotropins like BDNF. More about that later.

### Arousal in challenge and stress

Both challenges and stressors stimulate arousal that can be either beneficial for coping, or detrimental to coping, depending on the kind of arousal, its intensity, and its duration. During human evolution over the last 200 thousand years or so, we humans often encountered threats such as hefty beasts wishing to chew our legs. Such physical threats usually required major physical efforts and thus intense arousal that prepared us for huge energy expenditures. Fortunately, today most of us live in environments that are largely physically safe, but unfortunately, we still produce similar high-arousal stress responses. On the one hand, intense arousal in response to non-physical stressors seems unnecessary. But on the other hand, when we consider that the brain itself is a voracious consumer of energy, even coping that is largely mental may benefit from substantial physiological arousal— provided that the arousal is the proper type, and is not overdone. With that in mind, a high-arousal stress response may not be quite as serious a design flaw as it may initially seem to be.

But whether or not our arousal is helpful depends, in part, on the coping that is required and on the nature of the arousal itself. Consider a sequence beginning with either a challenge or with a stressor that, in either case, demands energy-rich responses. The sympathetic nervous system (sympathetic NS) relays stimulation from brain into the body in the form of signals that eventually reach the adrenal glands. The adrenals then release adrenaline (acting largely as a hormone, and sometimes called epinephrine), and noradrenaline (acting as both hormone and neurotransmitter, and sometimes called norepinephrine). Those hormones ask the liver to dump glucose and fatty acids into circulation to energize both brain (mostly by the glucose) and body (by both). Increases in heart rate and blood pressure enhance the distribution of those energy-generating molecules. Because of its role in increasing blood glucose, adrenaline is important even when only mental coping is required.

**Arousal in stress.** The components of arousal presented in the previous paragraph develop in response to either challenges or stressors. However, stressor-induced arousal includes additional components. In the brain, besides the arousing noradrenaline that is released during both challenge and stress, during stress the brain produces a flood of corticosteroid-releasing hormone (CRH). The CRH molecules that remain in the brain stimulate the amygdala to generate survival-relevant emotional responses. Those negative emotions and feelings of tension keep our attention focused on the looming threat, and they motivate us to cope with the developing disaster. Other CRH molecules abandon the brain, traveling the short step into the pituitary gland (pictured in Figure 1-2). The pituitary then releases other hormones that slap the endocrine system to attention, ultimately stimulating the release of cortisol from the adrenal glands. That sequence describes pituitary-adrenal-cortical arousal.

**Cortisol.** Cortisol is a major stress hormone. In the short-term and in moderate doses, stress-evoked cortisol can be beneficial. In the body, it (indirectly) supplies blood glucose and other energy-relevant molecules, thereby supporting the arousal efforts begun by the sympathetic NS with its adrenaline and noradrenaline. But some of the circulating cortisol crosses through the blood-brain barrier and enters the brain. In the brain, those cortisol molecules affect the functioning of neurons and even transcribe some of the genes within the neurons. When the cortisol response is moderate, short-term impacts such as increasing dopamine levels can aid in coping with the stress. And moderate cortisol levels can stimulate the hippocampi both to reassemble memories of past coping with similar threats, and to form new memories—memories that may aid in similar stressful situations in the future. Moderate cortisol can also energize the problem-solving activities of the prefrontal cortex and it can further stimulate the amygdala to activate the stress-relevant emotions that will, in turn, motivate coping and keep attention focused on the stressor (Mather & Lighthall, 2012; Schulkin et al., 1998). All those cortisol-stimulated responses can aid coping and even survival.

Unfortunately, if stress is intense or chronic, some enduring negative consequences follow from cortisol over-stimulating some neural structures, allowing otherwise benign neurochemicals to become toxic (e.g., expended neurotransmitters like glutamate) if they are released more rapidly than they can be eliminated. However, in both negative and positive ways, our diets have an impact on cortisol levels. For a positive example, cortisol base rate levels can be downregulated by the gut bacteria that we nurture with nutrient-rich diets, and/or diets that include sufficient prebiotics and probiotics. Those issues are discussed in Chapter 16 on the microbiome and Chapter 19 on toughening.

Both aging and stress accelerate the production and accumulation of waste within the brain. But in addition to bad stuff produced within the brain, as we age, the blood-brain barrier becomes more permeable because of the aging and subsequent inefficiency of the oligodendrocytes, the glia that should support the blood-brain barrier. Thus the aging brain is less effective in keeping toxins from entering our brains. Compounding that problem, with our aging the toxin-removal functions that are undertaken by the brain's microglia and glymphatic system become less effective.

Whether waste builds up from within-brain processes or sneaks in from outside, the constipation of brain waste products interferes with neural functions and degrades neural tissue (e.g., synapses decline and dendritic branches are pruned back; Xie et al., 2013). As attested in subsequent chapters, various nutrients are effective in encouraging efficiency in the brain's waste-removal processes. And specifically await Chapters 13 and 14 for some research on the impact of alcohol on brain-waste removal.

Both aging and high levels of stress-associated cortisol also affect genetic processes in the short term by regulating immediate short-term transcription of genes in neurons, and affecting the long-term epigenetic process of methylation (reducing transcription) and acetylation (enhancing transcription). For example, aging and stress indirectly cause methylation of the genes that create our favorite neurotransmitters, leading to shortages and thus to slower and less efficient transmission of impulses between sending and receiving neurons. But as noted in Chapter 19, both good nutrition and toughening activities can change the pattern of methylation toward that of younger individuals.

Chronic stress and aging both degrade control of cortisol, largely by reducing the brain's ability to detect circulating cortisol. Chronically high cortisol can then damage the brain even more, leading eventually to various symptoms of aging, including declining energy, muscle atrophy, suppression of the immune system, and suppression of the reproductive hormones. Worst of all, both reduced brain volume and cognitive decline in the elderly correspond with high cortisol levels, indicating that excessive cortisol may cause the brain atrophy that otherwise seems to be a natural consequence of normal aging (Lupien et al., 1998; Karlamangla et al., 2005).

Nutrition, bacteria, and toughening activities to the rescue! Besides the control of cortisol by diet and the microbiome, both described in subsequent chapters, toughening activities such as exercise, self-control activities, socializing (and others) similarly have calming impacts on cortisol responses. (Those issues are discussed mostly in Chapter 19 on toughening.)

**Homocysteine.** Homocysteine is an often-nasty amino acid that is produced naturally when tissue breaks down, but its production is accelerated by stress. In their review, Smith and Refsum (2021) note that elevated homocysteine levels correspond with over 100 diseases, including cardiovascular damage that degrades the inner lining of arteries, increasing risks for stroke. But most importantly for our interests, high homocysteine levels induce brain atrophy in even the healthy elderly, increasing the intolerance of stress and risks for Alzheimer's.

Because of that association with Alzheimer's development, the scientists who developed the *Food for the Brain* website believe that monitoring homocysteine levels is important in order to know one's Alzheimer's risk. The *Food for the Brain* organization itself provides cognitive tests that can indicate Alzheimer's vulnerabilities and they offer both dietary and lifestyle suggestions for minimizing those risks. Homocysteine is occasionally mentioned in some of the following chapters, and because of being influenced by levels of the B vitamins, it is discussed more extensively in Chapter 8.

**Myelin and white matter.** Recall from Chapter 1 that the white-matter parts of the brain consist of the long myelin-coated axons that inter-connect various neural structures. Newly created neurons require new myelin, and myelin upkeep and repair is needed for established neurons to maintain brain efficiency. Unfortunately, demand for myelin is balanced by supply only until around age 40. From then on myelin production and maintenance falls further and further behind. With aging and stress, those tracts of myelin-coated axons lose effectiveness in connecting different brain structures.

As with most other neural structures, good nutrition such as provided by the Mediterranean diet (Med; as discussed in Chapter 4) can improve the health of white matter and thus enhance the connectivity between structures. Similarly, the metals discussed in Chapter 10 can boost myelin, as can the B-vitamins of Chapter 8. It is the rapid deterioration of myelin that causes the neural-transmission problems of multiple sclerosis (Ziegler et al., 2010).

**Neurochemical decline.** With aging, our bodies also produce inadequate amounts of various important hormones and other neurochemicals such as the neurotropins and neurotransmitters described above. In fact, normal aging results in a slowing of protein synthesis generally—including especially some proteins associated with memory formation (Pavlopoulos et al., 2013). Important causes of such general decline are reduced amounts of the pituitary's human growth hormone (HGH) and decline of the brain's neurotropins. HGH normally maintains the health of bodily systems, including the muscles, the skin, and the immune system, and even in the brain; along with other important neurotropins HGH keeps neurons shinny and strong. Unfortunately, by age 80, HGH levels have declined to around 5% of youthful levels, and neurotropins like BDNF also decline substantially (Vitiello et al., 2006). Do not despair. As discussed throughout, but especially in Chapter 19 on toughening, the enhancement of the neurotropins by nutrition and toughening activities rebuilds brain tissue and resists age-associated cognitive decline.

**Cardiovascular decline.** Recall that brain health depends upon the health of the cardiovascular system (Jefferson et al., 2010). Unfortunately, the circulatory system is degraded by both stress and aging. Especially when stressors are extreme or chronic, the requirement for sustained arousal results in the release of various energy-supplying molecules that can contribute to the buildup of plaques throughout the cardiovascular system. And sustained arousal-produced high blood pressure can cause cardiovascular structural problems and clots that cause strokes and heart attacks. Because of the brain's voracious energy requirements, age- or stress-induced circulatory inefficiency degrades neural processing and cognitive abilities. The stiffening of arteries caused by the impacts of stress and normal aging can also cause spikes of blood pressure that result in cerebral micro-bleeding. An accumulation of those mini-strokes, rots our mental skills. (For even more discouraging details, see O'Rourke, 2008, and Waldstein et al., 2008.) Thus the nutrition discussed throughout that nourishes the cardiovascular system is good for brain and cognition.

**Even more shrinkage.** Besides stress and aging, other factors that degrade and shrink the various brain structures include depression, sedentary lifestyles, and a lack of mental stimulation. Even with the newest scanning techniques, the components of the shrinkage itself are not always easily identified. Specifically, shrinkage could develop from reduced vascularization (fewer capillaries), decreased size of neurons or fewer of them, less dendritic branching, reduced myelin, or fewer glial cells (Sherwin & Henry, 2008). Any of those factors would interfere with neural efficiency and account for problems in cognition, and every one of them is affected by nutrition.

## Cognitive abilities

**The good news.** The previous descriptions of physiological insults from stress and from aging seem to suggest an inevitable cognitive decline. And indeed, although population studies tend to support that conclusion, as mentioned briefly above, even as we age through and past our 70's many of us avoid the accumulations of β-amyloid, distorted tau proteins, and neurological deterioration that are the beginnings of Alzheimer's dementia (Harrington et al., 2021). Without those hallmarks of gloom, our cognitive capacities do not show nearly as much of the cognitive declines that we associate with normal aging. And (worth repeating from above), even when such physiological damage becomes evident (with modern scans etc.) substantial cognitive decline does not always follow—at least not immediately and perhaps not for many years.

Thus unless we have begun a slide toward dementia, our fluid intelligence can remain intact, and even in our dotage, we still retain much of the knowledge that each of us has accumulated across our lifetimes—our crystallized intelligence. At age 70 or so, we often know as much of things like vocabulary as we did at 50.

Another positive is that if we have developed areas of cognitive expertise and continue to use our expertise, it declines only very slowly. And some research suggests that some forms of wisdom even increase with age (Grossmann et al., 2012, but sometimes attributed to Pollyanna and colleagues).

**Then the bad news.** Various cognitive decrements result from the physiological deficits described above—deficits that are imposed by stress and, in many of us, by aging. The development of those cognitive decrements typically follows a time course that is the reverse of the developmental sequence, with the latest acquired capacities being the first to go.

Of importance for almost everything the brain does, the slowing of the brain's processing speed accounts for much of the cognitive decline associated with aging (Horn & Masunga, 2000). Modern research indicates that processing speed does not slow appreciably until after age 60 (von Krause et al., 2022), but with reaction-time tasks or with simple-but-timed cognitive tasks, people over 60 usually perform terribly in contrast to (say) typical 20-year olds. However, when no time limits are imposed on cognitive tasks involving complex problem solving, older people do as well (or almost as well) as do the young, with abilities often peaking on such measures at around age 50. Another mixed observation is that whereas *recall* of learned items declines substantially with age (like your best friend's name when you are trying to introduce her), performance on *recognition* tasks, such as identifying previously seen items, does not decline substantially with age (Parkin & Rosalind, 2000).

Deficits in memory formation and retrieval result from stress- and age-associated decline of the neurotropins like BDNF; when not in decline, those neurotropins sustain the brain, especially the hippocampi and cortical structures. Stress- and age-associated deficits in neurotransmitters such as acetylcholine pile on as well. It is especially episodic memories—memories of the events of our lives—that are negatively affected by insufficient acetylcholine.

Working memory, sometimes called the sketch pad of the mind, implies conscious mental processing—conscious thinking. Although several ideas can be processed by working memory, they are processed in sequence—not all at once. Working memory is adversely affected by the shrinkage of the cortex and the other physiological products of aging that many of us experience in our elderly years and that (probably) all of us will experience if we can just live long enough. When working memory itself shrinks, it means that fewer ideas can be held near-simultaneously in consciousness and that it is more difficult to keep from consciousness the intrusive thoughts and ideas that may interfere with the ongoing cognitive tasks (Horn & Masunga, 2000). That deficit of working memory and other age-related problems, such as slowed processing speed mean that as we age, we experience declining fluid intelligence and flawed executive functions. Fluid intelligence implies problem-solving, and the executive functions include choosing goals, organizing sub-goals, working with relevant information and ignoring irrelevant information, appropriately controlling impulses and emotions, and so on (Hess, 2005). However, such age-related deficits do not necessarily lead to dementia, such as Alzheimer's.

**Alzheimer's.** It will not afflict all of us, but Alzheimer's is centrally important. It is feared by the elderly more than any of the other potentially-lethal age-related diseases such as cancer and heart disease. That fear is justified by a fact from the Alzheimer's Association that one out of three American seniors dies with Alzheimer's or another dementia. Even more bad news recently published by the American Heart Association noted that in the last 30 years increases of 184% in deaths from Alzheimer's disease have greatly outpaced the 44% increases in deaths from cardiovascular diseases (Tsao et al., 2022).

My focus on brain health obviously implies far more than the avoidance of dementias, but for a moment, consider the four horsemen of Alzheimer's, or at least the four with the biggest horses. The first and most obvious physiological components are the between-neuron plaques created from misshapen β-amyloid protein (also called amyloid-β and sometimes abbreviated AB or Aβ). Produced by amyloid precursor protein, some research indicates that the plaques accumulate first in the limbic structures of the brain, subsequently spreading to cortical areas adjacent to the hippocampi (e.g., Lam, Takechi et al., 2021; Bhattacharyya et al., 2021). Other recent research suggests the plaques originate in multiple brain structures. Either way, once the plaques form, other proteins resulting from the accumulated β-amyloid cause the loss of nearby synapses.

Second, tangles that devastate cell functions form within neurons—tangles caused by misshapen tau proteins (technically phosphorylated tau). Those distorted tau proteins are then transmitted from neuron to neuron and from structure to structure within the brain in a manner resembling a spreading infection; recent research even shows how those twisted tau molecules are taken up by soon-to-be-kaput neurons.

Third, mental deterioration accelerates when the microglia of the brain's immune system fails to clear the β-amyloid (as they should). That highly activated immune response causes pockets of inflammation. With excessive inflammation, the microglia become even less capable of ridding the brain of β-amyloid and tau (Konttinen et al., 2019), so that further inflammation and neural damage results.

Fourth, with those developments, the mitochondria increase their production of energy and then, as a byproduct, increase their production of reactive oxygen molecules. That reactive oxygen damages the DNA of the mitochondria themselves and the DNA of the neurons and other cells that contain the mitochondria. Nothing works very well after that, but genetic damage is not the only genetic issue. The pattern of our inherited genes also affects our vulnerability to Alzheimer's. The *APOE-4* gene variant (allele) of the *APOE* gene increases that vulnerability by affecting dozens of other genetic processes in the brain, accelerating the physiological disasters outlined here. Those cumulative insults to brain tissue destroy synapses and kill neurons, ultimately leading to shrinkage of brain structures and to cognitive decline.

One of the lesser horsemen of Alzheimer's that is receiving exponentially increasing recognition is our microbiome—the gut bacteria that reside in our intestines. Those bacteria affect our brains, our cognitive capacities, and our moods (Kaplan et al., 2015). Because the health of the microbiome depends upon the nutrition we provide and because of the importance of the microbiome to brain, cognition, and to moods such as anxiety and depression, the microbiome has been assigned to its own Chapter 16.

Another issue relevant to our nutrition interests is the association of Alzheimer's with low levels of our favorite neurotropin BDNF (Qin et al., 2017). The shortage of BDNF may cause or exacerbate the cascade of negative impacts described above. Thus the contribution of various nutrients to BDNF (described in several subsequent chapters) directly implicates those nutrients in the prevention of Alzheimer's.

You can now see why defense against age- or stress-related cognitive decline and Alzheimer's might be accomplished by nutrients that nurture neurons and that have antioxidant and/or anti-inflammatory characteristics, or that maintain the health of our gut microbiome, or foster BDNF levels and assist in the removal of waste products. And some nutrients even directly reduce β-amyloid by affecting the brain's waste-removal systems.

Bredesen et al. (2016) have explored the question of what other identifiable factors may initiate Alzheimer's. In their relatively new theoretical perspective, they assert that excessive β-amyloid is produced to prevent neural damage within the brain—damage resulting both from toxins and waste on the one hand, and on the other hand from a lack of supporting elements such as adequate levels of hormones, neurotropins, and, most important for our interests, brain-healthy nutrition. According to that perspective, *any* physiological or neurochemical condition that threatens brain health encourages both β-amyloid accumulation and the additional damage to brain and cognition caused by that distorted protein.

Corresponding to that understanding of what initiates development of β-amyloid plaques, Bredesen and colleagues created a treatment protocol for people with mild cognitive impairment and early Alzheimer's. They first identify which of many possible causal elements may be threatening the brain health of each individual client. That analysis then leads to treatments that are individually designed to redress that unique array of elements. For example, appropriate dietary modifications and supplements could be recommended for possible deficiencies in insulin, or in BDNF, or vitamin D, or estrogen, or for excessive insulin, homocysteine, or glucose, etc. The approach of Bredesen et al. is not universally accepted, but there is supportive research, and it is intriguing.

**A final note.** Fortunately, neural damage from aging and stress is (at least somewhat) preventable and reversible. Positive neural health follows from lifestyle interventions that include physical exercise, mentally-challenging activities, nurturing and social activities, and meditation. In Chapter 19 and again in the final Chapter 20 I discuss relationships of those activities with appropriate nutrition.

In the meantime, knowing some of the ways that nutrition affects physiological processes that in turn affect mental capacities (e.g., repairing damage from reactive oxygen and from inflammation) opens hypotheses about how some nutrients may work their magic of preserving our mental capacities. In fact, some reviewers have reasonably short lists of nutrients that they believe to effectively resist cognitive decline. In the final chapter, I describe those lists as a kind of summary of the entire book.

Having said all of the above, it is certainly not the case that every physiological cause of (say) cognitive decline has an answer in some specific nutrient. But, as illustrated in subsequent chapters, many do.

# Chapter 3

# Nutrition research: the good, the bad, and the ugly

In the introduction, I mentioned some examples of nutrition research evolving from early certainty to recent contradictions. Some of those revisions are quite important, such as egg attitudes evolving from guaranteed heart attacks to current perspectives that daily eggs could be great for our brains and cognition. But contradictions or not, as in most scientific endeavors, nutrition researchers have been, and are, careful scientists. What happened? Or even more concerning, are similarly unreliable conclusions still flowing from current nutrition research?

Like nutrition itself, the answers are complex. And certainly, the answers are not all here, in this book. Nutrition science is clearly evolving. We can understand it better by examining the styles of research that provide the data, whether those data are flawed or golden.

## Nutrition research styles

**Cross-section research.** A substantial portion of nutrition research consists of studies that are snapshots at one moment. Often the research participants in such cross-section research report the kinds and amounts of food consumed over some recent interval, and the researchers correlate those amounts with some (hopefully) important outcome such as tests of memory capacity or hippocampal volume. The food questionnaires that are used are usually well-validated, so that responses to them reflect actual consumption; sometimes, they are even supplemented with interviews. Such correlations are informative and useful, but as the authors of such research readily acknowledge, by themselves those correlations cannot show that differences in nutrition *caused* the outcome at issue. Those limitations hold whether the outcome is health-related, such as cardiovascular health, or related to things we are most interested in, such as cognitive brilliance.

**Longitudinal research.** A more satisfying longitudinal approach assesses outcome measures such as cognitive capacity or brain structure at least twice, minimally once before and once after an interval of (often) between two and 30 years. For the longer time spans, the measures may be repeated at several-year intervals, sometimes with skilled interviewers insuring validity. Estimates are also made (often repeatedly) of the consumption of the key foods or nutrients during the entire span of months or years.

Even though collected by other researchers, the data from longitudinal studies (and cross-sectional research) are often made available for "mining"— checking for hypothetical relationships that may not have been considered when the research was originally conceived. For example, data sets from the Framingham heart study were originally collected to examine factors associated with cardiovascular disease, but are sometimes mined to test nutrition impacts on outcome variables such as vulnerabilities for cognitive decline or dementia. Similarly, the UK Biobank and other large cohorts of participants have provided data for subsequent analyses.

When *changes* in outcome measures (say of hippocampal size) are correlated with nutrition differences during those intervals (such as consuming more foods with omega 3 oils), in contrast to cross-sectional research, we can be somewhat more confident that nutrition has influenced changes in the outcome measures. However, as with the cross-section studies, the researchers who present longitudinal studies usually acknowledge that the direction of causality was not established with certainty by such research; it was still possible that cognitive brilliance led to eating more nuts, rather than the reverse.

Unfortunately, with either form of correlational research, despite the caution usually shown by the researchers themselves, articles often appear in more popular media with titles such as "Nut consumption delays Alzheimer's." Well, health and nutrition newsletters must write about something, and waiting until really solid research appears could mean waiting years rather than weeks. Thus because we people crave important dietary information, and because nutrition-news outlets crave readership, the cognitive whiplash we receive from contradictory nutrition information can result from the exaggerations of secondary sources more than from the research itself. Obviously, I would love to blame writers who see causes where only correlations abide, but nutrition writers need to accept only a small measure of shame. Most of us are more than capable of taking similar cognitive shortcuts on our own.

**Confounding factors.** Consider the findings by Vercambre et al. (2013) discussed more extensively in Chapter 7. The consumption of caffeinated coffee was measured for elderly women at risk for cognitive decline. There was a statistically significant correlation between coffee consumption and delayed cognitive decline across five years. Wow, the hypothetical headline reads: "coffee delays cognitive decline." Maybe it does, but some third factor(s) may account for the correlation between the coffee and delayed cognitive decline. Such "third" causal factors are called (here and for the rest of the book) *confounding* or *potentially-confounding* factors.

To illustrate a confounding factor that should be taken into account in the foregoing, consider the dimension of being well-read by staying up to date on news and current science. All kinds of news sources, including nutrition newsletters, tell us that moderate coffee consumption seems to enhance health. So, being well-read could, hypothetically, lead to drinking more coffee and it certainly leads to better scores on tests of cognition. Thus we have a correlation, because being well-read leads to both more coffee consumption and to higher cognitive scores. In this example, more coffee did not lead to higher cognition, nor did higher IQ lead to more coffee drinking, but there is still a positive correlation between coffee and cognition.

To personalize that issue, consider that your reading this book undoubtedly puts you into that well-read category, and that fact suggests your cognitive scores are higher than normal. Happily, those higher cognitive scores today predict slower cognitive decline in the future. (Yes, they really do!) And being well-read suggests that you already know a good portion of the content of this book—about what foods will lead to cognitive preservation, and that you act—at least sometimes—on that knowledge. Thus for you, being well-read causes the association between (on the one hand) cognitive preservation and (on the other) better nutrition over the last couple of years.

Naturally, conscientious researchers try to take potentially-confounding factors into account so that their possible impacts can be removed. They often use education level to substitute for being well-read or "smart." Using statistics, this is how that taking into account can be done. (This explanation is somewhat simplified, but skim it anyway if you feel a headache coming on.) Assume the likely possibility that the relationships outlined just above are all true. From the study data, our statistician can calculate the exact size of these relationships: the correlation of coffee consumption with cognitive scores; the correlation of education with cognitive scores, and the correlation of education with coffee consumption. Knowing those three numbers, with a little statistical magic our statistician and her computer can subtract the contribution of education to cognition and present us with a correlation between coffee and cognition that is not confounded with (or affected by) education level. In short, the result is a number designating the correlation of coffee with cognition "with education taken into account."

Although smart statisticians can solve the math part of the problem, the huge issue for the researchers is identifying and taking into account all of the possibly-confounding variables that could stink up their findings. The task can be daunting.

It certainly was daunting for the researchers who conducted this next study. Topiwala et al. (2017) designed their cross-sectional study to assess relationships between alcohol consumption across a 30-year span on the one hand, and on the other hand, brain volume at the end of that 30-year span. In a longitudinal component of the study, they also assessed relationships of alcohol consumption with repeatedly-measured cognitive changes across that span. These are the variables that they believed could either increase or decrease the *apparent* relationship between consuming alcohol on the one hand and brain structure and cognition on the other. Their list (from Topiwala et al., 2017, 3rd paragraph in "Study Design and Participants" section) was as follows:

> *Age, sex, education, smoking, social activity—such as attendance at clubs and visits with family/friends, physical activity, voluntary work— and component measures of the Framingham stroke risk score—such as blood pressure, smoking, history of cardiovascular events, cardiovascular drugs—were assessed by self report questionnaire. Social class was determined according to occupation at phase 3 (highest class=1, lowest=4). Drugs (number of psychotropic drugs reported as taken) and lifetime history of major depressive disorder (assessed by structured clinical interview for DSM IV) were assessed at the time of the scan. Information about personality traits was determined by questionnaire at phase 1 and included trait impulsivity (question: 'Are you hot-headed?').*

Obviously, Topiwala and her co-researchers were extremely conscientious. However, although their list is more extensive than most such lists in longitudinal research on nutrition impacts, the problem remains that even with a list of potential confounds as thorough as they provided, it is impossible to be sure that something important—perhaps crucially important—was not overlooked. In fact, as noted in Chapter 14, some omissions from the above list lead to questions about the interpretation of their results. Specifically, the results of the research showed that even modest amounts of alcohol provided no cognitive protection whatsoever, but that instead even modest amounts of alcohol correlated with brain shrinkage in vital neural structures. (If you consume any alcohol, do not panic; those findings are vastly qualified in Chapters 13 and 14.)

But before (nervously?) jumping ahead to Chapters 13 and 14, consider the potentially-confounding factors omitted from the long list, above. The specific alcoholic beverages consumed make a difference in outcomes, as do factors such as whether the alcohol is traditionally consumed with a meal or not, or in binge episodes or not, or by people in their 30s or people in their 70s. (Actually, as a spoiler for Chapter 14, research shows that all of those factors seem to be important in determining brain protection versus harm from modest alcohol consumption.) Obviously, making conclusions about impacts of nutrition on outcomes for brain and cognition is, at best, very risky business. But all is not lost.

**Animal research and randomized-control trials (to the rescue?).** Fortunately, correlational studies of food/nutrient consumption with brain health and cognitive outcomes are only one of the research arrows in the scientific quiver. Once correlational research shows a relationship between (say) cognitive preservation and an excess or deficiency of some nutrient, *randomized-control trials* often follow. Randomized-control trials randomly assign participants to experimental conditions and to appropriate control groups. Remember that such research is the model for the development of most modern pharmaceuticals, first using animals, and then people. When people are the participants in the research, the randomized-control trials are often conducted with double-blind procedures where neither the participant nor the researchers are aware of the participant's research condition.

As with pharmaceutical research, when nutritional impacts are assessed, initially that research usually employs animals—usually mice or rats. Some people are less than enthusiastic about nutrition research with rodents because of mistakenly assuming superiority (rather than some form of biological equivalence) to our fellow mammals. However, especially when the research animals have been genetically engineered with human genes inserted into their genome (e.g., transgenic mice or rats made susceptible to Alzheimer's) there are good reasons to value findings from such research. Even without genetic alterations, when an assortment of critters from rodents to fruit flies and even roundworms, show positive impacts from some nutrient or supplement, there are reasons to believe that animal cells are being impacted at a very basic level, and we humans cannot be excused from those effects. (The frequently-studied roundworms are more formally known as nematodes and even more formally as *C. elegans*. They have a whopping 302 neurons and a lifespan of two to three weeks. Thus cross-generational impacts are easily studied. You may not have wished to know that the *C.* stands for the genus name *Caenorhabditis*.)

**To be blind, or not.** There are a few limitations to the causal inferences we can make even from randomized-control trials with people. Consider one that randomly assigns a group of participants to control or experimental conditions for a year. People in the control group consume their normal diets; the experimental condition people consume the Med diet, with fish, olive oil, fruits, and veggies supplied by the researchers. The people in both conditions take a battery of cognitive tests at the study's beginning and end. Obviously, the participants must be aware of the nature of the research—that it is about whether diet may affect their cognition. (Even the people in the control condition would be aware, because of course all the participants were recruited for a study on nutrition.) Social psychologists (like me) know that the more costs that participants incur for being in a research project—costs from investments of time, or travel, or in food restrictions, or eating food items in undesirable quantities—the more invested they become in positive impacts for themselves and possibly for the study outcomes as well. Those expectations and motivations can bias the results—sometimes results assessed with methods (such as cognitive tests) that make perfectly transparent the expectations of the researchers.

However, although the true double-blind design common to pharmaceutical research may not always be possible when studying nutrition, it is much less likely that such awareness or accompanying expectations would affect physical measures such as body-mass index, or physiological assessments of neurochemistry, or neural structure, or blood flow in certain brain areas. Nutrients and placebos given in capsules also make double-blind nutrition studies possible.

But even when nutrition research takes the form of the gold standard—double-blind randomized-control trials with people—the results of such studies should be interpreted in view of the age, gender, overall health, and cognitive status of the participants. That is, we should know if the studied nutritional supplementation was beneficial to only women, or people over 60, or diabetics, or (most importantly for our interests) people already experiencing cognitive decline, etc. However, even with those limitations in mind, unlike correlational approaches, true randomized-control trials allow inferences of causality even without accounting for all the possibly-confounding variables.

**Elderly considerations.** Especially given that our interests are in the aging brain, we should also keep in mind the caution that nutrition studies of middle-aged persons and even of the "young old" may not apply to elderly people (Morley, 2004).

Research based on nutrition needs for younger people may not apply to the elderly in part because some nutrients are not absorbed as well in older people as they are in the young. And even after being absorbed, some nutrients are less effective in the elderly, especially if some age-related physiological progression has already passed some tipping point, or if receptor densities for that nutrient have declined (as happens frequently). A similar issue is that nutritional needs may change for older people simply because some needed substances that are manufactured in our bodies (such as vitamin D) may not be made in adequate quantities as we age. Thus although younger people may get plenty of such nutrients from a typical diet, older people may benefit greatly from dietary modifications or even (horrors!) supplements.

Besides randomized-control trials, another solid research approach is to investigate the nutrients already within the body by analyzing nutrients in the plasma of (usually) fasting individuals. That approach can offer unique perspectives. For example, in a study discussed in Chapter 8 on vitamins, Bowman et al. (2012) assessed 30 plasma biomarkers of common nutrients in elderly people; the researchers determined how clusters of those 30 nutrients corresponded with cognition. Such research has the feel of really sophisticated and advanced science, but ultimately the results are still correlations, not proven causal relationships.

**Reviews and meta-analyses.** Because of all of the limitations of interpretation of even the best of the gold-standard, double-blind, randomized-control trials, how can we be sure? One obvious approach is to review the body of research ourselves, trying to understand what experimental variables may account for the different outcomes reached by different studies. But the relevant research may consist of dozens of studies—sometimes even hundreds; most of us are not going to do that.

The approach taken here instead depends on reviews by experts—especially reviews published in major journals. Many of the reviews that I have used began with hundreds of possibly-relevant studies, with that list subsequently narrowed by assessments of relevance and quality. Often only a handful of studies remained to contribute to the conclusions. Typically the result was a meta-analysis that weighted each study by the number of participants and ultimately calculated how large an impact the diet or nutrition had on the outcome. Although several important individual studies are usually presented in each of the following chapters, I have also depended on such careful reviews by careful reviewers.

## Guiding principles for impacts of nutrition on brain

1) Almost anything (nutrient, exercise, or otherwise) that is good for the cardiovascular system is good for the brain. (E.g., cardiovascular risk factors are excellent predictors of progression from age-related mild cognitive impairment to dementia.)

2) Excessive blood sugar is harmful to the cardiovascular system and to the brain.

3)  Inflammation in the body usually harms the brain, and inflammation in the brain is really bad. Activities or nutrients that act as anti-inflammatories in brain *and/or body* are usually good for the brain.

4)  Antioxidants are usually good for the brain because antioxidants limit or reverse the oxidative stress caused by the overly reactive oxygen molecules (formally called reactive oxygen species) that are produced when our mitochondria release energy.

5)  Anything (like good sleep) that enhances the effectiveness of the brain's waste-clearing processes is good for brain. (Brain cleaning is accomplished by the brain's glymphatic system, its microglia, and sundry mechanisms yet unknown. Nutrition can affect the effectiveness of those cleaning processes. More later on that.)

6)  Maintaining a healthy gut microbiome maintains brain health. (We are poor hosts if we do not nourish our guests, even those who are bacteria.)

7)  Being obese, especially with too much belly fat, is bad for the brain, but being merely overweight in the elderly years may not be.

The following chapters will discuss the research that shows whether and how various dietary regimes and individual nutrients affect the brain, our cognitive capacities, and sometime even moods like depression. However, we cannot maximize brain health, cognitive capacities, or moods merely by wisely choosing our nutrition. Our informed selection of nutrients will benefit us more if those nutrients nourish a brain and body that is stimulated and exercised in a manner that corresponds with nature's design. Evolution did not favor slugs—at least not people who are slugs.

As you continue, remember that there is an appended Glossary for terms that may need elaborations beyond those given in the text.

Chapter 4

# Complete dietary plans for brain and cognition

Thinking about the Mediterranean diet (Med) makes me want to travel. But we need not travel for our food, because even during pandemics and winters the global transportation of food is one of the insufficiently-appreciated marvels of our modern age. At least it is a marvel for us denizens of developed countries. Other than cost, we have few believable excuses for avoiding diets that have proven to benefit brains and cognition.

Of the several major dietary plans that I review here, the Med is certainly best known. Although a substantial amount of sometimes-excellent research has assessed several of these diets, one need not commit to any of them in a religious fashion. Some variations of the diets reviewed below have been created to accommodate people who find strict adherence difficult, and some of the research studies of these diets consider levels of adherence, rather than dichotomizing participants into only adherents or delinquents. And the Med even has cultural variations to accommodate different traditions.

In later chapters, I review some of the specific nutrients that are components of the Med and its near relatives and that make positive contributions to brains, cognition, and resilience. By deconstructing the Med a bit in those chapters, we get a clearer view of how those great diets spin their magic webs. After determining *which* of the component nutrients seem to have positive impacts, in later chapters, I discuss in more detail *how* those mainstream components make their contributions. But having said that, keep in mind that modern nutritionists often suggest that we derive the most salutary benefits from combinations of nutrients rather than from nutrients in isolation. Looking forward, for example, Chapters 5 and 8 present research showing positive benefits to cognition from combinations of poly-unsaturated fatty acids and B vitamins, and Chapter 14 discusses benefits from consuming red wine with other nutrients.

**The notorious Western diet.** The five positive dietary plans reviewed below are essentially opposite to what is called the Western diet. As nutritionists define the Western, it consists of too many of the foods that we should minimize, and too few of the ones we should embrace. The list to minimize includes excessive red meat, processed meat, and any meats and dairy with saturated fat. Also minimized or excluded are highly refined foods, fried food, and foods with added sugar. And the Western has too few fruits, vegetables (hereafter simply veggies), whole grains, foods with fiber, and healthful fats. The foods of the Western increase oxidative stress and foster inflammation (Sodhi et al., 2021). Recall that both oxidative stress and inflammation are enemies of brain health. Thus it was not surprising that researchers who fed the Western to animals found that it impaired functioning of their hippocampi. Legal redress then became impossible because those poor creatures could not even remember their mistreatment.

**When the Western travels.** Support for the animal research arrived from Australian studies by Jacka et al. (2015). Elderly people aged 60 to 64 completed food questionnaires and contributed two MRI brain scans separated by four years. Across those four years, people whose diets were most like the Western had greater difficulties both learning and remembering.

Those cognitive processes depend upon the hippocampi, so it was not surprising that at both the study's beginning and end, lower volume of the left hippocampus corresponded with consumption of the Western (just as happened with the ill-fed animals mentioned above). In contrast, consumption of more of the "healthy/prudent" diet corresponded with enhanced left hippocampal volume. These relationships were independent of a large selection of potentially-confounding factors that were taken into account, including age, gender, education, occupation, depressive symptoms, medication, physical activity, smoking, hypertension and diabetes. Because the study by Jacka et al. was a correlational study, certainty that the Western caused those crummy outcomes is not possible, but the hippocampi are vital to memory formation, so we should pay attention; their health is not to be toyed with. And other studies support those findings.

In their Whitehall II population of over 5000 British residents, Ozawa et al. (2017) identified the components of an "inflammation diet"—a diet with great similarity to the Western. It consisted of those foods that enhanced levels of interleukin-6—one of the immune-system's signaling molecules that indicates the presence of general inflammation. The foods included in that inflammation diet consisted of the usual suspects in the Western—too much fried food, low levels of whole grains, but high quantities of iron-rich foods, including red and processed meat, peas, and legumes. (For health and for brain, dietary iron can vary from an essential ingredient to one that is detrimental, depending on age, gender, and other factors; more about that in Chapter 10.) After taking into account the potential confounds of age, sex, ethnicity, occupational status, education, and energy intake, Ozawa et al. showed that across the roughly six years of that prospective study the inflammation diet corresponded with significantly faster cognitive decline (both for reasoning and overall cognition). Those findings reinforce the observation that inflammation is one of the arch-enemies of brains and they support recommendations for the protection of brain and cognition from the anti-inflammatory nutrients discussed in several subsequent chapters. Beyond just brain impacts, a recent "*Harvard Health Letter*" listed 11 conditions (alphabetically) from asthma to weight gain, indicating that inflammation was the one hidden cause of all of them.

Other studies have focused on specific dietary components, such as the processed meats that are disparaged in literally all of the diets reviewed below. Iqbal et al. (2021) provided a huge review of studies conducted in 21 different countries—studies of unprocessed and processed meat consumption. They found processed meats to be universally bad for the cardiovascular system and life itself (mortality), without finding similar negative impacts from unprocessed red meat or poultry. That last phrase will be welcome for some of us, but keep in mind that the conscientious diets reviewed here want us to limit the reds anyway.

**The Mediterranean diet.** Of the five dietary approaches outlined briefly here, the Mediterranean (Med) is the best known and most researched. As succinctly described by Sánchez-Villegas et al. (2016, p. 1095):

> *The term Mediterranean diet refers to dietary patterns found in olive-growing areas of the Mediterranean region. Although some heterogeneity in traditional patterns of food consumption exists in these countries, there are also common features, such as consumption of abundant plant foods (e.g., high intake of fruits, nuts, vegetables, bread, pulses, potatoes, seeds, cereals, and pasta), fresh and varied fruits as the main and usual dessert, olive oil as the main source of fat and commonly used for salads and cooking, frequent consumption of fish, moderate wine consumption with meals, low amounts of meat (mainly poultry instead of beef and pork), and low to moderate consumption of dairy products.*

The extent of interest in this diet for neurodegenerative diseases (especially Alzheimer's and Parkinson's) is reflected in the book *The Role of the Mediterranean Diet in the Brain and Neurodegenerative Diseases*, edited by Farooqui & Farooqui, 2018). To illustrate the scope of coverage in that text, a sampling of chapter titles: "Contribution of Mediterranean diet in the prevention of Alzheimer's disease" (Panza et al., 2018; later cited liberally in this book); and (worthy of celebration!): "Red wine retards abeta [i.e., β-amyloid protein] deposition and neuroinflammation in Alzheimer's disease" (Dhir, 2018; his conclusions are discussed in Chapter 14).

Many recent longitudinal and cross-sectional studies using food frequency questionnaires have defined healthy diets as those that correspond most closely to the Med. Years of research shows that adherence to some form of the Med benefits the cardiovascular system and brain health, and even reduces osteoporosis. Studies directly relevant to our interests generally shown relationships between the Med-like diets and both cognition and scan-assessed volumes of various brain structures (e.g., Ballarini et al., 2021).

For another example, Prinelli et al. (2019) assessed 417 dementia-free participants aged 60 or more who participated in the "Swedish National study on Aging and Care." MRI scans assessed total brain volume and the integrity of the brain's white matter (i.e., assessments of lesions called "hyperintensities"). Food frequency questionnaires assessed consumption of 21 nutrients, leading to five nutrient consumption factors ultimately being extracted. Each of those factors was correlated with brain volume and white matter integrity. The components of nutrition that corresponded with brain volume and integrity corresponded closely with the components of the Med diet. Prinelli et al. (2019, p. 286) concluded that:

> *our findings suggest that optimal brain-health combinations of nutrients mainly from high intake of fruit, vegetables, legumes, olive and seed oils, fish, lean red meat, poultry and low in milk and dairy products, cream, butter, processed meat and offal, may help to maintain brain integrity (larger total brain volume and less white matter damage).*

**Med variations.** Over time and across cultures, the classical Med itself has changed somewhat. Some modifications have promoted fish consumption. And to accommodate dietary patterns in Greece, a Greek version was developed that limits poultry and promotes potatoes.

Another variation was created for meat-loving Australians by Wade et al. (2019). The authors noted that Aussies normally consume almost 100kg (220 pounds) of meat per person per year—an amount considered excessive by most nutritionists, and probably even by most American carnivores. Instead of their usual array of various meats, participants were given two to three servings (250g) of fresh lean pork each week (i.e., 1 to 1.5 pounds per week— less than half their normal meat consumption.) Participants in the study were randomly assigned to only eight weeks of that Med-Pork diet or to a control condition with a standard Low-Fat diet. After that eight-week period, the Med-Pork people and the Low-Fat folks switched conditions for another eight weeks. That is an especially powerful and efficient cross-over design, with each person serving as their own control. Not all cognitive measures should be expected to show dietary impacts in such a short time, and indeed most of the cognitive measures taken were not affected by those diets. An exception was that the Med-Pork resulted in faster cognitive processing speeds. That is not a trivial finding because declining cognitive processing speed is a major driver of cognitive aging, generally degrading cognitive abilities. The Med-Pork also led to better "emotional functioning."

Obviously, it would be lots more satisfying and convincing to see great cognitive effects from studies that last for years, with random assignments of many participants to well-chosen conditions. These next two studies fulfill those requirements. The participants in both studies had some cardiovascular risk factors.

Martinez-Lapiscina et al. (2013) randomly assigned 522 elderly Australians (mean age 75 at the study's end) to one of three dietary regimes. The first was the Med-Oil diet; for that diet, the normal Med diet was supplemented with additional extra-virgin olive oil. The Med-Nuts diet supplemented the Med with mixed nuts. The Low Fat Control condition counseled reducing dietary fats, but apparently was otherwise a usual diet. After maintaining those diets for 6.5 years, global cognitive performance was assessed with two quite-basic cognitive tests—the Mini-Mental State Examination and Clock Drawing Tests. (Unfortunately, those two tests are designed to detect substantial mental deficits, rather than to provide more refined cognitive assessments.) Even though the study was a randomized-control trial, lots of potentially-confounding factors were taken into account. Compared to Low-Fat Controls the participants in both of the Med-diet conditions had substantially and significantly higher scores on both cognitive measures. Compared to controls the mean effect sizes (combining the two cognitive measures) were Cohen's d = .56 for Med-Oil and d = .45 for Med-Nuts. (Those effect sizes describe the *size* of the difference on the cognitive measures between the Med diet people and the control people; see the Glossary for how to interpret effect sizes and how they contrast with statistical significance.) The apparent greater effectiveness of the Med-Oil compared to Med-Nuts was not statistically significant.

With many of the same researchers as in the previous study, Valls-Pedret et al. (2015) did a much better study, randomly assigning 447 cognitively healthy Spanish volunteers (mean age 71 at end) to the same three dietary regimes as in the previous Australian study. The dietary regimes lasted for an average of four years. The Med-Oil diet participants were given one liter of extra-virgin olive oil per week (seems a lot to me, but that is what was given, not necessarily consumed); the Med-Nuts people were allocated 30 grams of nuts per day, and as before, the Low Fat Control diet merely advised limiting dietary fats. In contrast to the basic cognitive measures of the prior study, in this study, the researchers used extensive and sophisticated cognitive assessments (e.g., several subscales from IQ tests). Another improvement over the previous study was that the cognitive tests were administered at the beginning and end of the dietary period. Thus change scores could be calculated for the cognitive measures of memory, frontal lobe functions (attention and executive functions), and for a global cognitive score. Potentially confounding factors were taken into account as in the previous study.

Despite the participants aging four years to a mean of 71 years, the participants in the two Med-diet conditions actually improved slightly on the *global memory measure*, in contrast to the expected (but small) declines for the Control participants; however, unlike the substantial and significant differences in other cognitive functions, those between-group differences in memory were not statistically significant.

As anticipated after aging four years, the Control participants declined on the composite measure of frontal lobe *executive functions*. In contrast, the Med-Oil participants improved substantially and did significantly better than the Controls (effect size of d = .50, $p$ = .003). The frontal lobe scores for the Med-Nuts participants were essentially unchanged across the four years and did not differ significantly from the Controls.

The *cognitive composite* score also declined substantially and significantly for the Control participants (for that decline, I calculated the effect size as approximately d = .40, $p$ < .05). In contrast, scores of the Med-Oil participants increased very slightly but differed significantly from the substantial decline of the Controls (effect size for the between-condition difference around d = .43, $p$ = .005). The very slight decline in global cognition for the Med-Nuts people was not statistically different from the more substantial decline of the Controls (but the effect-size for the between-group difference was d = .32). The authors' appropriate conclusion was that "in an older population, a Mediterranean diet supplemented with olive oil or nuts is associated with improved cognitive function" (Valls-Pedret et al., 2015, p. 1102). Other more recent studies give strong support to that conclusion for olive oil, both for cognitively normal elderly people and for those already experiencing some cognitive decline (Sakurai et al., 2021; Tsolaki et al., 2020).

Panza et al. (2018) also reviewed several studies of relationships between brain structures (based on MRI scans) and adherence to the Med diet and diets similar to the Med. Results showed that in general, the thickness and volume of various cortical areas correlated positively with adherence to those Med-style diets. The cortical areas that benefited most from the Med were structures of the left hemisphere—structures that are observed to shrink when Alzheimer's develops (and shown to be reduced with the Western diet as well). White-matter connectivity also benefited from adherence to the Med and related diets.

Panza and colleagues suggested that those physical benefits to the brain may have stemmed largely from improved vascular networks. Even though the studies they reviewed (and those reviewed just above) suggest that cognitive improvements are derived from olive oil, they speculated that it was the overall dietary approach rather than any specific nutrient that conveyed the observed benefits. In fact, as mentioned above, that idea is increasingly shared by nutritionists—that individual nutrients may be far less effective for brain and cognition than Med-like combinations of nutrients.

The most recent of the reviews of cognitive impacts from the Med, by Vinciguerra et al. (2020, p. 15), concluded similarly that beyond its proven reduction of cardiovascular disease and mortality that the Med reduces "the risk of development and progression of cognitive impairment." Furthermore, they note that the Med should be widely available because it can be tailored to fit the cultural habits of various countries and regions.

**The DASH diet**. DASH stands for "Dietary Approach to Stop Hypertension." The DASH diet emphasizes reduced salt intake to control blood pressure, and to minimize red meat the diet substitutes other forms of lean protein such as chicken, fish, and beans. Like the Med and closely-related diets, the DASH emphasizes fruits and vegetables and eliminates added sugars and fat. Because the DASH recommendations have been largely incorporated into the MIND, we consider it no more.

**The MIND diet.** The MIND diet is the awkwardly named "Mediterranean-DASH Intervention for Neurodegenerative Delay." Obviously, it seeks to combine elements of the Med and the DASH. Its noteworthy features are prescriptions of one daily serving of green leafy veggies, one other veg per day, three servings of whole grains, and some nuts, beans, berries, sea food, poultry, olive oil and wine. Berries and green leafy veggies are emphasized more than in other diets, and I love that as with the Med, wine is included. The MIND minimizes red meats, butter and margarine, pastries and sweets, fried/fast foods and (most cruel) cheese (but otherwise, dairy is not discouraged; Panza et al., 2018).

A longitudinal study by the National Institute of Health asked more than 900 adults (mostly women, average age 81) to complete food questionnaires and take lots of neurological tests across a span of 4.5 years (Morris et al., 2015). Those who followed the MIND diet most closely (top 1/3) had brains that functioned the equivalent of 7.5 years younger than those in the bottom 1/3, with 53% lower Alzheimer's risk. Even people who approximated the diet had reduced Alzheimer's risk by 35%. Alzheimer's risk reduction was achieved to a lesser degree by being in the top 1/3 in adhering to either the Med or DASH diets. The researchers controlled for age, sex, education, weight, physical activity, and cardiovascular health. That study is far from unique, with many other supportive studies. The review by Panza et al. (2018) and the summary by Moore et al. (2018) reached similar conclusions.

Dhana et al. (2021) determined the association of MIND diet with cognition, and asked specifically whether that relationship varied with the level of Alzheimer's-related brain pathology. Food questionnaires assessed adherence to the MIND. Cognitive scores were obtained from 19 detailed and thorough neuropsychological tests taken close to the time of the deaths of the participants. From those, a global cognitive score was compiled. Dhana and colleagues examined the autopsies of the brains of 569 elderly participants (average age 91 at death), especially assessing the hippocampi and various cortical structures. The pathology indicators included the nasty proteins β-amyloid and tau, and the plaques and tangles caused by distorted forms of those proteins.

As expected, more brain pathology correlated with lower cognitive scores ($\beta = -0.609$, $p<0.001$). However, also as anticipated, adherence to the MIND correlated with better cognitive scores ($\beta = .12$, $p = .003$), and with slower cognitive decline even after accounting for a host of potential confounds including age at death, sex, years of education, involvement with cognitive activities, exercise, total calories consumed, and variations of the Alzheimer's-related *APOE* gene. Most importantly, the (modest) level of that correlation of the MIND with cognitive preservation was not reduced at all when the scores for Alzheimer's pathology were taken into account. In other words, the cognitive benefits from the MIND were not only because it reduced brain pathology. Dhana et al. (2021, p. 690) concluded "that adherence to the MIND diet may ... contribute to building cognitive resilience in older adults."

A study of age of onset of Parkinson's by Metcalfe-Roach et al. (2021) used retrospective food frequency questionnaires to determine adherence to the MIND diet, the Med, or the Greek version of the Med diet. The 167 participants all had known dates of onset of their Parkinson's disease. Highly significant results showed that women in the upper third in adherence to the MIND had Parkinson's onset years later than those who adhered least to the MIND. For the men, adherence to the Greek Med diet made the most difference, with similar but not as spectacular results. Those in the top third in adherence to the Greek Med had Parkinson's onset several years later than the third of the men whose diets were least like the Greek Med. The authors concluded that we should consume a diet rich in fresh vegetables, whole grains, and healthy oils, but that we should limit our consumption of dairy products, red meat, added sugar, and processed foods.

**The Canadian Brain Health Food Guide.** These guidelines are like the MIND, except they recommend more fruit and veggies, and one rather than two servings of fish per week. Following a review of the diets that affect cognitive decline and Alzheimer's, Singh et al. (2014) noted a 36% reduction in Alzheimer's for followers of the Canadian guide.

**The Dietary Guidelines for Americans, 2015-2020, Eighth Edition**. Because the many editions seem to indicate rapid modifications, it may be best to see this plan electronically. For online access, visit: https://health.gov/dietary guidelines/2015/resources/2015-2020_Dietary_Guidelines.pdf.

The American guidelines emphasize veggies from colorful groups that are dark green, red and orange, and legumes, whole fruits, whole grains, low-fat dairy, and a variety of protein from fish, lean meat, poultry, eggs, nuts, seeds, and soy products. Oils should be included, but not saturated fats or transfats. Added sugar should be minimized, salt kept low, and women should have at most one alcoholic drink/day, and men at most two.

**Protein from animals or veggies.** Those diets and guidelines uniformly recommend lowering our typical high ratios of meat to veggies and fruit. Another form of support for that recommendation comes from those who study the "blue zones" where people reach extraordinary old ages. Those writers (e.g., Buettner, 2008) often note that instead of deriving much protein from animals (typically dead) that instead beans and whole grains are often main sources of proteins.

As you consider beans, note too that lentils are a type of bean that has received attention recently. In well-controlled random-assignment studies, lentils have shown dramatic impacts on lowering blood glucose and thus preventing diabetes. (As noted below, similar observations have been made for whole grain foods.) It is believed that when lentils are substituted for high glycemic-index foods that their blood glucose-controlling benefits are derived largely from their high content of polyphenols (Ganesan & Xu, 2017; polyphenols haunt Chapter 6; high glycemic index foods would include rice, potatoes, bread, and some fruits). Remember that in addition to directly benefiting the brain, that controlling blood glucose is also beneficial for the cardiovascular system, and that anything good for the cardiovascular system indirectly benefits the brain.

Perhaps deserving of more mention than received so far here, whole grains are major components of these major diets. Not only are whole grains laden with plant proteins, but apparently, because they are low in glycemic index they seem to inhibit the development of Type-2 diabetes. Martikainen et al. (2021) noted that one third of the people of Finland consume less than one serving of whole grains per day. They estimated that if Finnish people were to increase consumption to the recommended three to six servings, that reductions in Type-2 diabetes would result in vast savings in health, lives, and a billion Euros over the next 10 years.

**Fruit and veggies.** Obviously, all of the complex diets reviewed above emphasize consumption of the fruit and veggies that lead to brain health and to cognitive preservation. Researcher supports those specific relationships. For example, using a cross-section design, Nurk et al. (2010) studied over 2,000 Norwegians between 70 and 74 years old. Those participants completed food frequency questionnaires and took a large array of sophisticated cognitive tests. After taking into account an appropriately large array of potential confounds, including many foods and nutrients, consumption of each of the six food groups was correlated with the various cognitive measures. (Participants were assigned to categories of either "high intake" of each food group, or to "low or non-user"). The food groups were fruits, veggies, potatoes, grain products, mushrooms, and nuts. Those that corresponded with better cognition (at highly significant levels and with substantial effect sizes) were the separate categories of fruits and of veggies, with (in both cases) around 200 "low" users compared with over 1800 "high" users. The combination measure of fruits plus veggies showed very similar high correlations with the cognitive measures. (Mushrooms, discussed in Chapter 6 and elsewhere, were also associated with better cognitive scores.) The food groups that were not associated with better cognition were potatoes, grain products, and (surprisingly) nuts.

A more recent thorough review that similarly examined the fruit and veggie food groups was provided by Solfrizzi et al. (2017). Their emphasis was on those food groups that delayed cognitive decline and Alzheimer's. The studies they carefully selected were published from 2014 through 2016, often featuring thousands of participants. They concluded that consumption of oily fish by people over 65 led to greater cortical thickness in various brain areas, higher total gray matter, and improved cognition and memory. Results from consumption of fruits and veggies were mixed. But when the measure was the consumption of only veggies, the reviewed research showed veggie consumption to correlate with increased cortical thickness and cognitive preservation, especially when the veggies were leafy greens, as emphasized in the MIND. Similarly, when their combined measure of fruits plus veggies was examined, that measure also correlated with cognitive preservation. But Solfrizzi et al. noted that some studies of only fruit consumption showed *negative* correlations with both physiological measures such as cortical thickness and cognitive performance indicators. Solfrizzi et al. suggested that the negative relationship of some fruit with those dependent measures was due to the high glycemic index (see Glossary if needed) of some fruits, and the neurological decrements caused by high blood glucose levels. More coverage of the benefits from diets rich in fruit and veggies is offered in Chapter 6.

**A brief summary and glance ahead.** There are far more commonalities than differences between the main dietary approaches reviewed above, and obviously, the Med, the MIND, DASH, and the similar diets sketched above are very effective for preserving brain and cognition. On the other hand, more recent diets such as Keto, Paleo, calorie-restricting, and fasting diets have far fewer elements in common with those five diets. Their popularity is recent, and so is research evaluating them. I discuss that research and their possible benefits later, in Chapter 17.

Chapter 5

# Fats

Reaching back to the mid-20th Century, chefs and grandmothers knew that various foods should be sizzled in bacon fat, and that real quality in pastries and pie crusts depended on lard—lots of it. But those culinary traditions changed dramatically between then and later decades, with fat acquiring evil connotations. Cooking with bacon fat and lard gave way to buying foods labeled "low fat" or even "fat free." Products that proudly wore those new labels ranged from crackers to milk and things like yogurt and ice cream that were made with milk. The meat we searched for was lean, and adding the melted butter to the popcorn became a moral issue. Besides worms and protein derived from insects, by the early 21st century fats had become our most-avoided food group.

But times have changed again. Modern approaches to fats are more nuanced because we know that the various fats we consume are vastly different from each other in benefits to our health, even the health of our brains and cognitive functions. Instead of condemning fats, today the pendulum of dietary concerns swings against added sugar, carbohydrates in high-glycemic foods, and even carbohydrates in general. Thus we begin.

**Saturation.** The impacts that fats have on our bodies depend largely on their degree of "saturation." Saturated fatty acids are saturated by virtue of keeping all the hydrogen molecules they can carry. Those saturated fats are found in meat, dairy, and in coconut and palm oils. Like transfats, they are solid at room temperature, and like transfats they should be limited in our diets. Transfats occur in small amounts in some foods naturally (especially beef and dairy), but most of the transfats in food were created by a process of adding hydrogen to unsaturated fatty acids. That process solidified those liquid fats and extended their shelf life, but it also made them awful for the cardiovascular system; thus, adding them during food processing is discouraged in most countries, and illegal in some.

Consider (and consume) the unsaturated fats. Monounsaturated fatty acids (hereafter just "monos") have lost (but presumably do not search for) one pair of hydrogen molecules, whereas polyunsaturated fatty acids ("polys") have been especially careless, having lost two or more pairs of hydrogen molecules. Both the monos and the polys are liquid at room temperature, and both are way better for us than saturated fats and transfats.

**Fat studies.** Some studies have examined the relative impacts of those categories (i.e., saturated, mono, and poly fats) on cognitive outcomes. One described (at the time) as the most detailed and powerful study of dietary fats on health, included over 125,000 nurses from the Nurses' Health Study. The study lasted up to 32 years (Wang et al., 2016). The Nurses' Health Study was about deaths, not cognitive capacity, but one of the included death categories was neurodegenerative diseases. When compared with the same number of calories from carbohydrates, every 5% increase in *saturated fats* was associated with an 8% *increase* in overall mortality. Substituting *poly fats* (Omegas 3 and 6 mostly) and *mono fats* for carbohydrates led to (respectively) 11% and 19% mortality *reduction*. Substituting the polys (especially) for the saturated fats also led to reduced neurodegenerative diseases. Although those data are correlational, by themselves they are strongly suggestive and supported by much of the research on specific fats that is presented below.

One of the research issues to keep in mind when consuming this type of research is the level of habitual consumption of the food or nutrient in the population supplying the participants. For example, elderly Japanese people consume less fat, and especially less saturated fat than typical Americans. Thus the study of elderly Japanese that found overall fat consumption to correlate positively with cognition does not strongly imply that similar relationships would hold for Americans (Sakurai et al., 2021).

**The monos: olive oil.** Olive oil is usually thought of as one of the monounsaturated fats, and although that is largely correct, olive oil is actually a complex food that also contains beneficial polyphenols (discussed in Chapter 6) and some of the poly oils (e.g., several of the omega's) as well; it even has some saturated fats, but not enough to be concerning. Perhaps because of that complexity, olive oil is a star, considered by some to be the ingredient that provides the magic in the Med diet. Olive oil earned that recognition largely by lowering LDL (bad cholesterol), and by controlling blood pressure, strokes, and inflammation. But far more importantly from our perspective, it supports brain integrity and cognition.

One of the causal paths between olive oil and cognition was explored by Zamroziewicz et al. (2017). To assess whether the various categories of fats corresponded with the organization of neural networks, blood assays of monos and saturated fats were taken from 99 middle-aged adults. Higher blood levels of monos were associated with higher IQ, and as shown by fMRIs, the mono levels also correlated with better "intrinsic connectivity" of the dorsal attention network. (Functional MRIs are brain scans that assess activity in a working brain, rather than the volume or integrity of brain or other structures derived from MRIs.) A well-integrated dorsal attention network (affectionately known as DAN) is vital for intelligence. The authors suggested that it is olive oil's benevolent impact on the organization of such networks that explains the positive correlations found between monos and IQ. Do not lose that most important research finding in the array of lesser facts: higher intake of olive oil and (presumably) other monos apparently makes us smarter. (At least it does if the causal arrow flies in the proper direction). The main component of olive oil is oleic acid, but given the complexity of olive oil (composed also of other oils and some polyphenols) it has been difficult to establish which of the components is responsible for its cognitive benefits.

My enthusiasm for olives notwithstanding, keep in mind that for all the spiffy scientific look of that research, it is still a correlational finding that could have resulted from smarter people choosing more mono fats than saturated fats. (You do, don't you?)

But even though the relationships in that Zamroziewicz et al. study were correlational, credibility is gained from supportive randomized-control trials—even those using critters. For example, Lauretti et al. (2017) enrolled transgenic Alzheimer's mice in their research. Those star-crossed creatures had genes that predisposed them to accumulate β-amyloid plaques and to develop dementia. To (attempt to) redress that unjust treatment, half of the mice received daily supplemental olive oil. Compared to controls on a normal diet, the olive-oiled rodents had better brain autophagy (i.e., better removal of dead cells, β-amyloid, and other disgusting residue) resulting in reduced plaques between neurons and fewer tangles within them. Versus the controls, the well-oiled mice showed "dramatic" positive differences in the appearance and function of their neurons. Benefits to their neurons undoubtedly resulted too from the observed higher levels of synaptophysin, a protein that, as the name suggests, builds synapses (and would have constructed synapses in those rodents if the neurons had been allowed to remain in their original local). As normally follows those positive physiological modifications, the olive-oiled mice were lots smarter too.

With that supportive research, it seems much more likely that the correlations between plasma mono levels on the one hand and cognition and neural connectivity on the other (from the study of elderly people by Zamroziewicz et al.) were actually because the monos caused those great results. Perhaps a celebratory swig of olive oil is in order!

Excessive heating degrades olive oil, especially olive oil in its purist "extra virgin" form. That heating problem is common to the other mono oils as well. Olive oil that is *not* extra virgin is more resistant to degradation by heat and so is better for cooking, but it seems unlikely that typical cooks will buy low quality olive oil to resolve that issue. (Canola oil, also often used for cooking, is a mono that is similarly acclaimed by some (but not all) nutritionists; it is somewhat suspect because after being extracted from rape seeds it is *very* highly processed.) Other healthful monos are found in safflower seeds, nuts, peanuts, and avocados. (See Chapter 16 for exciting impacts of avocados on the microbiome.)

**The omegas.** The omega 3s and omega 6s are polyunsaturated fatty acids. In the research literature the polys are often referred to by their pleasant-sounding acronym of PUFAs. But the omega 9s are monounsaturated. Each of the omegas is usually written with an "s" as I did in the subtitle, because some have components. Although the three omegas are important for overall health and for brain health, their impacts differ. I begin with some notes on the two we know least about.

Omega 6 converts to arachidonic acid (AA) and gamma-lenolenic acid (GLA); for our purposes, there is no need to remember those. In contrast to the anti-inflammatory functions of the omega 3s, the omega 6s are at least somewhat inflammatory, and that aspect of omega 6s seems to benefit some immune system responses. Nevertheless, modern nutritionists suggest that the omega 6s should be limited in our diets and balanced with equal (or almost equal) amounts of omega 3s. That balance is not easily achieved, however, because the omega 6s are much more prevalent in our modern diets, with some estimates that a typical American diet has up to 15 times more omega 6s than omega 3s. To keep that balance closer to the ratio typically recommended, nutritionists suggest that we consume fatty fish that are high in omega 3s (like salmon) once or twice per week or (gads!) resort to omega 3 supplements. The foods with unhealthy concentrations of omega 6s are some refined cooking oils and some of the usual suspects: processed snack foods, and processed and fatty meats.

The components of omega 9 are oleic acid and erucic acid. Those components are found in avocados, nuts, peanuts, and especially olive oil. In fact, olive oil is well over 50% oleic acid. Because oleic acid is one of the omega 9 fatty acids, in general all of the great results from olive oil that are outlined above apply as well to omega 9s. Thus omega 9s are antioxidants that are also thought to lower blood pressure, reduce insulin resistance and promote healthy blood glucose levels, but the ample research literature on impacts of olive oil (and of oleic acid) on cognition essentially substitutes for similar research on omega 9s.

More research attention has been focused on the omega 3s than the other omega fatty acids. Two major omega 3 components are DHA (the unpronounceable docosahexaenolic acid) and EPA (not the Environmental Protection Agency, but the equally-difficult eicosapentaenoic acid; you can see why nutritionists tend to use their acronyms rather than formal names). EPA is recommended by professional organizations such as the American Heart Association and American Diabetes Association for its positive impact on cardiovascular health and glucose management. But of course, if the components of omega 3s benefit the cardiovascular system and glucose metabolism, then besides anticipated benefits to brain and cognition, they may contribute to longevity. Let us see.

Recall that Zamroziewicz et al. (2017) assessed mono levels in blood, finding positive impacts on cognition. McBurney et al. (2021) used a similar approach. They studied the omega 3 levels in red blood cells of the elderly participants of the Framingham cohort (who have been studied for cardiovascular issues for decades). After taking into account the potential confounds, death from all causes was lower in the elderly people with the highest omega 3 levels (the top fifth). They lived almost five years longer than those in the bottom fifth. The authors also noted that Japanese people, who outlive Americans by several years, also had average omega 3 blood levels that were even higher than the Americans in the top fifth in the study. Keep in mind that those were not direct assessments of brain function, but nevertheless, we remain aware that deceased brains score zero on cognitive tests.

**Impacts of omega 3s on cognition.** First, I review some studies from the substantial research showing that omega 3s have physiological impacts on our brains. I will conclude the section with less-definitive reviews and meta-analyses that addressed whether we might become (even minor) stable geniuses from consuming copious quantities of omega 3s.

Omega 3 fatty acids affect brains by stabilizing neural cell membranes, suppressing inflammation, eliminating β-amyloid, and supporting the brain's mitochondrial functions by improving glucose delivery and metabolism. Amen et al. (2017) noted that when people were scanned by fMRIs while doing various cognitive tasks, that increased brain blood flow corresponded with blood levels of omega 3s, illustrating one of the many possible causal avenues between omega 3s and cognitive performance.

After noting the effectiveness of omega 3s for restoring cognitive abilities in both mice and people following stressful situations, Hennebelle et al. (2014) suggested such cognitive restoration probably followed from omega 3s' anti-inflammatory activities and regulation of neurotransmitters. The net impacts of those functions are to build and maintain synapses, especially for those neurons in and around the hippocampi that use glutamate for neurotransmission. The omega 3s also have positive impacts on the brain-cleaning activities of the microglia.

Several recent reviews of longitudinal, cross-sectional, and randomized-control trials provide mixed support for the expectations that the great physiological impacts of the omega 3s should translate into great cognitive impacts. For example, the extensive review by Avallone et al. (2019) concluded that only the correlational studies showed that higher omega 3 consumption preserves cognition and decreases the risk of Parkinson's disease. But unfortunately, even in the context of those findings, Avallone and colleagues found no substantial support from the randomized-control trials they reviewed. Furthermore, they came to similar null conclusions in their review of randomized-control trials of omega 3 impacts on both mood and severe depression.

Rangel-Huerta and Gil (2018, p. 17) also came to null conclusions from their equally extensive review of randomized-control trials. They stated that "it is still unclear if [omega 3s] can improve cognitive development or prevent cognitive decline in young or older adults." In the most recent of the reviews of possible cognitive impacts, after considering 38 randomized-control trials, Brainard et al. (2020) concluded that omega 3 fatty acids apparently had no substantial impact on cognitive decline.

The lack of any confirming evidence from the randomized-control trials is surprising, especially in light of the research that shows *how* the omega 3s can have positive brain impacts. However, hope was not dashed completely. Even after their tepid review of those mixed results Avallone and colleagues suggested that the strengths of the longitudinal research should not be ignored. They noted that the randomized-control trials of nutrients are often necessarily conducted in spans of months, rather than the years (or even lifetimes) such as is done by some of the longitudinal and cross-sectional studies.

Another (weak) possible explanation for the inconsistent results from different research styles is the likelihood that nutrients like the omega 3s benefit brain and cognition only in the presence of sufficient levels of some other nutrients or neurochemicals. As an illustration of that approach, Jernerén et al. (2019) studied the impacts of omega 3s while taking into account levels of homocysteine in plasma. Homocysteine is not only an indicator of stress, but also regarded by Jernerén et al. as a marker of B vitamin status. For six months, 171 patients with mild to moderate Alzheimer's dementia were randomly assigned to a placebo control condition or to receive the components of omega 3 (1.7 grams/day of DHA and .6 grams/day of EPA). The statistically significant interactions showed that in patients with low levels of plasma homocysteine (indicating low stress and adequate vitamin B levels) supplementation with the omega 3 components increased cognitive performance as assessed by several tests administered at the beginning and end of that 6-month study. Jernerén et al. concluded that vitamin B vitamin levels must be adequate in order to obtain cognitive benefits from omega 3s. In fact, the likelihood of interactions of the omega 3s with the B vitamins was supported by Oulhaj et al. (2016). They showed that cognitive decline was delayed by enhanced B vitamins only when omega 3 levels were above the mean. (Details of the Oulhaj et al. study are presented in Chapter 8.)

Great sources of those healthy omega 3s are ocean fish, especially salmon, with walnuts and soy contributing some. The omega 3s and other polys are also found in and extracted from sunflower seeds, flax seeds, corn, and cottonseed, but those sources actually provide combinations of monos and polys and mixes of omega 6s with omega 3s. Omega 3s are also readily available in inexpensive supplements from fish oil and flaxseed. Those supplements seem to have no negative side effects.

**Summary.** Await Chapter 17 for thoughts about brain and cognitive impacts from diets that are high in fats versus those with normal amounts.

Of course, we should *replace* unwholesome fats with more nutritious ones, rather than adding new fat calories to the diet. My summary assessment is that the foregoing tells us unequivocally that olive oil should be one of the oils of choice in our diets, and although the omega 3s have not (yet) been proven beyond a reasonable shadow to benefit cognition and mood, other health indicators suggest we should include them too.

Remember that salmon is almost always on the menu at the local steak house, and that double veggies are typically permitted to replace the fries. And choose olive oil for the salad.

Chapter 6

# Phytonutrients

When you next enjoy a holiday dinner with the family, as you survey the many veggie dishes that will (hopefully) attend the table, consider using the term phytonutrients. Doing so will establish your bonafide as a learned sophisticate, even though the term means nothing more than plant-derived nutrients. If confronted with unappreciative responses from the gathering, mention that the term "phytonutrients" is often used interchangeably with "phytochemicals." Your desirability as a future dinner guest may now be assured.

The phytonutrients bolster the immune systems of their host plants, defending against potential pathogens, including bacteria, viruses, and fungi. After we people consume those plants, the phytonutrients generally enhance our health by serving as both antioxidants and anti-inflammatories. Brightly colored fruits and veggies typically have high phytonutrient concentrations. That is the reason your mother insisted you eat both your veggies and the daily apple with the skin intact. Besides giving us our mitochondria, (see Chapter 15) mothers often give excellent advice.

The phytonutrients we consume are especially beneficial to our brains. For example, in their review of the neuroprotection conferred by phytonutrients Naoi et al. (2019) note that diets rich in bioactive phytonutrients may delay onset and retard the progress of several neurodegenerative disorders, including Alzheimer's and Parkinson's. Those protective functions rely on phytonutrients opposing oxidative stress, suppressing inflammation, supporting mitochondria, and restoring important and well-loved neurotropins like BDNF. They also regulate cell death, and prevent the accumulation of the deformed proteins such as the $\beta$-amyloid and tau that we associate with Alzheimer's dementia.

Major sub-divisions of phytonutrients described below are the polyphenols and the carotenoids. Each of those sub-divisions is in turn further subdivided. For example, the ever-popular flavonoids comprise a sub-category of the polyphenols. The sub-categories in turn subsume other sub-categories (e.g., flavanols and flavonols) and literally hundreds of individual phytonutrients. Those many nutrients are introduced only briefly here because our overarching mission is to understand only known impacts on brain and cognition. Thus I mention some of the individual foods that supply those important phytonutrients, especially if those foods or supplements are popular or have research-confirmed impacts on brain and cognition. For example, in Chapter 7, I give special attention to coffee, tea, and caffeine because they are consumed around the world and are the subjects of reams of research, and because they have impacts on cognition, states of alertness, and moods. Besides, they have interesting phytonutrients.

## Polyphenols, flavonoids, and carotenoids

**Polyphenols.** Although they can be synthesized, polyphenols are plant-based compounds containing several (the "poly" part of the term) phenol structures. The impacts of specific polyphenols are determined by the individual nature of the phenol structures, and their quantity. All of the things said above about the good results we obtain from consuming phytonutrients apply especially to the polyphenols; happily, there are over 500 kinds of bioactive polyphenols. Their antioxidant and anti-inflammatory activities are legendary. Some, nutrients, such as the spices like cinnamon that benefit us via their polyphenols, are reviewed in other chapters.

High levels of polyphenols populate the Mediterranean and the MIND diets. Polyphenols are found in fruits, veggies, and whole grains and they are found in olive oil with the highest concentrations in extra virgin olive oils. Some other foods rich in polyphenols include grapes, apples, pears, cherries and berries. (Recall that berries are emphasized especially in the MIND diet.) For each 100 grams (roughly ¼ pound) of any of those fruits, one obtains 200 to 300mgs of polyphenols. If that meal is accompanied by a glass of red wine, then we gain around 100mgs more, and with a cup of coffee or tea afterward, another 100mgs is added. But more about those beverages later.

**Flavonoids.** As noted above, flavonoids are one of the important sub-categories of polyphenols, with hundreds of separate compounds assigned to six flavonoid sub-categories that look and sound confusingly alike. Along with another sub-category of phytonutrients, the carotenoids discussed below, flavonoids provide the vivid colors in fruits and in some vegetables.

Recent research by Holland et al. (2020) provides major support for the hypothesis that positive cognitive impacts result from consuming high levels of flavonoids. (Holland et al. actually studied flavon*ols*, a subgroup of flavo*noids*.) The 921 elderly participants who were initially free from dementia (at age 81) were given annual neurological exams and a validated food frequency questionnaire for six years. During that time, 24% developed Alzheimer's dementia. (That is a frightening number, especially for the elderly.) Even after controlling for the potentially-confounding factors of age, sex, education, participation in cognitive and physical activities, and the *APOE-4* gene (the genetic variant that increases Alzheimer's vulnerability), the fifth of the participants consuming the least flavonols were twice as likely to have developed Alzheimer's as the fifth with the most flavonols. That is, the hazard ratio was an astonishing HR = .52 for total flavonol consumption. (Hazard ratios are much like risk ratios; an HR of .52 means that for every 52 people developing dementia in the high flavonol condition, there were 100 in the group with low flavonol consumption; see the Glossary if more is needed).

Four specific subcategories of flavonols were also associated with reduced incidences of Alzheimer's; they were kaempferol (HR = .49), isorhamnetin (HR = .62), and myricetin (HR = .62) and perhaps most important, quercetin (HR = .69). Certainly, those are not household names, but the better-known quercetin is thought to contribute to the delay of Alzheimer's—delay associated with *Ginkgo biloba* (discussed in Chapter 12) and with red wine (discussed in Chapter 14).

A similar study of the "Framingham offspring cohort" of 2800 participants who were on average 60 years old at onset were followed across almost 20 years by Shistar et al. (2020). Food intake questionnaires were administered at 5-year intervals. Bad cognitive outcomes were classified as Alzheimer's-related dementia. Compared with the lowest 15% in flavonol intake, those in the highest 40% of flavonols had half the incidence of Alzheimer's-related dementias (HR = .54, $p = 0.003$). Higher intake of anthocyanins (another flavonoid subtype found in red, blue and purple berries and grapes) also provided even better protection against Alzheimer's-related dementias (HR = .24, $p < 0.001$). Given the odd division of 40% of participants in the "high" flavonol category compared with 15% of the participants considered low in those nutrients, the logical conclusion seems to be that for people between 60 and 80 years old being very low in consumption of flavonoids is really dangerous for cognitive preservation.

In fact, those correlational relationships are so surprisingly large that we certainly need confirmation from studies that can determine causal directions. Happily, the supportive randomized-control trials reviewed below do exactly that. Some of those studies show impacts from flavonoids from cacao, so first, let us consider, cacao, cocoa and chocolate.

Chocolate is a wonderful by-product of cacao. Cacao is the relatively raw product of the cacao bean. The more common term, cocoa, designates the cooked or processed form of cacao, and even the bean itself is called a cocoa bean after it has been processed. Although the two forms taste similar and can be substituted for each other in baking, it is cacao—the relatively raw product—that is especially high in flavonoids that are both antioxidants and anti-inflammatories. Unfortunately, it is the less nutritious cocoa that finds its way into the typical chocolate bar that we pick up in the rest stop to keep us alert during our trip home.

These next two randomized-control trials by Neshatdoust et al. (2017) assessed flavonoids derived from fruit and veggies (Study 1) and from cocoa (Study 2). The fine quality of the research and importance of the findings deserves thorough coverage. The well-chosen dependent measures assessed both cognitive changes and serum measures of the essential neurotropin BDNF. (Serum BDNF levels correspond with brain concentrations, and remember, BDNF maintains and grows neurons.)

In Study I, the 154 participants (aged 26 to 70) were randomly assigned to one of three conditions: either a control condition featuring "own habitual diet" or to the high or the low flavonoid conditions. The flavonoids were provided in fruit and veggies supplied by the researchers. The participants in the two flavonoid conditions consumed an average of three servings per day for 18 weeks, but whereas the fruits and veggies selected for the high flavonoid participants supplied over 15mg per 100 grams, the less generous fruits and veggies for the low flavonoid group supplied fewer than 5mg of flavonoids per 100 grams.

The cognitive components that were assessed for both Studies I and II included measures of executive function, episodic and spatial memory, working memory, attention, and processing speed—a thorough and admirable array that used different forms of the tests at each administration and that took 90 minutes each time. For Study I the cognitive measures were assessed at baseline, at six weeks, 12 weeks, and at the study's end at 18 weeks.

At 12-weeks and at the study's end at 18-weeks, the high flavonoid group substantially and significantly outperformed the other two groups on the cognitive assessments ($p < .01$) with the low flavonoid and control groups remarkably similar to each other. Although the authors did not offer an effect size for the relative cognitive brilliance of the high flavonoid group, from their figures, it appears to be around $d = .23$ (the Glossary provides an explanation of effect size). Did your mother tell you that besides making you grow, eating your fruits and veggies would make you smarter too?

Levels of the great neurotropin BDNF were assessed from serum. Relative to the diet-as-usual control condition, serum BDNF levels were higher at six weeks, 12 weeks, and 18 weeks for both the low and high flavonoid groups. But BDNF levels for the high flavonoid group were uniformly highest at each measurement interval ($p < .026$ for the interaction of condition by time). As predicted, higher baseline BDNF levels corresponded with better scores on those sophisticated cognitive measures, even after taking into account the possible confounding variables of age, gender, BMI, waist circumference, and blood pressure.

Using a cross-over design in Study II, Neshatdoust et al. randomly assigned 40 older participants (aged 62 to 75 years) to one of two flavonol conditions. Unlike the fruit and veggies of Study 1, the flavonol was delivered in daily chocolate drinks made with cocoa. (Now we're talking!) The high flavonol drinks had 494 mg of flavonols whereas the daily cocoa drinks in the low condition supplied only 23 mg.

After spending four weeks consuming either high or low levels of flavonols, the participants took four weeks off (a "washout period") before switching to four weeks of the other flavonol condition. Thus such crossover designs are quite powerful because each participant serves as their own control by (in this case) receiving four weeks of high flavonols and four weeks of low, either in that order or in the reverse order.

At the study's end, relative to the low flavonol condition, the high flavonol condition led to higher global cognitive performance assessed by the sophisticated and extensive test batteries ($p < .01$, with my estimated effect size of d = .35). High flavonol also led to very substantially *higher serum BDNF levels* ($p = <0.001$) and as predicted, those BDNF increases correlated with improvements in global cognitive performance. Regarding both studies, Nashatdoust and colleagues concluded that flavonoids have their positive impact on global cognitive function at least in part by up-regulating levels of BDNF. The research certainly supports those conclusions at a surprising (for me) level given dietary modifications that lasted only 18 weeks (Study 1) or just four weeks (Study 2).

In their review of both short-term and long-term impacts from cocoa, Socci et al. (2017) noted that in studies ranging from five days to three months using (mostly) elderly people, cocoa resulted in both short-term and long-term improvements in attention, processing speed, working memory, and verbal fluency. Those impacts were most pronounced in people who had begun to show some cognitive decline.

The solid affirmation from those studies and reviews of flavonoid impacts on cognition and on delaying Alzheimer's has led to recent research efforts to understand how flavonoids have those profound impacts. Obviously, flavonoid encouragement of the great neurotropin BDNF plays an important role, but others have emphasized the antioxidant and anti-inflammatory impacts of the flavonoids. For example, Ruan et al. (2018) noted that flavonoids enhance levels of the antioxidant NAD+ and thus increase the vital sirtuins. (Await discussion of NAD+ and sirtuins in Chapter 15 or, if feeling impatient, see the Glossary.) Still, others note the transformation of flavonoids by the organisms of our gut microbiome into various neuroprotective compounds. (For more on that topic, see the Chapter 16 discussion of the microbiome, and see Hole & Williams, 2020.)

We gain insights into how flavonoids have their great long-term impacts by observing their short-term impacts. Researchers at Loma Linda University Adventist Health Sciences Center (2018) found that dark chocolate (70% cacao) consumption upregulates several immune-system indicators, including T- cell activation, and it transcribes genes that affect various neuron functions. Other research shows remarkable short-term cognitive performance impacts right after consuming cacao, and perhaps accounting for that, increased blood flow in the hippocampi. In turn, the increased brain blood flow is undoubtedly related to the impacts of cacao on nitric oxide (NO), a key regulator of cardiovascular dilation (and the mechanism for action by erectile dysfunction medications—suggesting that substituting cacao ... but I am just speculating here, so never mind).

In a recent paper using yet another powerful cross-over design with high or low flavonols from cocoa given to the same participants at different times, Gratton et al. (2020) then subjected their participants to high carbon dioxide levels—a procedure that causes compensatory increases in cerebral blood flow. Their title serves as a brief summary: "Dietary flavonols improve cerebral cortical oxygenation and cognition in healthy adults." Compared to low flavonol, in response to the carbon dioxide procedure, the high flavonol consumption increased cerebral blood flow in areas of the prefrontal cortex, and cognitive performance was better after the high flavonol, but only when the cognitive test was complex.

In their review titled "Botanicals and phytochemicals active on cognitive decline..." Cicero et al. (2018) identified cacao as one of the six nutrients that current research literature supports for inhibiting cognitive decline. In that review, they identified various flavonoid receptors on neurons. The many kinds of receptors that are sensitive to cacao are also receptors for an opioid, for the wonderful neurotropin BDNF, for both estrogen and testosterone, and for several neurotransmitters including calming GABA. That sentence alone identifies various causal paths available for flavonoids to affect major brain processes.

Remember that besides cocoa and (even better) cacao, other good sources of flavonoids include colored fruits, veggies, broccoli, tomatoes, teas, and red wine. The benefits of flavonoids account for the recommendations in the Med and MIND diets discussed in Chapter 4 to have lots of those fruits and veggies and the meal-time glass of red wine, and (as emphasized by the MIND) to consume berries, especially blueberries.

**Resveratrols.** These comprise another sub-category of polyphenols found in concentration in grapes and made famous by the hope (mine included) that the modest amount found in red wine (in addition to the flavonoids) will keep us young and healthy. Red wine is often invoked to explain the "French paradox"—that even after the French soak their food in butter they avoid cardiovascular problems due to their red wine consumption. Perhaps, but reserve judgment until after you read more about resveratrol and red wine in Chapter 14.

Beyond that hypothetical French paradox, resveratrols (there are many types) have a wide range of positive health benefits. Resveratrol has proven to be an effective anti-cancer agent in both *in vivo* and *in vitro* studies—effective in inhibiting all stages of cancer. The resveratrols are also anti-inflammatory, and perhaps largely because of that feature, they are also cardioprotective, and neuroprotective. Supplements for resveratrol are available, but those have poor solubility and thus poor bio-availability. Therefore it is best to get them from healthy diets, such as prescribed by the Med and MIND (perhaps including the recommended moderate nip or red wine).

**Carotenoids.** These are another group of phytonutrients. They are distinct from the polyphenols and flavonoids mentioned above, but like those other excessively large categories, there are lots of them—over 750 different carotenoids. Along with flavonoids, they provide some of the vivid colors found in some fruits and vegetables. Although the colors of the flavonoids are varied, including the blue of blueberries, etc., carotenoids specialize in bright yellows, oranges, and reds—yes, like carrots and tomatoes. The carotenoid (and flavonoid) pigments play an important role in the health of the plants that have them, and in we folks who eat them as well. (One sees titles in sources like the Massachusetts General Hospital's bulletin *Mind, Mood and Memory* (July, 2017) such as "Plant power: pigments in fruits and vegetables boost cognition.") Both major types of carotenoids, the carotenes (orange in color), and the xanthophylls (yellow), are also major antioxidants.

Some carotenoids like the well-known beta-carotene (but also including some you will probably forget, like alpha-carotene, and beta-cryptoxanthin) can be converted to the essential vitamin A. Vitamin A is a great antioxidant that maintains the health of eyes and the immune-system, and although it may be helpful for brain and cognition, its roles there remain essentially unstudied.

Other carotenoids like lycopene (and also lutein, zeaxanthin, and astaxanthin) do not convert to vitamin A, but they still may make major contributions. For example, lycopene is thought to preserve mental agility and eye health. In fact, Feeney et al. (2017) did analyses of the amounts of both lutein and zeaxanthin in the plasma of 4,076 adults aged 50 years or older who participated in the Irish Longitudinal Study on Ageing. After accounting for the potential confounding by demographic and socioeconomic factors, health conditions, and health behaviors, Feeney and colleagues found that both lutein and zeaxanthin were independently associated with better global cognition, memory, and executive function, and that higher plasma zeaxanthin was associated with faster speed of cognitive processing.

A supportive study by Zamroziewicz et al. (2016) examined the correspondences of lutein levels (assessed from plasma) and both cognition and brain structure assessed by MRI scans. Note that luteins are one of many xanthophylls and that the xanthophylls accumulate in neural tissue (as we age) and are, in turn, a subclass of carotenoids. Because of their increasing concentrations in human brains with our aging, the xanthophylls are major suspects for delaying cognitive decline. But of the many carotenoids in the brain the luteins are the most prevalent, and thus potentially the most important. Clearly, the luteins convey some neuroprotection. The title of the paper by Zamroziewicz et al. summarizes their finding that "Parahippocampal cortex mediates the relationship between lutein and crystallized intelligence in healthy, older adults." That conclusion depended on the positive correlations between lutein levels, parahippocampal size, and measures of crystallized intelligence. But as always, we seek confirmation of causal directions from the randomized-control trials.

Nouchi et al. (2020) noted that there had been a few recent randomized-control trials, but their meta-analysis was the first to assess impacts on cognition from *any* carotenoid. From an initial selection of 1095 relevant studies, only seven studies met their criteria of being randomized-control trials with placebo control conditions. Five studied lutein. Nouchi et al. concluded that 10mg/day of lutein for a period of 12 months improved various cognitive functions in adults. The recent review by Mitra et al. (2021) supported those conclusions and noted that the diets of the elderly typically include insufficient amounts of lutein. Unfortunately, the review by Nouchi et al. found only one of two relevant studies of astaxanthin showing positive results. They concluded that astaxanthin impacts on cognitive function are uncertain. Thus I continue with a focus on lutein.

One of the proven means for lutein having its positive impacts is by increasing brain levels of the esteemed neurotropin BDNF. Lutein is known for its positive impacts on the health of eyes as well as brain. In a well-constricted randomized-control trial, but with only 21 participants per condition, in a 6-month period Stringham et al. (2016) showed that lutein significantly increased ($p = .02$) BDNF in both retina and brain. The BDNF increases in those two areas were highly correlated.

Not many randomized-control trials of quality have tested the many hundreds of carotenoids that we should consider in our diets. Without those tests of specific ingredients, it does appear that we shall be required to eat 10 pounds or so per day to consume all those thought to bring major brain/cognitive benefits. Exaggerations notwithstanding, clearly eating the highly colored fruits and veggies emphasized in the MIND diet is in order, but failing that, some supplements are available, such as those for lutein. By the way, tomatoes are celebrated for their lycopene, and when they are cooked, especially with olive oil, the load of lycopene is enhanced.

**Mushrooms.** If they are to find a home somewhere, I believe they belong in a chapter on phytonutrients. As detailed below, there are reasons to expect that consuming mushrooms will preserve cognition, and indeed research supports those expectations.

Recall from Chapter 4 that in a large study of over 2000 elderly Norwegians, Nurk et al. (2010) examined the correspondences of various food groups with a sophisticated array of cognitive measures. Surprisingly, one of those food groups was mushrooms. After taking into account a large array of potential confounds, the fourth of those participants having "high" mushroom intake were significantly superior in cognition to the three-fourths having "none-to-low" mushroom consumption. Remarkably, that relationship was a doses-response linear correlation with increasing mushroom consumption leading to increasing cognition scores.

Mushrooms impacts are derived at least in part from high amounts of two powerful antioxidants: ergothioneine and glutathione (those are not household names, but important ones). Glutathione, sometimes called the "master antioxidant," is made in our bodies, but those supplies are supplemented by our nutrition. Because the antioxidant functions of glutathione are crucially important, it receives frequent mention in subsequent chapters. Unfortunately, it declines dramatically with aging. Ergothioneine receives less subsequent mention, but it has been found to be low in various cognitive disorders, including mild cognitive impairment and "frailty" (Teruya et al., 2021). In their recent research on the nutrients in red blood cells, Teruya et al. found that both ergothioneine and glutathione were also deficient in people with dementia, in contrast to higher levels in normal controls. Certainly, such facts are not proof that declines in those antioxidants cause dementia or that boosting levels by eating mushrooms will delay cognitive decline, but mushrooms are also conscientious providers of another important nutrient: spermidine (await Chapter 12 for more about that).

The wild porcini species have the most ergothioneine and glutathione, but most types of mushrooms are higher in those two antioxidants than most other foods. In support of the potential importance of mushrooms in our diets Kalaras et al. (2017) noted that countries with the most mushroom consumption, like France and Italy, have the least neurodegenerative disease.

Although nothing is proven by such correlations, it is curious that someone even thought to suggest that relationship (while ignoring the possibility that speaking French or Italian ... never mind). (Besides all the foregoing, mushrooms can be delicious.)

**Summary.** If there is a reasonable conclusion to this diverse chapter, it is simply to remember and take seriously those admonitions from our childhood to eat our fruit and veggies, at least occasionally including berries, mushrooms, and tomatoes. And go for the pretty ones with the bright colors. Consider too that even though not recommended by our moms as a health food, that adding some chocolate (or even better, powdered cacao) to our daily coffee could make us brilliant. It is not expensive. I recently purchased (mail order) a pound of cacao powder for around $8. I have not previously considered brownies to be health foods, but now ...

Chapter 7

# Caffeine, tea, and coffee

Even Garfield, the comic-strip cat of my morning paper, cannot face his day without his coffee. The hero of "Adam at Home," a nearby strip, is similarly addicted; the caffeine monkey on his back hangs on full time. We joke about it, but coffee begins each day for over half of American adults, and many of us consider it to be essential. Google tells us (when we ask) that, on average, we coffee drinkers consume over three cups per day. Many who avoid coffee seek out tea and other caffeinated vehicles in the form of energy drinks, soft drinks, and chocolate. We drink (and eat) lots of caffeine.

But having said that, keep in mind that studying caffeine is quite different than studying coffee, or tea. Thus the possible benefits to brain and cognition from caffeine tell us little about the benefits from tea and coffee, largely because both tea and coffee have important phytonutrients besides caffeine. We begin with caffeine.

**Caffeine.** Caffeine research lacks consistency. Some of the apparently well-done studies that I review briefly below, for example, had huge numbers of participants, but their results sometimes pointed in different directions. A resolution will surely follow ... eventually.

There are substantial reasons to anticipate benefits to the brain and to cognition from caffeine. The primary one is that research on caffeine is remarkably consistent in showing that soon after consuming caffeine, most people show cognitive enhancement, including problem-solving capacities and consolidation of long-term memories, and they show increased physical endurance as well (Borota et al., 2014).

One of the most likely mechanisms for those impacts is caffeine's stimulation of energy production by the mitochondria throughout the body, including the mitochondria in the neurons of the brain. Another mechanism for caffeine's impacts, noted by Gardener et al. (2021) and described in a study summarized more thoroughly below, was that such impacts may stem from the blocking of adenosine receptors, thereby preventing the neuromodulator adenosine from slowing neural activity and relaxing us. Usually, when nutrients provide such consistent short-term impacts, then long-term consumption yields corresponding long-term benefits. Another reason to anticipate such benefits from caffeine is that animal research usually shows such positive long-term impacts (e.g., Zapata et al., 2019). Ultimately through various means caffeine seems to decrease accumulations of the nasty forms of β-amyloid and tau proteins. Those physiological benefits should surely lead to positive long-term impacts on cognition.

Despite hopeful expectations, reviews of research with people sometimes come to negative or null conclusions. For example, in a meta-analysis of many studies totaling over 500,000 European people, Zhou et al. (2018) found neither cognitive benefit nor harm from years of consumption of caffeine, whether from coffee, tea, or caffeine from other sources. Because of the huge total number of participants in the many studies in that review, the detection of even very small effects was possible, so it is especially significant that none were found.

But wait! Analyzing data from the Women's Health Initiative Study, Driscoll et al. (2016) noted that of the 6,467 women studied across a 10-year span that 388 received a dementia diagnosis. The authors took into account an appropriately large set of potentially-confounding factors, including hormone therapy, age, race, education, body mass index, sleep quality, depression, hypertension, cardiovascular disease, diabetes, smoking, and alcohol. With those factors accounted for, Driscoll et al. noted that compared to the women consuming below median amounts of caffeine (mean daily intake of 64mg), those in the upper half of caffeine consumption (mean intake of 261mg) had a much lower hazard ratio for developing any type of dementia (HR = .74, $p$ = .04) and an identical hazard ratio for displaying *any* cognitive impairment (hazard ratio also HR = .74, $p$ = .005); those substantial hazard ratios mean that either the probability of dementia or the probability of cognitive impairment was 26% lower for the half of the participants with above-average caffeine consumption. Unfortunately, we know little about the sources of the caffeine in that study, nor do we know about the beverages in the many studies in that vast null review by Zhou and colleagues.

In support of positive long-term impacts of caffeine on cognition, Vercambre et al. (2013) studied 2475 elderly women participants in the Women's Antioxidant Cardiovascular Study. The women were all over age 65 and had already been identified as having vascular disorders that put them at high risk for cognitive decline. Caffeine intake from all sources was assessed at baseline (1995–1996), and cognitive decline was assessed over five years by multiple cognitive tests of verbal memory, category fluency, and global cognition.

Vercambre et al. took into account a huge list of potential confounds that included demographic, health, and lifestyle factors. They were particularly conscientious in accounting for dietary factors, including even supplements of individual vitamins. The principle finding was that during the five years of the study, caffeine intake slowed the cognitive decline of those elderly and vulnerable women. At the study's end those in the top quintile (upper 1/5) in caffeine intake (at over 371mg/day) were cognitively sharper, appearing to be seven years younger (cognitively, $p$=0.006) than those in the bottom fifth in caffeine consumption. (However, it appeared that the effect was due to consumption of caffeinated coffee rather than to other caffeine sources).

As we reach down to molecular levels to understand caffeine, consider the relationship of caffeine to the crucially-important enzyme you may not yet know that goes by the catchy initials—NMNAT2 (known technically and awkwardly as nicotinamide mononucleotide adenylyl transferase 2). Recent research identifies NMNAT2 as absolutely crucial for the maintenance of neurons, and especially for the maintenance of the axons of brain neurons. NMNAT2 also guards against the accumulation of the distorted tau protein molecules associated with Alzheimer's. Deficiencies of NMNAT2 are found in several neurodegenerative conditions, including amyotrophic lateral sclerosis (aka: Lou Gehrig's disease), Alzheimer's, Parkinson's, and Huntington's diseases.

Ali et al. (2017) searched for molecules that would stimulate NMNAT2 production, discovering that among the several found that caffeine was especially effective, so that supplying extra caffeine resulted in the restoration of normal cognitive function in mice genetically predisposed to produce insufficient levels of NMNAT2. (Chapter 15 on mitochondria features more about dietary impacts on nicotinamide molecules.)

Although much of the foregoing suggests the likelihood of positive impacts on cognition from caffeine, the occasional null and negative results remain bothersome. Let us attempt to resolve those inconsistencies.

**Some resolutions for caffeine.** Fulton et al. (2018) provided a major review of genetic impacts on caffeine processing. Of the 26 studies included, half were randomized-control trials, allowing causal inferences. The review showed that people differ greatly in how quickly they metabolize caffeine, with faster metabolism corresponding with a greater liking for coffee and greater consumption. Perhaps those genetic tendencies affect research outcomes, depending on how participants are recruited or enrolled for studies on caffeine.

Another factor that could modify research outcomes is the age of participants. Recall that aging reduces mitochondrial efficiency, disposing reductions in both mental and physical energy. Given caffeine's stimulation of mitochondria, it is logical that caffeine may have more substantial and more positive impacts in the elderly. Indeed correlational research by Beydoun et al. (2014) of the Baltimore Longitudinal Study of Aging cohort found that caffeine intake corresponded with better global cognitive performance for participants over age 70, but not for participants who were younger.

But I suspect that one of the largest contributors to the inconsistencies between various caffeine studies with humans is simply that caffeine sources are often unknown and thus unreported in the published research. Most of the caffeine undoubtedly comes from the consumption of either tea or coffee, but those two beverages each bring different combinations of ingredients "to the table." And they are certainly different than caffeine added to soft drinks and different than the caffeine administered in research directly to either critters or humans. Some of the other ingredients in tea and coffee are certainly neuroprotective, whereas others can be counter-protective (as are some of the components of unfiltered coffee). Thus we must look separately at impacts from added caffeine, or impacts from tea, or coffee, and even at impacts from coffee prepared in different ways.

**Tea**. Worldwide, more tea is consumed than any other caffeinated beverage. As this section begins, note that the caffeine load in a typical cup of tea is about half that of coffee, whether the tea is one of the typical black or green teas, or the maté favored in parts of South America.

Much excellent research affirms that tea is simply good for brain and body. For example, in a sample of over 2000 older Norwegians (aged 70 to 74), Nurk et al. (2009) looked at the joint and separate correlations of long-term consumption of tea, wine, and chocolate with cognition. Unfortunately, the cognitive assessments were made only once, but were excellent measures. After taking into account the various potentially-confounding factors of nutrition, health, and education, the consumption of tea corresponded with better cognition in a linear fashion (i.e., more tea, better cognition).

That (and similar) research has spawned major longitudinal and cross-sectional studies supporting the benefits of tea for the brain and cognition. Recent research by Zhang, Yang et al. (2021) assessed cognitive impacts from tea (and from coffee, and the combination of tea and coffee together) in over 365 thousand people comprising the UK Biobank cohort. The participants were all over 60. That vast number of participants and the sophistication of the analyses allowed a detailed look at the amount of protection against dementia (over 5,000 developed dementia during the study) and stroke (over 10,000 cases) during a median duration of 11.4 years. Due to the quality and importance of the findings, this study will receive a closer look here and at appropriate spots below. The long list of potential confounds taken into account included sex, age, ethnicity, income, body mass index, physical activity, alcohol status, smoking status, diet pattern, consumption of sugar-sweetened beverages, high- and low-density lipoprotein, and health histories of cancer, diabetes, arterial disease, and hypertension.

Zhang, Yang et al. (2021, p. 2) noted:

> *"that (1) the separate and combined intake of tea and coffee were associated with lower risk of stroke, ischemic stroke, dementia, and*

*vascular dementia; (2) participants who reported drinking 2 to 3 cups of coffee with [here "with" means "in addition to"] 2 to 3 cups of tea per day were associated with about 30% lower risk of stroke and dementia; (3) the combination of coffee and tea seemed to correlate with lower risk of stroke and dementia compared to coffee or tea separately; and (4) intake of coffee alone or in combination with tea was associated with lower risk of poststroke dementia.*

In this section, I emphasize the findings by Zhang, Yang et al. for tea. Compared to those who drank no tea, risks were lowest for those drinking three to five cups per day for both dementia (a 28% reduction, indicating a hazard ratio of HR = .72, $p$ = 0.002) and stroke (a 32% reduction; HR = .68, $p <$ 0.001). However, daily tea drinking provided benefits at amounts only up to a point. Consumption beyond nine cups of tea per day actually increased probabilities for stroke and dementia (i.e., HR's over 1.00).

**Protection from moderate tea consumption.** Although the two studies sketched above were correlational, they are supported by many studies that reveal causal impacts from randomized-control trials. Some of that causal research has used human cells *in vitro*, but most of them have used mice or rats. Often those rodents were transgenic—having been given (without consent) genes that disposed them to develop Alzheimer's or some other neurodegenerative affliction.

Lacking opposing thumbs, most rodents have difficulties with teacups, so the tea extracts studied were typically added to drinking water. The principle beneficial nutrient in tea is the important polyphenol known ungracefully as epigallocatechin-3-gallate, but mercifully almost always written as EGCG. The many fortunate critters volunteering for the various studies showed that EGCG extended their lives, redressed damage to liver and kidneys, reduced inflammation and oxidative stress, reduced cholesterol, and otherwise benefited cardiovascular function. But there were also more direct impacts on brains and cognition.

Rezai-Zadeh et al. (2008) summarized their research in their title: "Green tea … EGCG reduces β-amyloid mediated cognitive impairment and modulates tau pathology in Alzheimer's transgenic mice." That is a magnificent finding, based on the observation that tea helps the brain to clear itself of the two notoriously nasty proteins of Alzheimer's—β amyloid and tau. I celebrate that finding, but keep in mind that although those mice had been given human genes to dispose them to develop Alzheimer's, not everything that seems to help Mickey and friends resist Alzheimer's has proven to be effective for people who are not mice. Nevertheless, the β-amyloid reduction was 50% (versus controls on a regular diet), with similar reductions in the ugly tau protein. Those physiological improvements were reflected in superior cognition (maze running—infrequent in research with people). The authors appropriately suggested that supplementation with EGCG was potentially safe and effective for reducing the potential for Alzheimer's disease.

Other research has supported those observations of EGCG-caused reductions in both β-amyloid and tau accumulations in cortex, hippocampi, and adjacent structures (e.g., Niu et al., 2013, with rats; Walker et al., 2015, with mice). EGCG also preserves the active life of a principle cancer-destroying protein (simply known as P53) that, although produced in our bodies, is otherwise short-lived (Zhao et al., 2021). And EGCG and other tea-derived catechin flavonoids have recently been shown to relax blood vessels, thereby reducing blood pressure, ultimately benefiting brains (Redford et al., 2021). The flavonoids of tea also provide neuroprotection as antioxidants and anti-inflammatories; furthermore, they enhance insulin effectiveness, reducing the potential for developing Type-2 diabetes.

Finally, an important avenue for EGCG to have those great physiological impacts is by affecting the epigenetic processes (i.e., methylation and acetylation) that regulate long-term genetic transcription, and specifically to affect transcription of some of the genes that affect Alzheimer's (Momtaz et al., 2018). Preliminary research by Li et al. (2019) showed tea drinkers to have better white-matter connectivity than non-drinkers.

In summary, the tea research is convincing: drinking tea fosters brain health and cognitive preservation, and the physiological research shows how our brains benefit from the tea's EGCG and related flavonoids.

**Coffee.** Even though mortality is not our primary concern, several recent studies show positive impacts of coffee on longevity. For example, in a huge correlational study, Park et al. (2017) enrolled 215 thousand US participants who were between 45 and 75 years old at the start. In the 16 years of the study, there were over 58 thousand deaths. Data were adjusted for the potential confounds of age, sex, ethnicity, smoking, education, diseases, physical exercise, and alcohol consumption. Compared to non-coffee drinkers, there were 18% fewer deaths (i.e., HR = .82) for moderate drinkers (2-4 cups) of both caffeinated *and decaf coffee.*

In an even more humongous correlational study of over 521 thousand participants, Gunter et al. (2017) found that participants in the highest quartile of coffee consumption had significantly lower all-cause mortality with a hazard ratio of HR = .88 ($p < .001$) for men and HR = .93 ($p = .009$) for women. And closer to our main concerns, the hazard ratio for cerebrovascular disease was HR = .70 ($p = 0.002$).

Focusing on cognitive decline, a major review and meta-analysis of nine longitudinal studies by Liu et al. (2016) found that compared to drinking less than one cup, that drinking one to two cups of coffee per day reduced the probability for cognitive decline or for dementia, including Alzheimer's.

But I return here to the 11-year study by Zhang, Yang et al. (2021) outlined above. Recall that the impacts of consuming tea, or coffee, or the combination of tea and coffee together were assessed for over 365 thousand people in the UK Biobank cohort. Although their findings for coffee were not quite as impressive as those mentioned above for tea, moderate levels of coffee alone were clearly effective for preventing stroke and dementia. Compared with the study participants who did not drink coffee, drinking two to three cups of coffee led to the best hazard ratios of between HR = .80 and HR = .90.

But as with tea, too much coffee increases risks. Specifically, consumption of five or more cups per day increased risks for dementia in a dose-response fashion, with even more coffee (beyond five cups) leading to even more risk; similarly, stroke risks increased at over six cups per day. A subsequent analysis of the data from that same UK Biobank cohort led Pham et al. (2021) to conclude that for those consuming over six cups of coffee per day, the probability of dementia dramatically increased by 53%.

Because of the huge number of participants, Zhang, Yang, and colleagues were able to examine separately impacts for coffee drinkers of instant (160 thousand), ground (63 thousand), and decaf (57 thousand) coffee. Although they had no data on the potentially-important methods of preparation of the ground coffee, Zhang, Yang et al. concluded that the best protection was obtained from ground coffee, with the least protection from decaf. More about that issue later.

**Protection from moderate coffee consumption.** Gardener et al. (2021) provided a unique human longitudinal study that examined coffee impacts on the brain and cognition. Participants were 227 Aussies enrolled in the Australian Imaging Biomarkers and Lifestyle study. Participants were 70 years old and cognitively normal at the start of the 10 ½ year study. Coffee consumption was assessed by a food frequency questionnaire that unfortunately provided no data on the potentially important variables of preparation method or whether the consumed coffee was caffeinated or decaf.

To study rates of cognitive decline, tests were administered at 18-month intervals. The extensive tests assessed episodic memory, recognition memory, executive function, language, attention, and processing speed, and Gardener and colleagues included a test specifically designed to detect early signs of impending Alzheimer's.

Pet scans to assess β-amyloid levels (for 60 of the participants) and MRIs scans to assess brain structure (for 51 participants) were similarly done at 18-month intervals. Many potentially confounding variables were taken into account including age, genetic vulnerability (the Alzheimer's-disposing *APOE-4* allele), sex, education level, and energy intake.

The null findings were that over the entire span of 10 ½ years coffee consumption did *not* defend against gray matter atrophy, nor did coffee protect white matter, or hippocampal volume. But on the bright side (for coffee drinkers) compared with high and medium coffee drinkers, participants in the third with the least coffee performed poorly on the test that detected early signs of Alzheimer's. Corresponding with that finding, higher coffee consumption also correlated with lower β-amyloid accumulation.

Gardener et al. concluded that an increase in coffee consumption from one cup per day to two, over an 18-month period, could result in a lesser decline in executive function of 8%, and in a 5% decline in cerebral β-amyloid accumulation. From that small increase in coffee consumption, those were not trivial impacts. Obviously, over the entire 10 ½ year span, coffee could be a major factor protecting brain and cognition.

**Paths for benefits from coffee.** Actually, it is logical that coffee should benefit brain, because coffee has loads of antioxidants, polyphenols, and beneficial phenolics. Thus long-term benefits from coffee are probably not due to its caffeine, and in fact other research supports that conclusion, because decaf and caffeinated coffee sometimes both show long-term benefits, (as in the study by Park et al., 2017, mentioned above, that showed enhanced longevity from consumption of either kind).

To support the conclusion that coffee's benefits do not come from its caffeine, some recent research on telomeres shows opposite impacts from caffeine (negative) versus coffee (very positive). Remember that by protecting our chromosomes from genetic mutations and other evils, it is generally believed that longer telomeres portend a longer and healthier life. In a cross-sectional study, Tucker (2017) assessed the telomeres of 5826 adults from the National Health and Nutrition Examination Survey. After controlling for age, gender, race, marital status, education, housing, smoking, BMI, physical activity, and alcohol consumption, coffee intake was positively related to telomere length ($p = 0.0013$). Isn't that great (if you drink coffee, that is)! On the other hand, when caffeine from all sources was assessed, telomeres became shorter with more caffeine consumed ($p = 0.0005$). It is interesting that for telomeres, coffee is good and caffeine bad. A more recent study by González-Domínguez et al. (2021; more thoroughly reviewed in Chapter 16) noted a similar "caffeine paradox," finding correlations indicating that biomarkers (in blood) of coffee protected against cognitive decline, whereas biomarkers of caffeine had opposite impacts.

Another important factor that may contribute to inconsistent coffee research is that benefits and even harms follow from the way that the coffee is prepared. In a recent paper titled "Plasma metabolite biomarkers of boiled and filtered coffee intake and their association with type-2 diabetes risk" Shi, Brunius et al. (2019) noted that boiled coffee, like most espresso and French press brews that are not passed through paper filters, has harmful diterpines—molecules that degrade the cardiovascular system and increase the risks for developing type-2 diabetes. When the diterpine molecules are filtered out by passing the coffee through paper filters, the brew is transformed from a net health negative to a positive.

Tverdal et al. (2020) supported that conclusion with a massive study of over 500,000 Norwegian coffee drinkers aged from 20 to 79. It has been known for over three decades that unfiltered coffee contains around 30 times the level of cholesterol-raising substances compared to filtered coffee. Tverdal et al. assessed whether those differences made substantial differences in deaths from cardiovascular diseases, so coffee preparation methods were taken into account in a longitudinal study that lasted a mean of 20 years. By the study's conclusion 46,341 participants had died, with ¼ of those dying from cardiovascular disease. After taking into account the possible contributing factors of smoking, education, physical activity, height, weight, blood pressure, and cholesterol, drinking filtered coffee resulted in a 15% reduction in deaths from all causes, compared to not drinking coffee. As we consider the cardiovascular deaths, remember that anything that boosts cardiovascular function is good for the brain and good for cognition. Compared to abstaining from coffee, for filtered coffee drinkers, there was a 12% reduction in cardiovascular-related deaths for men and a 20% reduced risk of cardiovascular-caused deaths for women. Compared to abstainers, younger people who drank *un*filtered coffee experienced neither more nor fewer cardiovascular deaths. However, men over age 60 suffered higher cardiovascular death rates from drinking unfiltered coffee.

**Tea and coffee together.** The findings for tea and for coffee very strongly suggest that both support cognitive preservation. Because caffeine is a major ingredient in both beverages, we can question whether their affects on brain and cognition are due to caffeine or other nutrients common to both, or whether tea and coffee each offer unique benefits. To address that issue, I first return to the Zhang, Yang et al. (2021) research on the 365 thousand British people of the Biobank cohort to consider the joint impacts of tea and coffee.

The Biobank people who drank two to four cups of tea *and* two to three cups of coffee each day resisted strokes and dementia with a great hazard ratio of

HR = .65. Not only did they resist neuropathologies better than non-drinkers of coffee and tea, but they resisted better than those who drank *either* tea or coffee—even better than the people who drank the ideal amounts of either of those two beverages. For their sakes, we can hope those "double-dippers" did not then attend theater performances with long-delayed intermissions. Compared to drinkers of only tea or only coffee, the hazard ratios for those drinking both were HR = .89 for both stroke and for ischemic stroke, HR = .92 for dementia and HR = .82 for vascular dementia (all statistically significantly at $p < .001$). Those improved odds of avoiding neuropathologies ranging from 8% to 18% were not huge, but remember those modest improvements were over and above the improvements in risk for drinking ideal amounts of either tea or coffee.

Recall too that the data from the Zhang, Yang et al. study showed that daily drinking of more than five cups of coffee or nine cups of tea per day is counter-protective, leading to greater rather than lesser probabilities for neuropathology. Yet benefits from consumption of *both* coffee and tea are not eliminated until daily consumption exceeds 16 total cups. That and the substantial hazard ratio of HR = .65 for dementia (with an ideal total of five cups of *both* tea and coffee) show that coffee and tea consumption had additive impacts, leading Zhang, Yang et al. (and logic) to strongly suggest that they each contributed unique bioactive ingredients to cognitive preservation.

**Summary.** Anything that promotes general health (and delays death) is usually good for the health of the brain too. But those benefits from caffeine are uncertain; there is still much to learn about long-term caffeine impacts. However, research evidence is strong that long-term consumption of tea benefits the brain and cognition. Although evidence supports such benefits from both decaf and caffeinated coffee, the evidence is stronger for caffeinated coffee, as long as it is filtered. Add tea, and filtered coffee to the diet that already features olive oil, some omega 3's (from fish or supplements), and loads of phytonutrient-loaded fruits and veggies. Cacao too perhaps added to the coffee. Enjoy!

Chapter 8

# Vitamins through the Bs

To multivitamin or not to multivitamin? A couple of my health newsletters report that half of all adult Americans (and 70% of adults over 65) take a supplement for vitamins and minerals. Those same newsletters often add that such supplements show no proven health benefits. Instead, they suggest we should consume the healthy phytonutrient- and vitamin-rich diets that nutritionists often recommend. My most recent newsletter from the Icahn School of Medicine at Mount Sinai (2022, p. 1) noted that although some vitamin supplements (such as vitamin D) may benefit seniors, "the U.S. Preventive Services Task Force (USPSTF) has concluded that evidence is insufficient for determining the benefits and harms of most single or paired and multivitamin supplements." But as you must suspect, the USPSTF focus was, as usual, on cancer, cardiovascular disease, and death. Before accepting those conservative conclusions, we should question whether they apply to brain health and cognitive preservation, and especially whether they really apply to people who may be approaching ancient.

But even if those supplement-disparaging opinions were relevant to our specific interests, remember that nutrition-rich diets like the Med and the MIND, supplying berries, fresh fruits, green leafies and other veggies, fish, and even red wine, are not available to everyone. We are not all wealthy, and instead of those recommended foods, many of us are forced to seek out the nutrition-deficient "fast foods" that provide less-expensive calories. And even with sufficient wealth, there are "food deserts" without the well-stocked groceries and fresh produce that allow healthful diets in all seasons.

Consider too that supplement needs depend on our age. As we approach elderly some of our body's structural maintenance and repair requirements become both urgent and nutrition-demanding. Unfortunately, those needs for additional nutrition arise just as our aging digestive systems may be less able to absorb nutrients from our food.

Stressors too influence physiological demands that may be unmet with normal levels of dietary nutrients. It has long been known that chronic stress promotes inflammation, fosters destructive free radicals, and increases homocysteine and C-reactive protein (e.g., Blake-Mortimer et al., 1998; more about those proteins later). Those unwelcome products of stress threaten the health of body and brain, but the vitamins we consume, especially vitamins C and D and the B vitamins, play a role in restoring bodily integrity.

Unfortunately, that restoration of integrity is not accomplished easily because stress also robs us of vitamin C, and reduces absorption of the B vitamins. Thus both stress and aging create a potential role for supplements.

**Research issues.** Consistent with the summaries that attempt to persuade us to forego supplements, randomized control trials of vitamin impacts on cognition tend to produce equivocal results—results that can dampen enthusiasm for supplements. But as with the field of economics, with nutrition science there is usually an "on the other hand." In this instance, on the other hand, positive results frequently emerge from correlational studies that compare the cognitive capacities of people who consume various supplements with people who do not. Naturally, at first we should question the correlational studies for all the reasons discussed in Chapter 3—suspecting that smarter people may simply choose both supplements and better nutrition (rather than the reverse) or that some confounding variable like exercise or adequate sleep may account for the correlations. But quite possibly, it may be that the null-results of many of the randomized-control trials are simply misleading. The randomized-control trials are often weak because they are too time-limited, spanning only weeks or months, whereas the correlational studies sometimes span decades. Furthermore, confidence in the correlational studies is often supported by other research that shows *how* the specific nutrients enhance cognition by working their magic on our neurons, our neurochemistry, and even on our genes. As in many scientific fields, our ultimate conclusions should depend upon evidence derived from all of the relevant and valid research approaches.

An interesting and useful research approach is to assess nutrients in combination, as illustrated by the next two studies. Mazidi et al. (2017) compared nutrient consumption with telomere length. (Remember that telomeres are the caps on our chromosomes that protect them from damage.) From over 10,000 US citizens (mean age 44) they assessed daily intake of 60 nutrients including vitamins, minerals and other bioactive compounds. Three nutrition factors were identified from a factor analysis. Of those three factors, the one defined by higher mineral and vitamin consumption was associated with longer telomeres. That is only a correlational result, but given the association of longer telomeres with longevity, perhaps it is not extravagant to invest the small amount of cash needed for a daily vitamin/mineral supplement, even if it is usually better for us to obtain those nutrients from balanced diets.

Another research approach by Bowman et al. (2012) examined nutrients and their biomarkers in blood plasma, rather than depending upon food consumption questionnaires from research participants. Bowman et al. searched for patterns among the blood biomarkers of 30 nutrients in the plasma of 104 elderly participants (mean age 87) from the Oregon Brain Aging Study cohort. Assessments of those blood-born molecules overcome the potential problems of individuals possibly miss-remembering their own consumption patterns—problems that worry some consumers of nutrition research. After controlling for potentially confounding factors including age, sex, blood pressure, body mass index, etc., three nutrition clusters emerged from the patterns of inter-correlations of those blood-born nutrients. Somewhat like the factor identified in the prior study by Mazidi et al., one cluster was based on positive correlations between vitamins C, D, E, and some of the B vitamins (including B-1, B-2, B-6, B-9, and B-12). A second cluster was characterized by levels of omega 3 fatty acids, and the third featured transfats. (The finding that two of the clusters were based on fats highlights the importance of selecting the healthy dietary fats emphasized in Chapter 5.) MRI brain scans and a variety of cognitive functions were assessed. Higher cognitive scores corresponded with higher omega 3 concentrations but with lower transfats. Supporting the findings of the study described above by Mazidi et al., higher vitamin scores also correlated positively with cognition, but with the bonus that more vitamins also correlated with greater brain volume.

Despite the scientific precision of the studies by Mazidi et al. and by Bowman et al., those relationships were still correlational, leaving causality somewhat uncertain. But the results illustrate the wisdom of looking at impacts of combinations of nutrients rather than single nutrients. Following that observation, as we examine the B vitamins below, a substantial portion of the research focused on vitamin combinations. And some studies examined combinations of vitamins with other foods. For example, the study reported in Chapter 7 by Vercambre et al. (2013) that found positive impacts of caffeinated coffee on cognition also noted that those impacts were greatest for people using vitamin B supplementation (interaction $p = 0.02$).

**Potency and recommended amounts.** In order to provide some information about costs and potency of typical vitamin/mineral supplements, in the sections below, I will mention the percentage of recommended daily allowances (hereafter RDA) in the multi-vitamin consumed by my wife and me. Like the multivitamin supplements sold by many retailers, ours seems to mimic the formulations of other recognizable brands. It is formulated for "Adult 50+" and is both inexpensive and common, costing (like similar ones) less than US $.10/per pill. At that price, we do not worry over much about whether it is cost-effective. If we exchanged that expense for carrots or green leafy veggies, as is sometimes recommended, the few bits we would bring home would hardly supplement a decent salad.

In addition to the RDA of vitamins, occasionally, I also mention quantities in milligrams (mg—1/1000 gram) or micrograms (mcg—1/1,000,000 gram).

Another measure that occasionally sneaks onto multi-vitamin labels is the IU or "international unit," explained briefly in the glossary, but being somewhat goofy it is not mentioned often here. Some of the RDA amounts in our multi are odd quantities (e.g., 131% of the RDA of vitamin B-2); I assume those odd amounts are derived from assessing amounts actually in the batch that our pills came from.

But what exactly are the RDAs—the recommended daily allowances? RDAs are essentially the same as the RDIs (reference daily intake) that are often used on supplement labels, apparently to add a dose of confusion. But for our purposes, do not bother about the distinction. Over almost eight decades, the RDA amounts have evolved. The original RDAs were created at the time of World War II as measures of the minimal amount of a nutrient required to prevent diseases that would result from deficiencies. Today RDAs estimate the amount required to meet the needs of 97.5% of a specific population that is defined by age and sex. Modern dietary literature may also include the difficult-to-determine upper tolerable limit that can be consumed daily by 97.5% of people in that age-and-sex defined population—consumed without causing overdose problems.

Keep in mind that those who describe these measures (and the several others identified by other easily-confused letter combinations) often add caveats that optimal levels have not yet been scientifically identified for any nutrient at any life stage. Furthermore, remember that insofar as real data were used to determine RDAs (however approximately), that those determinations were made for general health and for avoiding deficiency diseases. Sufficient amounts for the health of bone, muscle, skin, or eyes may be quite different from ideal amounts for brain and cognition. Finally, as mentioned several times, as our bodies slide toward the elderly, our absorption capacities decrease for some nutrients, and yet we often need more of them.

Besides age, other individual differences in capacity to absorb and process some nutrients can certainly exist, as noted by a friend who needed huge vitamin D supplements to bring his D levels into a normal range. Attending to hints of such conditions can be part of taking charge of our own health care.

### Specific vitamins

Because our topic is the wellbeing of brain and cognition, only the vitamins known to foster those impacts are extensively reviewed in this chapter and the next.

**Vitamin A.** Because vitamin A is a powerful antioxidant, besides its positive impacts on vision and eyes, it should have measurable impacts on brain and cognition. However, those vitamin A impacts remain essentially unstudied. Enough said for now.

**The B Vitamins.** Even though the B vitamins range from B-1 to B-12, there are only eight of them. The B vitamins listed immediately below in this brief introduction are the ones that apparently survived predation by nutritionists, or the habitat loss (etc.) that eliminated the others. The Bs are all water soluble, and even though several are frequently found in the same foods, they are all chemically distinct. As noted in the short descriptions below, collectively, they seem to be important for everything the body requires for the growth and maintenance of cell structure and metabolism.

Vitamin B-1 (thiamin) contributes to healthy myelin on neural axons. We get it mostly from fruits and veggies. Our basic multivitamin supplies 125% of RDA.

Vitamin B-2 (riboflavin) is especially vital for normal cell growth and function, but when neuroscientists write about the Bs that influence brain and cognition, B-2 receives scant mention. Foods rich in B-2 include milk, meat, eggs, nuts, *enriched* flour, and green vegetables. Our multi has 131% of RDA.

Vitamin B-3 (niacin) regulates the energy metabolism of the mitochondria and therefore is essential for adequate brain function. It is found in meat, fish, poultry and whole grains. Our multi has 125% of RDA.

Vitamin B-5 (pantothenic acid) has direct impacts on the brain by influencing neural transmission, the health of the adrenal cortex, and production of the neurotransmitter acetylcholine. Its impact on acetylcholine is crucial. Recall that because acetylcholine is vital to adequate hippocampal function, deficits degrade memory formation and retrieval. We get B-5 from chicken, beef, potatoes, grains, tomatoes, egg yolk, and broccoli. Our multi has 200% of the RDA.

Vitamin B-6 (pyridoxine) influences the production of the hormone adrenaline and has major impacts on brain and cognition by affecting several of our most beloved neurotransmitters, including serotonin, noradrenaline, and dopamine. By enhancing serotonin levels, it builds resistance to depression and controls aggression and impulsiveness (Berman et al., 2009). (Note too that depression is a risk factor for dementia; Burton et al., 2013.) By maintaining levels of noradrenaline, B-6 indirectly assists in maintaining attention and concentration, and resisting depression and fatigue (Wallenstein, 2003). By maintaining dopamine, B-6 enhances states of motivation and positive moods, while resisting the age-associated shrinkage of the prefrontal cortex (LeDoux, 2002). Obviously, B-6 is not a vitamin to be ignored. Find it in *fortified* cereals, organ meats, and *fortified* soy-based foods. Our multi has 176% of the RDA.

Vitamin B-9 (folate, or the synthetic form: folic acid) regulates fatty acid metabolism in the brain. It is involved in both making and repairing DNA and thus, it plays a vital role in cell division and growth. Another of its vital functions is to facilitate the methylation of genes. In those roles, folate is so important that deficiencies (that, unfortunately, are too common) are harmful to spinal development in fetuses. Folate is found in dark leafy veggies, whole grains and *fortified* cereals and breads. Our multi has 208% of the RDA.

Vitamin B-12 is known by the seldom-seen term cobalamin, but on your multi-vitamin container, it may be listed as either cyanocobalamin or methylcobalamin. B-12 is crucially important because it influences fatty acid and amino acid metabolism in all tissues. Along with B-9, B-12 also plays a vital role in DNA synthesis and regulation, and it is involved in the synthesis of the neurotransmitters serotonin, noradrenaline, and dopamine. It plays a major role in fostering the vital antioxidant glutathione and in controlling predatory homocysteine (discussed more fully below). Perhaps as a result of those functions, at least in some critters, it plays a role in protecting neurons from the toxic impacts of $\beta$-amyloid (Lam, Kervin et al., 2021).

Vitamin B-12 is found in meat, fish, and poultry and *fortified* cereals, and because of those limited sources it is *not* possible to obtain sufficient quantities of B-12 from a vegetarian or vegan diet. Good meat sources for B-12 and for most of the other Bs include turkey, tuna and liver, and good veggie sources include beans, whole grains, potatoes, bananas, and chili peppers. (Be careful of the peppers.) Our multi has 25mcg—an amount listed as 1042% of RDA. Certainly, in absolute terms that is a tiny amount, but on the other hand, it is way over the recommended amount. Given the importance of vitamin B-12, as indicated by some of the following research, perhaps a generous over-supply is a good thing.

In the following paragraphs, I will consistently include the name of the B-vitamin in addition to the B-vitamin number only for those that have commonly-recognized names.

**Homocysteine.** Homocysteine was introduced in Chapter 2, but because some of the next research focuses on the control of homocysteine by B vitamins, I provide some additional notes here. Recall that homocysteine is an often-nasty amino acid that (among other evil deeds described by Smith & Refsum, 2021) increases with stress, causes cardiovascular damage, renal problems, brain atrophy, and increases the potential for Alzheimer's. Not previously mentioned was that the carnivores among us need to remain conscious that homocysteine levels also increase with high levels of meat consumption. However, because homocysteine levels are downregulated by vitamin B-9 (folate) and vitamin B-12, the potential for Alzheimer's may be reduced by enhanced levels of those two B-vitamins. Thus it seems likely that extra B vitamins could benefit especially the carnivores among us.

**Impacts of the B vitamins.** Although whole grains and cereals naturally have substantial levels of several of the important B-vitamins, after those vitamin-laden grains are refined the vitamin concentrations are substantially reduced. Because the vitamin Bs are so vital, but not easily obtained from veggies, the enrichment of flour with some of the Bs is mandated by law in some countries (such as the US, but relevant to research cited below, not the UK or Ireland). The Bs that are added to enriched flour are vitamin B-1 (thiamine), vitamin B-2 (riboflavin), vitamin B-3 (niacin), and most importantly, vitamin B-9 (folate). In fact, it was the observation that deficiencies of folate lead to neural tube defects in human embryos that led to B-vitamin flour-enrichment mandates. In countries where those mandates exist, they have led to substantial reductions in children born with neural-tube defects. In addition, B-vitamin supplements are usually suggested for pregnant women and sometimes for the elderly, because the elderly may not absorb the Bs as well as younger people.

Now consider a handful of studies that support the Bowman et al. (2012) finding of the importance of the B vitamins for both brain and cognition (especially in the elderly). Fliton et al. (2019) provided a cross-sectional study of middle-aged participants from both the UK's National Child Development Study (NCDS) and from a study of twins called TwinsUK. Nutrition intake was assessed from the 4400 NCDS participants, whereas serum levels of homocysteine and B vitamins were assessed from the blood plasma of the 1177 TwinsUK participants. In both cases, the intent was to assess specific nutrients that were believed to retard the progression of dementia. The many cognitive tests that were administered were factor analyzed, resulting in two "dementia-sensitive" cognitive factors of "visuospatial associative memory" and "verbal semantic memory." Performance on both cognitive measures was significantly higher for those NCDS participants who had greater intake of B vitamins, ($p < 0.001$), and support for the benefits of higher B-vitamin consumption was confirmed by the serum analysis of the TwinsUK participants. In the serum of those participants, both high levels of B vitamins and low homocysteine levels corresponded with better visuospatial associative memory performance ($p < 0.05$). Fliton et al. concluded that vitamin supplements provide an affordable means for maintaining cognitive health.

Other random-assignment studies support the conclusions by Fliton et al. that vitamin supplements preserve cognition. For example, de Jager et al. (2012) studied more than 250 adults who were over 70 years old and who had already shown evidence of mild cognitive impairment. Those participants were randomly assigned to 24 months of receiving either a placebo or a daily B-vitamin combination of vitamin B-6, vitamin B-9 (folate), and vitamin B-12. Cognition, MRI scans of brain volume, and blood levels of homocysteine were assessed. Across the 24 months, the homocysteine levels dropped 30% in the

B vitamin condition relative to the placebo condition, and the B vitamin regime had substantial positive impacts on the cognitive measures, especially for half of the participants who were initially high in homocysteine. The cognitive measures that benefited from the B vitamins included global cognition ($p < 0.001$), episodic memory ($p = 0.001$) and semantic memory ($p <$ 05). Because a common (but not necessarily-universal) feature of aging is some cognitive decline, B vitamin *supplements* may be a wise (and certainly inexpensive) investment for cognitive preservation for most of us.

Given the evidence that the Bs preserve cognition, they must have measurable brain impacts too. I mentioned in Chapter 2 that although the hippocampi and the prefrontal cortex shrink at the alarming rate of around 1% per year in the elderly, that the entire brain also atrophies, but at the lesser rate of around 0.2% per year in the elderly. But shrinkage tends to be faster in people experiencing mild cognitive impairment (about half of whom eventually develop Alzheimer's). In a separate paper, Smith et al. (2010) presented the results of the brain scans of those elderly participants who showed mild cognitive impairment and who had participated in the study (described above) by de Jager et al. (2012). Recall from the de Jager et al. description that for 24 months all the participants received either a placebo or a triple-B-vitamin combination. The mean brain atrophy for the placebo-group participants was extraordinarily high at 1.08% per year. That atrophy level is several times higher than normal, and obviously awful, but probably not unexpected given the mild cognitive impairment and the elderly status (all over 70) of the participants. In contrast, the annual atrophy rate for the participants receiving the B-vitamin supplements was significantly less (though still grim), at 0.76% ($p = .001$ for between-condition differences). And as expected, greater atrophy was associated with lower final cognitive tests. An even later analysis of those data by Douaud et al. (2013) found substantially reduced cerebral atrophy from that 24-month B vitamin treatment, specifically in structures surrounding the hippocampi. Finding those impacts only in participants with above-the-mean levels of homocysteine led Douaud et al. to conclude that the positive impacts of vitamin Bs on brain structure depends upon their lowering of homocysteine.

I offer two modest caveats for the interpretation of those results. The first is that because the UK does not mandate flour enrichment, the UK base rates of B vitamin consumption are probably substantially lower than in countries with flour enrichment, such as the US. Thus the impacts of the vitamin B supplements may have been greater in that UK research than they would be in countries that mandate enrichment. Second, recall that the participants in those two studies were included because they already showed evidence of mild cognitive impairment. Some nutritionists believe that vitamin B supplements do not have similarly noticeably positive impacts for cognitively-normal people.

Those two caveats notwithstanding, the studies reviewed above show that homocysteine levels are controlled by supplements containing some combination of vitamin B-6, vitamin B-9 (folate) and vitamin B-12—control that would benefit cognition in people with and without mild cognitive impairment. Furthermore, I reiterate previous comments that we are all aging, with the normal consequences of some cognitive decline and neural atrophy from some combinations of genetic mutations, oxidative damage, inflammation, the dwindling of neurotransmitters (or their receptors), reduced neurotropins (or receptors), lower production of myelin, high levels of homocysteine, etc. Add to that observation that as we age, some of the B vitamins we need are not absorbed as well as when we were younger.

**Vitamin B reviews.** Fortunately, several major reviews support the findings of positive impacts of the Bs on brain and cognition. Fenech (2017) reviewed the current literature on vitamin impacts on age-associated brain atrophy, cognitive decline, and dementia. The review emphasized randomized-control trials, but Fenech went beyond reporting the major relationships to include analyses of *how* the studied nutrients affect cognitive decline and Alzheimer's dementia. (Both the studies described above by Smith et al., 2010, and by de Jager et al., 2012 were included in the Fenech review.) Fenech concluded that of the B vitamins, B-6, B-9 (folate), and B-12, had positive impacts on brain health, certainly in part by suppressing potentially brain-damaging homocysteine levels.

Another thorough contemporary review by Moore et al. (2018) supported the importance of vitamin Bs for brain and cognition. Moore et al. concluded that of the various possible dietary approaches to slowing cognitive decline, and possibly reducing the risk of depression, that the evidence is strongest for positive impacts from vitamin B-2 (riboflavin), vitamin B-6, vitamin B-9 (folate), and vitamin B-12.

The most recent review by Wang et al. (2021) located 95 relevant studies with a total of 46 thousand participants. Fortunately, over ¼ of the studies were randomized-control trials. Studies lasting over 12 months (but not the shorter studies) found that compared to placebos, vitamin B supplements slowed cognitive decline only in non-demented participants. That observation does not rule out, however, that B vitamins may benefit cognition in those merely experiencing cognitive decline. When Wang et al. assessed individual B vitamins, they noted no major impacts on cognitive decline and dementia from either vitamin B-6 or vitamin B-12.

Instead, Wang et al. noted that the really strong impacts on cognition preservation were found from folate (B-9) and from lower levels of homocysteine. Specifically, folate deficiencies corresponded with cognitive decline (with odds ratio of OR = 1.26) and with dementia (with a much higher OR = 1.76); and high homocysteine levels corresponded with both cognitive decline (OR = 1.19) and with dementia (OR = 2.09). (All of the cited OR's were statistically significant).

Thus although Wang et al. posit a starring role for only folate (vitamin B-9), Fenech (and others noted above) concluded that several of the B vitamins have positive impacts on cognition. Add to those inconsistencies that another review by McCleery et al. (2018) of just vitamin B impacts on cognition found no measurable impacts in people with mild cognitive impairment. Perhaps we can be more tolerant of such inconsistencies by considering the recurrent theme of interactions between nutrients and between specific nutrients and other factors. Some of those interactions are elaborated below, but first, consider the most obvious factor that perhaps we should expect general positive impacts of various B vitamins on cognition only in individuals (or populations) with chronically low base rates of vitamin B consumption (e.g., those countries without B-fortified flour). Observations of such interactions should help us to be tolerant of some inconsistencies in this literature.

## Interactions

**Interactions with omegas and homocysteine.** Recall the observation from Chapter 5 that positive cognitive impacts from the B vitamins depended upon participants having adequate levels of omega 3 fatty acids. In the relevant study, Oulhaj et al. (2016) conducted a 2-year randomized-control trial in 266 people age 70 and older with mild cognitive impairment (MCI). Initial assessments were made of cognitive status (by clinical ratings, tests of global cognition, etc.). Oulhaj et al. also assessed plasma levels of homocysteine, and the two major components of omega 3 (DHA and EPA) . Across the two years of the study, the B vitamin treatment consisted of vitamin B-6, vitamin B-9 (folate) and vitamin B-12. However, the statistically significant impacts of the B vitamins on the cognitive measures depended on levels of those two components of omega 3s, with higher concentrations of DHA  having the greater impact. But the crucial point, illustrating the importance of interactions between nutrients, is that the Bs had no positive impact on cognition when omega 3s were low.

Similarly, the research reviewed above by Douaud et al. showed impacts by several of the B vitamins only when homocysteine levels were too high.

**Interactions of Bs with alcohol, coffee and the *APOE gene.*** It is not only age that inhibits the absorption of the vitamin Bs. Ethanol—the alcohol we drink—inhibits absorption of most Bs, including B-1 (thiamine), B-2 (riboflavin), B-3 (niacin), B-7 (biotin), and B-9 (folate). Therefore, people who consume alcohol regularly constitute another group that might benefit from B-vitamin supplements. (Alcohol is discussed more extensively in Chapters 13 and 14.)

Consider too that although some meats supply B vitamins, being carnivorous also has the less salutary effect of boosting our homocysteine levels (and depressing cardiovascular health). As with people who consume alcohol, perhaps voracious carnivores might also benefit from B supplements to control homocysteine.

Another interaction that suggests benefits from B supplements was noted by Vercambre et al. (2013) and discussed in Chapter 7. They found that the positive impacts of caffeinated coffee on cognition were greatest in people taking vitamin B supplements.

To illustrate the interaction of B vitamins with the genes we carry, studies reviewed by Fenech showed that vitamin B-12 seems *especially* effective for brain health among people who carry an evil copy of the *APOE* gene—*APOE-4*—the allele that potentiates Alzheimer's dementia. With that in mind, Fenech noted that some nutrition interventions that are intended to slow cognitive decline may have positive impacts only in people who are cursed with one or two copies of that despised *APOE-4* genetic variation.

# Other vitamins and their interactions

In the previous chapter, I noted the study by Bowman et al. (2012) that showed that it may be useful to assess clusters or combinations of nutrients (from blood analyses, for the Bowman et al. study) rather than individual nutrients, and, as emphasized by Fenech (2017) to focus especially on interactions between nutrients.

### Vitamins C, E, and multivitamins

Using an analysis spanning 11 years Basambombo et al. (2017) studied the self-reported consumption patterns of vitamin C and vitamin E separately or in combination with multivitamins. Participants were almost 5300 people who were all over 65. Basambombo et al. adjusted their data for the potential confounds of age, sex, education, and a typical list of health indicators (e.g., diabetes, cardiovascular issues etc.) and health-relevant behaviors (e.g., smoking and exercise). After those adjustments, compared with participants who did not take any supplemental vitamins, the substantial hazard ratios for those taking vitamins E and/or C plus multivitamins were HR = .78 (statistically significant) for cognitive impairment. The hazard ratios of HR = .83 for Alzheimer's, and HR = .86 for all-cause dementia were strong trends (that were not statistically significant), similarly suggesting neuroprotection from those vitamins. Those hazard ratios mean that compared to those not taking multivitamin supplements with either E or C during the 11 years of the study, the group taking the supplements had 22% fewer cases of cognitive impairment, 17% fewer people with Alzheimer's, and 14% fewer cases of all-cause dementia. Causation is not determined by such data, but multivitamins are very inexpensive and certainly not harmful.

Both vitamins C and E are powerful antioxidants, and for that reason, they are sometimes studied together. For example, Mock et al. (2017) reviewed the research on impacts on cognition from combined C and E. They noted that research with rodents has shown that combinations of vitamin C and vitamin E prevent both age-associated cognitive deficits and deficits associated with high homocysteine levels, apparently by the vitamins reducing oxidative damage.

Fortunately, there are supportive studies with non-rodent humans. The first did not examine the C and E combination, but instead examined whether either vitamin C or E alone could affect levels of the nasty inflammation indicator we know as C-reactive protein. Just by itself, inflammation in any part of the body is usually harmful to the brain, but the accompanying C-reactive protein is especially harmful to the cardiovascular system. Block et al. (2008) randomly assigned 396 adults to one of three groups. For two months, the groups received either a placebo, or 1000mg of vitamin C per day, or over 500mg of vitamin E per day. (For both vitamins, those are more than 10 times the RDA, and close to the "upper limits" of 1200mg for vitamin C and 600mg for E.) Compared with the placebo condition, vitamin C significantly reduced levels of C-reactive protein, but only in people with above-average levels of C-reactive protein at the study's beginning. The reduction for that group was a substantial 25% ($p = 0.02$) versus a 17% reduction for the entire vitamin C group. Vitamin E had no significant affects on levels of C-reactive protein. The study did not assess cognition, but the inflammation-brain relationship is important, so control of inflammation is vital for resisting cognitive decline.

Although impacts from vitamin E in that study were not substantial, from his extensive review Fenech (2017) concluded that both C and E repair oxidative damage to DNA. That repair may be especially important in the brain; brain levels of vitamins C and vitamin B-9 (folate) are considerably higher than normal blood levels, indicating high brain requirements for those vitamins.

Sources of vitamin E are veggie oils, cereals, nuts, fruits, veggies, and meats. My multi has 167% of RDA. You know that the best sources for vitamin C are citrus, tomatoes and other fruit, and you may know the vitamin C-linked origin of calling British sailors (and others) "limeys." If not, Google can tell you. The RDA estimates for C are 90mg; my inexpensive multi for old folks has exactly that amount.

### Vitamin D

Although more precisely named vitamin D3, and even more precisely 25(OH)D3, hereafter I use merely "vitamin D." Also, technically, vitamin D is really a hormone rather than a classical vitamin, and that has implications noted below.

If you were to Google "vitamin D deficiency" you would find essentially the same facts that you may have learned eons ago in junior-high health class. You would re-discover that vitamin D is known as a vital ingredient for bone development, for preventing osteoporosis, and most importantly, for preventing the not-commonly-seen soft-bone disease called rickets. Addressing those problems has led to vitamin D supplements in milk and in a few other commodities. Unfortunately, as with most vitamins the role of vitamin D in cognitive preservation and neurological function receives only scant mention.

But even with fortified milk, diet alone may not supply adequate amounts of vitamin D, and some nutritionists estimate that Americans get only 1/3 of their daily requirement from diet alone. Fortunately, like other hormones, vitamin D is manufactured in our bodies, but unlike other hormones, vitamin D is manufactured only when our skin is exposure to sunlight or other ultraviolet light sources. But even with that in-body supply chain, typical estimates are that around one billion people worldwide suffer from vitamin D deficiency, with a substantial portion of deficient people in *developed* countries (e.g., Anjum et al., 2018). In northern climates deficiencies result from people staying indoors, or covering their skin, particularly during the darker winter months. People with darker skin are also less able to manufacture sun-stimulated vitamin D, and some (but not all) research finds that even applying sunblock reduces our bodies' ability to create it. But it is not only reduced exposure to sunlight that causes deficiencies. As we age, we become less able to synthesize vitamin D, and to compound that problem, with aging, we become less sensitive to the smaller amounts we do manage to make, due to diminishing densities of vitamin D receptors. Thus despite the frequently published reservations about supplements, supplements of vitamin D are often recommended for general health and well-being, especially for the elderly.

Those deficiencies are relevant for us because vitamin D really does have major impacts on brain and cognition. D'Amelio and Quacquarelli (2020) begin their review of the relevant research by reviewing studies using transgenic rats disposed to develop Alzheimer's. When those unfortunate creatures were given a diet deficient in vitamin D, they suffered accelerated cognitive deterioration, compared to transgenic rats on a normal diet.

Mice were not excused from similar research. Transgenic Alzheimer's mice given diets with deficient vitamin D produced more β-amyloid protein and thus developed more between-neuron plaques. But do not despair that the only future awaiting those mice was institutionalized memory care. Increasing their dietary vitamin D reduced the plaques and enhanced the clearance of the β-amyloid from their little brains. And as we would expect, those positive brain impacts enhanced the cognitive performance of those diminutive research volunteers. *In-vitro* cultures of cortical neurons exposed to vitamin D show similar reductions in nasty β-amyloid protein.

Consider people. Substantial support for vitamin D's positive brain impacts is provided by correlational research with humans. Goodwill and Szoeke (2017) provided a meta-analysis of impacts of vitamin D on cognition. They included 26 cross-sectional and longitudinal studies that assessed both cognitively normal people and patients with impaired cognition. In those studies, higher vitamin D levels corresponded with better cognitive performance (with hazard ratios of HR = .75, indicating 25% fewer cases of cognitive decline in the higher vitamin D groups). Of course, those were correlational studies. Unfortunately, the three randomized-control trials in their meta-analysis failed to show substantial or significant impacts on cognition from vitamin D supplements versus placebos. The conclusion they offered (and the similar one from the review by D'Amelio & Quacquarelli, 2020) was that the results from the random-assignment studies did not justify recommending Vitamin D as a treatment for Alzheimer's. Indeed irrefutable proof of effectiveness *in humans* is lacking, but not all reviewers agree that treatment for Alzheimer's with vitamin D is ineffective.

Some support for positive vitamin D impacts comes from physiological studies. For example, Al-Amin et al. (2019) reviewed data from a large community sample of 1663 individuals showing that low levels of vitamin D in serum was associated with a lower hippocampal volume. Their study first identified 56 Korean elders who had all received a diagnosis of mild cognitive impairment. After accounting for the usual array of potentially contributing factors (ranging from age, education, and physical activity to various health indicators), the people in the top 50% of serum vitamin D had higher cognitive scores on all of the tests and significantly larger hippocampal volume ($p = .013$). They also showed better connectivity of hippocampi with other brain structures.

Other reasons for hope for some relief from Alzheimer's from vitamin D treatments are based on more fine-grained observations of how vitamin D affects neurochemistry, neural structures, and neural functions. For example, Mayne and Burne (2019) noted that vitamin D supports the synthesis of both neurotransmitters and neurotropins, and also affects cell differentiation, intracellular calcium homeostasis, and the protection of neural tissue from oxidative damage. Vitamin D also helps to control inflammation. And vitamin D inhibits β-amyloid production and aids in its removal. Those impacts result from activated vitamin D receptors stimulating the expression of genes that influence those various effects.

After surveying all of that compelling evidence, Mayne and Burne concluded that vitamin D was a likely candidate for preserving cognitive capacity in normal and healthy adults. Similarly, following their survey of the literature, Patel and Shah (2017) added that vitamin D supplements could both reduce the potential for Alzheimer's and slow its progression.

Given its apparent benefits, how do we obtain sufficient quantities? Food sources are oily fish and some fortified foods such as milk and cereals. But because so few foods are rich sources of vitamin D, the primary sources for most people are either creating it subcutaneously in response to sunlight or from taking supplements. If one has minimal exposure to sunlight, only

15mcgs from food and/or supplements are recommended for most adults, with 20mcgs recommended for adults over 70. My multivitamin supplies around 12.5mcgs, but vitamin D capsules with varying amounts are also easily available and inexpensive. (I take one listed as 50mcg, taking that huge amount because I am old, but each costs only US $.05.) However, excessive amounts of vitamin D are potentially harmful, especially for amounts approaching 10 times RDAs; the tolerable upper limit (safe for 97.5% of people) is assessed to be 100mcg.

### Vitamin K

Vitamin K (formally phylloquinone) is known primarily for its contribution to blood coagulation. But vitamins are never simple. Vitamin K itself has several vitamers (not a typo: vitamers are vitamin variations.) Of the vitamers of vitamin K, Menaquinone-4 (MK-4), is the most prevalent in both humans and rodents, and so when vitamers of K are isolated, MK-4 is the one most studied. The research shows that MK-4 prevents both oxidative damage and inflammation in *in vitro* studies, and in mouse studies depletion of MK-4 correlates with poor cognitive performance. However, most vitamin K research identifies the vitamin studied merely as vitamin K or phylloquinone.

Alisi et al. (2019) provided a recent review of the research testing the hypothesis that vitamin K may enhance brain structures, brain processes, and cognition. They noted that various studies show that vitamin K defends neurons from damage and death caused by excessive β-amyloid. In support of positive impacts, they cite six cross-sectional population studies showing that especially in older populations, low vitamin K levels correspond with poor cognitive performance (a seventh study of middle-aged people found only null results). In another study published one year after the Alisi et al. review, Kiely et al. (2020) assessed cognitive performance in 500 older (all 64 or more) Irish adults. After controlling for sex, age, body mass index, triglycerides and blood pressure they examined the correlations of both serum and dietary vitamin K levels with cognition. Higher levels of K assessed by both measures significantly and independently predicted better cognitive function, even after controlling for inflammation. (That later finding shows that some of vitamin K's positive impacts on cognition are apparently independent of its positive role in suppressing inflammation.)

Several health conditions benefit from reducing blood coagulation. Thus people who need to reduce coagulation often receive medications called vitamin K antagonists (e.g., warfarin or coumarin derivatives). Findings of brain abnormalities in warfarin-exposed newborns led to suspicions that K antagonists may damage brains and degrade cognition, even in adults. That hypothesis was confirmed in studies showing K antagonists degraded rat cognition, and those studies led in turn to research with people taking those blood-thinners. Indeed, the studies reviewed by Alisi et al. suggested that vitamin K antagonists have negative impacts on visual memory, verbal fluency and brain volume. In patients with atrial fibrillation who take anti-coagulants to prevent strokes, tests of vitamin K antagonists versus other blood thinners found worse cognitive outcomes with the K antagonists. Although nothing is proven about the value of simple vitamin K supplements from such research, clearly reducing the body's vitamin K levels is detrimental to cognitive brilliance. Alisi et al. concluded that although the association of deficiencies in vitamin K with cognitive decline is "not definitive," the evidence is strong that vitamin K improves cognitive performance.

Vitamin K is found in various kinds of green leafy veggies, including spinach, kale, chard, parsley, and green leaf lettuce. Brussels sprouts and broccoli have some too. My multivitamin has only 25% of the RDA (at 30mcg). That is probably ok if I eat wisely, but I note that it is the lowest % of RDA for any of the vitamins included in my pill. That could be an indicator of either the manufacturer's low regard for the importance of K, or a belief that most of us get all we need from normal diets.

### Summaries of vitamin impacts

Concluding his thorough review of impacts of vitamins on cognitive processes, Fenech (2017) noted that beyond the strong evidence that cognitive health is promoted by the Mediterranean diet, flavonoids, omega 3 oils, and unsaturated fats, that positive impacts on brain and cognition are also promoted by an assortment of vitamins including vitamin B-9 (folate), vitamin B-12, vitamin A (and β-carotene), and vitamin C, vitamin D, and vitamin E. He noted that a meta-analysis of 106 studies of vitamin levels in plasma showed vitamin deficits in people with Alzheimer's. Specifically, compared with healthy controls, the Alzheimer's participants had lower plasma levels of vitamins A (–14%), B-9 (folate; –21%), B-12 (–12%), C (–33%), D (–27%), and E (–18%). Those observations were supported in turn by another meta-analysis included in his review—a meta-analysis of 43 prospective studies, showing that the relative risk for dementia was decreased with the Mediterranean diet (risk ratio of RR = .69, $p < .0001$), by higher intake of vitamin E (RR = .80, $p < .05$), and by more of the combination of vitamins B-6, B-9 (folate), and B-12 (RR = 0.72, $p < .05$; risk ratios differ only slightly from hazard ratios; for clarification, peruse the Glossary). Fenech noted that other lesser-studied vitamins may also contribute to cognitive health, including vitamin B-1 (thiamin), vitamin B-3 (niacin), and vitamin K.

Another thorough review published three years later reached similar conclusions. Mielech et al. (2020) noted that deficiencies in vitamin A, the vitamin Bs, vitamin C, vitamin D, and vitamin E seemed to increase the risk of Alzheimer's, and that diets rich in vitamins A, D, C, B-6, B-9, B-12, and supplements with high levels of vitamin E may decrease that risk.

Almost all of the studies contributing to the meta-analyses and the reviews above were correlational. Unfortunately, no matter how conscientiously researchers account for potentially-confounding factors, correlational studies alone cannot definitively establish that vitamins mitigate brain deterioration and cognitive decline. However, in the case of every single one of the vitamins mentioned above in the brief summary, we know at least some of the intervening physiological paths between vitamins on the one hand and neurochemistry or brain structure or brain function on the other. In other words, we know how the vitamins we consume accomplish their magic. Supplements of at least multivitamins could be in order.

Chapter 10

# Galvanizing metals

Galvanized metals—usually steel or iron—are coated with zinc to prevent rusting. Other than iron and zinc being two of the most important metals our bodies require, that statement is completely irrelevant to the content of this chapter. Magnesium is the third of the three metals discussed below. All three make major contributions to brain, cognition, and resilience.

## Iron

Whether we are pumping it or consuming it, we are vulnerable to problems of either too little or too much iron. In their review of research on iron deficiency in the young, Pivina et al. (2019) noted that 25% of the world's population suffers from anemia with at least half of that due to iron deficiency. Although upwards of 60% of the iron in our bodies is in the blood's hemoglobin, iron is a vital component of all our cells.

Adequate iron is essential for brain development in the young. During development, iron deficiencies degrade neurotransmitter balances, myelin production, and the building of new synapses, ultimately damaging both cognitive abilities and psychomotor development. Iron deficiencies may even contribute to attention-deficit/hyperactivity disorder (ADHD) and autism.

Because iron levels are reduced by menstrual bleeding, ovulating females are prone to experience the energy deficits that result from anemia—deficits that can also include degraded cognition. And of course degraded cognition from iron deficits can occur in both males and females, and at any age. Those deficits in adults can usually be remedied with supplements (not necessarily iron supplements, but potentially including vitamin B-12, etc.) or dietary modifications.

On the other hand, iron surpluses can cause a different set of problems in older people of both genders. Because of those age-related differences, the multivitamin supplements designed for people who are younger than 50 usually include iron, whereas the supplements formulated for those of us over 50 sometimes announce prominently that iron has been excluded.

Naturally, iron processing in our bodies is regulated by our genes. In their search through a huge data set for the genes associated with healthy aging and longevity, Timmers et al. (2020) noted the crucial impact on aging that is due to the genes that regulate iron metabolism, such as the genes that (indirectly) produce hemoglobin. Unfortunately, the body's ability to adequately regulate and process iron declines with age. Excess iron then accumulates in various tissues, with that excess contributing to oxidative stress, infection-control problems, and even damage to our beloved mitochondria. Timmers et al. concluded that high blood iron levels reduce our healthy years of life by fostering those various types of age-related damage. Furthermore, they suggested that for the elderly, the poor health consequences from over-indulging in red meat may be due largely to red meat increasing blood iron levels, rather than from the saturated fat.

Although causal direction is not established by these next correlations, excess iron accumulates especially in the brains of people experiencing the neurodegenerative diseases of Alzheimer's, Parkinson's, multiple sclerosis, and even in people with only mild cognitive impairment. In both mild cognitive impairment and Alzheimer's, more iron in some brain structures correlates with more severe cognitive deficits (Du et al., 2018).

Research by Shi, Li et al. (2019) found similar relationships even in cognitively-normal people. They studied diet and cognition in 4852 elderly Chinese adults. The cognitive measures included delayed word recall, backwards counting, and serial subtraction. Food consumption assessments were carefully made during multiple home visits by the research team. A well-chosen host of potentially-confounding variables were taken into account, including health indicators such as blood pressure, diabetes, and stroke; social factors included education, income, and urban-rural environment; and health-related behaviors included physical activity, smoking, and alcohol consumption.

Those elderly participants were divided into quintiles (i.e., fifths) based on their iron consumption. The elderly participants with the highest iron intake were 30% more likely to be classified as poor in cognition compared to people in the quintile with the least iron consumption. For them, extra iron was clearly not a plus. However, for the elderly participants who were overweight (i.e., BMI of over 24) too much iron became an even more severe issue. That is, for the overweight participants, the odds ratio for poor cognitive function for the high iron quintile was OR = 3.01 (compared to the quintile with the lowest iron intake). That extremely high odds ratio means that the overweight people in the high iron quintile were three times as likely to have poor cognition compared with the people in the low iron quintile group. (Poor cognition was defined as having cognition scores in the bottom 20% of all participants.)

It seems apparent that with problems from insufficient iron in the young and from too much iron in older people that more thoughtful regulation strategies are required for iron than for many other nutrients. There are many possible causes of unwelcome iron levels at any age. These can range from generally poor diets to vitamin B-12 deficiencies, stomach acid imbalances, minor bleeding from taking aspirin or similar anti-inflammatory drugs, genetic predispositions, etc. The increased dangers from iron over-abundance in the elderly should not be interpreted to mean that iron supplements should be avoided by all older people. It depends. Informed decisions about adding or deleting iron supplements should be made with knowledge from health checkups that inform about current hemoglobin levels and other features of the health profile.

## Zinc

Zinc is essential for everything important in the body. The functions it supports include DNA synthesis and the epigenetic functions of acetylation (sensitizing) and methylation (desensitizing) of specific genes. Zinc is crucial for cell reproduction, cell survival, and health. Wessels et al. (2017) emphasized the role of zinc in enhancing immune function. That important impact has resulted in zinc being marketed in various forms as an over-the-counter remedy for respiratory illnesses, etc. For our concerns with brain and cognition, zinc is essential for the production and regulation of neurotransmitters including serotonin, noradrenalin, dopamine, glutamate, and GABA. Thus zinc insufficiency should be one of the usual suspects for causing conditions that can result from neurotransmitter deficits—conditions such as cognitive impairment or depression. I deal with the relationship of zinc with depression in Chapter 18.

Two other recent reviews of randomized-control trials of zinc supplements have concluded that zinc deficiencies may contribute to Alzheimer's (Piao et al., 2017; Wessels et al., 2017). In their recent (and highly recommended) review of zinc impacts on brain, emotion, and cognition, Piao et al. cite research showing that zinc-restricted diets affect transgenic mice (destined to develop Alzheimer's) by enhancing both β-amyloid plaques and tau tangles. Zinc-deprived animals also showed impaired learning and memory, and they responded to stressors as if they were depressed. Piao et al. 2017, p. 383) concluded their review by noting that "zinc treatment will be beneficial for neuronal diseases and emerges as a new target of research for therapy of different mood disorders and neurodegenerative diseases."

Subsequent to that detailed review, Squitti et al. (2020) reviewed research specifically testing the effectiveness of zinc supplementation for treating Alzheimer's. They noted that although the research was not yet conclusive, that with no side effects from zinc treatments that zinc showed potential for improving cognition.

Besides zinc's role in building and regulating neurotransmitters and their receptors (especially glutamate and GABA), the ways that zinc reduces the potential for depression and cognitive decline are not all understood, but zinc also regulates various important genes, and is anti-inflammatory. Most importantly, by combining with various polyphenols, including those found in coffee, tea, and red wine, zinc forms synergistic combinations that seem necessary to derive the antioxidant impacts from those phytochemicals. Thus besides the more direct contribution of zinc molecules to life and health, adequate zinc levels are essential for us to benefit from other important nutrients (Ward et al., 2018). The secondary source that led me to the Ward et al. research had the intriguing title "Can chocolate, tea, coffee and zinc help make you more healthy?" The answer provided was "yes."

Wessels et al. observed that although in the past it was thought that zinc deficiency was rare, it is now known to affect about two billion people, especially in developing countries where it is the 5th leading cause of the loss of healthy years of life. Even in developed countries, zinc deficiencies affect 20% to 30% of the elderly population (estimates differ). But should our zinc come from supplements? With both immune-system weakness and inflammation being chronic problems for the elderly, zinc supplementation for older people may be especially important for health maintenance. My inexpensive multi contains 11mg or 100% of RDA—an appropriate level given zinc's importance.

Besides zinc's availability in multivitamins and in across-the-counter supplements at the local drug store, zinc is found naturally in brewer's yeast, fish, soy, liver, spinach, red meat and egg yolk. (As for the brewer's yeast source, for very mysterious reasons people in and from New Zealand and Australia seem to like the noxious foods called vegemite and marmite; people from other countries wisely disdain those yeast-based foods.) Note that not many veggies were in that list of food sources, leading to concerns that zinc deficiencies could follow from vegetarian diets. I keep my egg consumption up for the protein and the essential choline, and that, along with my multi, should take care of keeping my zinc topped up as well.

### Magnesium

Like iron and zinc, magnesium is required for hundreds of vital enzymes, proteins, and neurochemicals. Because it performs functions in various brain structures and builds vital neurochemistry, magnesium is one of the usual suspects for nutrition that supports mood and cognition.

To illustrate the causal paths that the relevant research has taken, I begin with two randomized-control trials designed to enhance the brain health and cognitive ability of various critters. Slutsky et al. (2010) added magnesium to the drinking water of the fortunate half of their randomly assigned rats. Using rat-appropriate cognitive tests (e.g., maze solutions rather than word recall) the additional magnesium enhanced learning, working memory, and both short- and long-term memory in both the young and the older rats. Accounting for those cognitive gains, the magnesium-condition rats had higher levels of a synapses-building protein (i.e., synaptophysin) and more synapses in their hippocampi.

Huang et al. (2018) explored similar hypotheses with transgenic mice disposed to develop Alzheimer's. First, note that as detailed in Chapter 19, when we humans engage in cognitively challenging activities, we develop resistance to age-related cognitive decline and to dementia. Previous research had shown that transgenic mice also benefited cognitively from environmental enrichment. Huang et al. assigned young pre-dementia mice (3 months old) and mice already showing cognitive deterioration (12 months old) to either environmental enrichment, or to magnesium supplements alone, or to a combination of enrichment plus magnesium. For both young and old mice, the combination of enrichment plus magnesium improved cognition and spatial memory more than either treatment alone. As with the rats of the Slutsky et al. research, those fortunate mice also showed enhanced synaptic development in their hippocampi. The benefits from such randomized-control trials clearly show causal links from magnesium to brain and cognition. But we really want to see similar impacts from magnesium in people.

Kirkland et al. (2018) conducted a major review that included previous meta-analyses of magnesium research along with recent individual studies. Their review assessed the therapeutic value of magnesium for various conditions, including migraine, depression, chronic pain, anxiety, and stroke. They concluded that magnesium therapies are useful for migraine and depression, that the data suggest a protective effect for chronic pain, anxiety, and stroke, but that more research is needed to be *sure* of a therapeutic effect on Alzheimer's and Parkinson's. Thus I review some even more recent supportive research.

**Interactions of magnesium and vitamin D.** Recall that some vitamin D is manufactured in our bodies. Magnesium plays a crucial role in vitamin D biosynthesis and metabolism, and deficiencies in either D or magnesium lead to poor cognition. Choosing a representative sample of almost 2500 older adults over age 60, Peeri et al. (2020) examined the interaction of magnesium and vitamin D. The participants were drawn from the US National Health and Nutrition Survey conducted from 2011 to 2014. Cognitive assessments were based on the Digit Symbol Substitution Test, a well-established measure of executive function and processing speed. Cognitive impairment was defined as having a score in the lowest quartile (i.e., lowest 25%) on the Digit Symbol test. As is appropriate for a hormone, vitamin D was measured in blood serum, but magnesium was assessed by analyzing each person's diet. The potentially-confounding factors that were taken into account showed that cognitive impairment corresponded with being significantly older, *not* consuming alcohol, having less education, and not exercising ($p < .01$ in all cases). Subsequent analyses adjusted for those variables.

As predicted, higher levels of serum vitamin D corresponded significantly with better cognition ($p = .05$). Higher magnesium intake also corresponded with higher cognitive scores, although that relationship was strongest for women, physically active participants, and those with sufficient vitamin D levels ($p < 0.01$). The very large number of participants in the research justified the authors' conclusion that magnesium may improve cognitive function in older adults, especially in those with sufficient levels of vitamin D. Thus, as noted frequently before, it is often combinations of nutrients or interactions between nutrients that are more important that single-nutrient impacts.

**Magnesium and dementia.** A much longer and larger longitudinal study of over 12 thousand elderly participants drawn from the Atherosclerosis Risk in Communities Study was conducted across a 24-year span by Alam et al. (2020). Serum magnesium levels were assessed initially from 1990–1992. Across the 24-year span, 2519 cases of dementia were recorded. The researchers adjusted the magnesium-dementia relationship by taking into account a thorough list of potential-confounding variables. That list included genetic predispositions for Alzheimer's (the *APOE-4* gene allele), age, sex, race, education, smoking status, drinking, heart disease, blood pressure, waist-to-hip ratio, aspects of diet and plasma levels of C-reactive protein, plasma levels of potassium, sodium, and calcium, and health issues including diabetes, heart disease, stroke history, cholesterol, blood pressure and various medications related to those health issues. After taking those many factors into account, low levels of magnesium assessed at the study's beginning still corresponded with dementia. Specifically, there was a 24% increased risk of dementia (i.e., RR = 1.24) for participants in the quintile (20%) with the least magnesium compared to the top magnesium quintile. (In other terms, for every 100 cases of dementia in the high magnesium group, there were 124 individuals with dementia in the low magnesium group.) Perhaps a more meaningful measure of magnesium (i.e., more than a single assessment at the beginning) would have yielded even stronger relationships between magnesium and cognition; or perhaps not.

Some nutritionists note that over half of Americans are deficient in magnesium—a real problem, given its proven importance. Food sources include the usually-great-for-you dark leafy greens, nuts, seeds, and fish. Dark chocolate sneaks into that list too, but unfortunately, not red wine. My multi has a mere 50mg, corresponding with only 13% of RDA. That is certainly not great, but I have occasional dark chocolate, and nuts almost every day, so maybe I'm ok, but bring on the spinach anyway.

Chapter 11

# Spices

Some spices have been cultural mainstays for millennia, either as food or for their medicinal value. We tend to celebrate them and use them metaphorically in expressions such as "the spice of life," "spicy food," or even the "spice girls." The four featured in this chapter were chosen only because each has inspired research that has shown either promise or strong evidence of positive impacts on brain and cognition.

Even though some herbs such as basil and rosemary show up in spice sections of the local grocery, herbs and spices are different. Spices have stronger flavors than herbs by virtue of being the portions of plants with high concentrations of essential oils. I mention this here because at the chapter's end, I comment briefly on basil, an herb showing promise for brain and cognition.

### Turmeric and curcumin

Turmeric is such a cherished spice, valued for thousands of years for its flavor in Indian curries and its rich yellow-orange color, but credited as well with medicinal and healing qualities. The main component of turmeric is curcumin, a polyphenol that has well-established anti-inflammatory and antioxidant impacts. For centuries turmeric (hereafter just "curcumin") has been used for relief of digestive problems, arthritic conditions, and age-related cognitive decline, but here I evaluate only research on its impact on cognition. I begin with brief coverage of a pair of indecisive randomized-control trials, both of which were important enough to be included in the three up-to-date research reviews that follow. The two randomized-control trials remind us that we can learn even from studies that show modest impacts.

A 12-month study by Rainey-Smith et al. (2016) of 96 older adults showed that compared to placebo, curcumin had essentially no positive impacts on cognitive measures at 12 months, even though the cognitive measures were based on a large and sophisticated battery of tests. Subsequently, with only 40 participants, Small et al. (2018) conducted a longer 18-month randomized-control trial in an attempt to find those elusive curcumin-cognition impacts, and to assess possible effects of curcumin on the accumulation of the nasty forms of the proteins tau and β-amyloid. The 40 participants, who were all over 50 years old and cognitively normal, received either 90mg of curcumin or a placebo twice daily for 18 months. The cognitive assessments that were made at 6-month intervals showed few between-group effects on the cognitive measures. Although pet scans showed significantly less β-amyloid in hypothalamic structures of the curcumin-condition participants, the meaning of the hypothalamic reduction is suggestive, but uncertain without similar β-amyloid reductions in other structures (Dcruz et al., 2018).

With those two individual studies showing inconsistent results, I turn to the three major recent reviews. For each review, the search began with reams of studies culled from multiple databases, but in all three reviews, the authors ultimately considered only those studies that fit stringent but reasonable criteria. In the first of the three reviews, Voulgaropoulou et al. (2019) chose 20 randomized-control trials using animals (mice and rats, with one primate study) and five studies of humans (including the two studies described above). Voulgaropoulou et al. noted that the animal research did not show that curcumin enhanced cognition in "normal" animals; nevertheless, they concluded that curcumin can prevent or even reverse cognitive decline caused by pathological conditions. Curcumin's positive impacts apparently result from its anti-inflammatory and antioxidant properties and, most importantly, from its ability to directly reduce β-amyloid plaques.

Regarding only the five human randomized-control trials, Voulgaropoulou et al. noted that the results were mixed for people already experiencing cognitive impairments, but they attributed those equivocal results to the limited number of published studies. Nevertheless, they concluded that like the research with animals, the human studies showed that rather than improving cognition in cognitively normal people that curcumin could prevent cognitive decline, or slow decline once it had begun.

For the second of the three reviews, Sarker and Franks (2018) examined both animal and human randomized-control trials that showed the impacts of curcumin on age-associated cognitive decline. Sarker and Franks offered a positive conclusion similar to that of Voulgaropoulou et al. They too noted that the 15 animal studies of normal aging showed conclusively that curcumin could slow age-associated cognitive decline. That conclusion seems to suggest that healthy-but-aging populations could benefit from additional curcumin. Furthermore, like Voulgaropoulou et al., they emphasized that the animal research shows positive impacts of curcumin curtailing inflammation, resisting oxidative stress, and directly reducing β-amyloid—all impacts that should indeed slow age-related cognitive decline.

*In vitro* research found that curcumin protected neurons against excessive (and thus potentially damaging) neurotransmitter levels and preserved mitochondrial functioning (Grabowska et al., 2017).

It is not surprising that the conclusions by Sarker and Franks that were based on the five human studies were similar to the conclusions of Voulgaropoulou et al. because four of the five studies were common to both reviews. However, Saker and Franks were somewhat more conservative, suggesting that whereas the use of curcumin as a therapy for cognitive decline holds some promise, that curcumin's effectiveness remains unproven. Nevertheless, because of curcumin's positive impacts on inflammation, oxidative stress, and β-amyloid, Sarker & Franks anticipate that future studies will show curcumin to be effective for cognitive preservation in aging people.

In the third of the curcumin-cognition reviews, Zhu et al. (2018) assessed only studies with humans. They identified six appropriately-rigorous randomized-control trials, but those six included the five reviewed by Voulgaropoulou et al. plus one of schizophrenics that spanned only eight weeks. Even though Zhu et al. reviewed the same research as Voulgaropoulou et al., Zhu et al. (2018, p. 524) concluded that curcumin seemed to benefit the normal and healthy elderly, perhaps not merely by stabilizing cognition, but by improving it as well. They noted that "curcumin appears to be more effective in improving cognitive function in the elderly than in improving symptoms of AD [Alzheimer's dementia] and schizophrenia."

Although strong conclusions of curcumin's efficacy are not possible from only the randomized-control trials with people, the reviewers all suggested, albeit weakly, that curcumin supplementation seems to be good for cognitive endurance. And research shows no ill effects from normal levels of curcumin supplements. On the positive side, the animal research shows clearly that small hairy creatures gain cognitive capacity from adding curcumin to their diets. Nevertheless, enthusiastic endorsement at this time seems risky.

Turmeric supplements cost around $.30 to $.50/capsul for the typically-recommended doses. If you choose to add such supplements to your diet, note that curcumin is not easily absorbed, and because of that, some preparations enhance bio-availability with additives like pepper.

### Cinnamon and sodium benzoate

Anderson et al. (2013) noted that cinnamon was introduced into Egypt in 2000 BC, and received numerous biblical references. Could that be a recommendation? Perhaps it should, because in more modern times research has shown positive impacts on various bodily functions that in turn affect brain and cognition. The research presented by Anderson et al. assessed whether cinnamon could counter problems caused in rats fed a Western-style diet that was high in both fat and fructose. Those diminutive volunteers were randomly assigned to a control diet or to the Western diet with or without supplemental cinnamon. The cinnamon improved performance on several cognitive tests (mazes) and reduced levels of the precursors for the nasty Alzheimer's-associated proteins β-amyloid and tau. A major impact was cinnamon improving insulin sensitivity in body and brain, substantially countering the negative impacts of the Western diet. Other research has shown that cinnamon also benefited rodent brains that were injured (not by accident, of course; Yulug et al., 2018).

A primary metabolite of cinnamon is sodium benzoate, a food preservative added to many foods to extend shelf life. In a pair of extraordinarily thorough papers, Modi et al. (2015) and Modi et al. (2016) noted that various brain structures show increased levels of sodium benzoate after cinnamon is consumed and metabolized. Previous research had shown that sodium benzoate was an antioxidant with anti-inflammatory properties, an immune-system modulator, and a contributor to neural health and growth. It may also extend brain shelf life, but there is no real data on that.

Modi et al. (2016) assessed the impacts of both cinnamon and sodium benzoate on cell cultures of hippocampal neurons. Both substances increased the functioning of CREB, a transcription factor affecting various crucially-important genes that regulate neural activity, synaptic formation, and synaptic plasticity. Other reviewers have noted cinnamon's reduction of the tau tangles in *in vitro* formulations—tangles linked with Alzheimer's dementia (Momtaz et al., 2018). Although substances that stimulate neural plasticity in cell cultures often fail to show similar impacts in live brains, Modi et al. (2015) also reviewed tests of the affects of cinnamon and sodium benzoate on the brains and the cognitive skills of living mice. After a month of feeding those two nutrients, the positive impacts were that both spatial learning and memory capacity increased in the "poor learning" mice to the level normally seen in "good learning" mice. The intact brains of those lucky creatures showed impacts like those seen in the *in vitro* cell cultures. That is, through the genetic impacts mentioned above, both substances enhanced the establishment of new synapses and the general plasticity of hippocampal neurons—all modifications that explain how the cinnamon and sodium benzoate enhanced cognition. Other research reviewed by Modi et al. (2016) showed positive impacts from cinnamon and sodium benzoate in reducing cognitive deterioration in transgenic mice destined to experience Alzheimer's. Momtaz et al. concluded that those positive cognitive effects were due to cinnamon reducing β-amyloid plaques and tau tangles, and to enhancing the memorable neurotransmitter acetylcholine.

Although rodent cognition is of great concern to us all, my search for recent relevant papers assessing cinnamon impacts on humans yielded little. Given the substantial and meaningful research with critters, the lack of equally substantial research literature with human participants is curious. I offer nothing except the speculation that with the frequent addition of sodium benzoate to our human foods, further supplementation with either cinnamon or sodium benzoate may not offer additional benefits. Nevertheless, I shall continue to add small amounts of cinnamon to my coffee. (*After* the coffee is filtered though, because ground cinnamon thoroughly plugs paper filters; obviously I've tried that.) There is no cinnamon in my vitamin supplement.

### Ginger and 6-gingerol

The use of ginger also has roots deep into past millennia, with some evidence of the trade and use of ginger as long ago as 7000 years—way before the pyramids. Ginger has been used in traditional cooking as an herb and a spice, but it serves also as a component of traditional medicines. Its active ingredient is 6-gingerol. It has been used for conditions from indigestion to diabetes, migraine, and nausea—especially to control the nausea associated with pregnancy and motion sickness. My own recent "research" fits that pattern; I used it to quell nausea on a small boat heaving (yes heaving, not merely rocking) on heavy ocean swells. Despite the unfortunate outcome, I have not lost faith in ginger, and anyway real research supports its efficacy in various medicinal roles.

This research review begins with an unusual and important randomized-control trial. (After the modest results reviewed above for turmeric and for cinnamon, prepare for surprise.) This study is unusual because it used human participants rather than animals, and important because the results pertain to our interests in attention and cognition. For two months Saenghong et al. (2012), assessed the impacts of daily doses of placebos or dietary ginger extract (400mg or 800mg) on 60 randomly assigned middle-aged Thai women.

At the beginning of the 2-month study by Saenghong et al. and at one-month intervals, the women completed an extensive computerized battery of cognitive and memory tests. The tests included recognition and memory of words and pictures, various attention-measuring tasks, and measures of reaction time. The test battery was thorough. EEG measures of brain electrical activity were also made three times at those same one-month intervals while the women experienced the "auditory oddball" paradigm. In the "oddball" attention is assessed by the size of the P-300 EEG wave that follows the "oddball" sound in a sequence of repeated sounds. (See "oddball" in the glossary if unnaturally curious for even more information).

The results of the cognitive and memory tests were spectacular. Without my detailing differences between the 800mg and the 400mg conditions, or the differences between assessments at one month versus two, Saenghong et al. concluded that supplementation with ginger improved performance in all of the domains of attention and cognitive processing, with the strongest impacts on the attention measures.

Some of the physiological impacts noted by Saenghong et al. that can contribute to attention and cognition were increased levels of the neurotransmitters noradrenaline, dopamine, and serotonin. And by suppressing cholinesterase (the enzyme that degrades acetylcholine), ginger indirectly increased levels of acetylcholine, the neurotransmitter vital for learning and memory.

I discovered that study by Saenghong et al. through an extensive review by Sahardi and Makpol (2019)—a review that specifically assessed ginger's impacts on neural degeneration. Sahardi and Makpol noted that ginger was antibacterial, and protected against cancer. More important for our interests, they noted ginger's potential to be neuroprotective by reducing β-amyloid accumulation and by reducing oxidative stress and inflammation in people (and rats) who were diabetic. Most importantly, in mice it was noted that ginger increased levels of the wonderful neurotropin BDNF; many good things in the brain follow from that.

Besides ginger boosting acetylcholine levels in normal animals, it had similar impacts in transgenic Alzheimer's rats. Those unfortunate creatures also showed improved maze learning and (in at least one study) ginger completely eliminated β-amyloid plaques. And in studies of transgenic Parkinson's mice, ginger extracts improved the health of the brain's astrocytes and microglia, they enhanced the expression of the important neurotropin NGF (neural growth factor), and most importantly, the ginger protected dopamine-producing neurons. Those impacts apparently resulted from ginger inhibiting reactive oxygen molecules and reducing brain inflammation. Although the dosage levels of ginger given to the animals in typical studies of both Alzheimer's and Parkinson's rodents were many times greater than the doses in the very impressive study by Saenghong et al. with real people, that human study too was impressive.

As a summary of ginger's impacts, note that the research with relatively high doses for animals has shown absolutely convincing positive results for brain and cognition. For myself, having not previously considered ginger, except for its sometimes-effective use to suppress nausea, I am surprised by the consistency and power of its impacts in the animal research. We should certainly pay attention when research shows ginger to increase neurotransmitters and neurotropins, attenuate inflammation, control oxidation, and even eliminate β-amyloid accumulations in an Alzheimer's brain—even one that was previously in a mouse. However, as is often the case, some questions remain concerning application of those findings to us humans. The results from ginger supplementation in the study by Saenghong et al. (2012) with Thai women suggests strongly that we people should indeed expect spectacular results—both physical and cognitive—from ginger abstracts. But I would endorse those findings with more enthusiasm if a moderate number of supportive human research studies had been published in the decade since 2012.

Ginger root supplements are inexpensive at around $.10 per 500mg capsule, and some supplement manufacturers combine ginger with turmeric. If supportive research confirms the promise of ginger, at such a price ginger is a bargain. I have begun to add a couple of thin slices of ginger root (easy to find and very inexpensive in grocery stores) to the tea that I brew, finding that it adds a hint of ginger flavor and (equally important) supports my illusion that I am growing smarter.

## Saffron

Iran is by far the leading saffron-producing country. I have seen saffron harvested (though not in Iran). It must be among the most tedious jobs possible. Saffron has traditionally been used mostly for keeping depression at bay, and thus may be of great benefit to the people who must harvest it. But in this chapter, I consider only the evidence for its prowess in defending our cognitive capacities, saving review of the quite-encouraging depression research for Chapter 18.

The review by Marx et al. (2019) included animal research that showed saffron to be a regulator of neurotransmitters, the immune system, inflammation, oxidative stress, pituitary-adrenal-cortical arousal (and thus cortisol), and neurotropins, including our esteemed BDNF. Thus expectations are justified for major cognitive impacts in us humans. Cicero et al. (2018) noted its effectiveness, based on its antioxidant impacts and on lessening the impact of acetylcholinesterase (the enzyme that degrades acetylcholine), thereby enhancing acetylcholine levels and potentially, the memory capacities that depend upon that neurotransmitter. Their review of two randomized-control trials showed improvements in patients with Alzheimer's on various cognitive measures from saffron (versus placebo) administered for 16 weeks in the first study and for one year in the second. Another of the reviewed randomized-control trials indicated cognitive improvements in people with only mild cognitive impairment. The more recent review by Ayati et al. (2020) searched both English-language and Chinese databases for randomized-control trials that assessed effects on mild cognitive impairment and dementia, finding only four that met their criteria. All four indicated improvement on cognitive tests appropriate for Alzheimer's patients. Similar conclusions were reached by Avgerinos et al. (2020) based on the five randomized-control trials of people with Alzheimer's that met their criteria. On various cognitive tests, the saffron treatments proved to be superior to placebos and equal in effectiveness to conventional Alzheimer's medicine. (Note, however, that the final phrase is a weak endorsement because those conventional medicines are not very effective at all.)

Saffron's effectiveness for slowing cognitive decline in people who already show decline and in people with Alzheimer's is well established by those recent reviews. However, delaying age-related cognitive decline in pre-clinical populations is not supported by those research results.

### The herb (not spice) basil

Razazan et al. (2021) conducted an extensive "virtual screening" of over 100 thousand compounds in a search for some that might be effective activators of a neuron receptor known by the catchy name "free fatty acid receptor 2" (and usually written as FFAR2). Activation of the FFAR2s is normally achieved by metabolites produced in the gut by active members of the microbiome. (More about such processes in Chapter 16.) Activated FFAR2s inhibit the buildup of the nasty Alzheimer's-causing form of the β-amyloid protein, and those activated receptors facilitate the removal of expired neurons.

Razazan et al. determined that fenchol, the compound that gives basil its aromatic scent, was an activator of the FFAR2s. As anticipated, giving fenchol to various critters did indeed result in the clearing of β-amyloid. Those tantalizing results lead to expectations that either basil itself or some form of the fenchol could inhibit the development of Alzheimer's. But the relevant research has just begun.

**Summary for spices.** None of the spices reviewed above seem to have any potential for harm, so consider them even if some showed only tepid evidence for cognitive support. The recent reviews all suggested the likelihood that turmeric and its derivative, curcumin, preserve cognition in older peoples, and that cinnamon and its sodium benzoate have similar potential. Given what we know of their substantial impacts on the underlying physiology, such expectations are well justified.

Although there was only one randomized-control trial with ginger showing real cognitive enhancement (for Thai women), at this point, the evidence for cognitive preservation (rather than enhancement) is strong for ginger. And like ginger, saffron has shown physiological impacts on neurotransmitters, neurotropins, the immune system, inflammation, and oxidative stress. It too should be good for all of us even though it has, to date, proven impacts only in people already experiencing cognitive decline. Saffron and turmeric were nominated by Cicero et al. (2018) as two of the seven most likely of the phytochemicals to alleviate cognitive decline. That is a noteworthy endorsement. And happily, all of saffron's great physiological impacts seem to be similarly effective for alleviating depression. Await Chapter 18 for more about that.

# Chapter 12

# Nutraceuticals including choline and spermidine

"Nutraceutical" was initially unrecognized by my spell check. The term combines elements of "nutrition" with "pharmaceutical." Thus nutraceutical substances are credited with, and may actually have, some curative or medicinal impacts. A related term, "nootropic," implies the capacity to enhance memory; the similar term "cognitive enhancer" means ... well ... cognitive enhancer. Besides some nutraceuticals being nootropics and cognitive enhancers, some are described as "micronutrients," and terms like "herbal medicines" or "natural supplements" or even "dietary supplements" are, rightly or wrongly, sometimes used instead. Substances that wear those labels usually have active ingredients that were not elaborately created in labs, but rather extracted (however elaborately) from plants, or consumed as a part of those host plants (like the caffeine from coffee and tea or the nicotine from tobacco).

Obviously, some nutraceuticals have already been described in previous chapters, without the fancy label having been applied. They are the vitamins, nutrients, and micronutrients derived directly from our food or through action of our microbiome. We are more likely to apply the nutraceutical term to those that have ancient roots, especially those derived from the Ayurvedic traditions of India and from Chinese traditional medicine. One can learn much more about the varieties of substances considered to be nutraceuticals from Napoletano et al. (2020). Here I review several that did not fit into prior chapters but that have been studied extensively or that have been shown to have major impacts on brain, cognition, or resilience.

Because many nutraceuticals used in the US are not officially marketed as drugs with established claims of efficacy, they are not certified by or regulated by agencies such as the US Food and Drug Administration. Without such certification, the purveyors of the nutraceuticals are discouraged from making specific health claims, but on the other hand the lack of regulation naturally leads to such claims—sometimes false. When untrue claims of purity or potency are exposed, as happens occasionally, the overly-hyped assurances are (usually) withdrawn (e.g., Calderone, 2018). Another issue complicating nutraceutical acceptance is that some people associate them with other "traditional medicines" known to be useless (rhino horn or pangolin scales anyone?). But here we put all that behind us and study evaluations of a few of the promising nutraceuticals by (hopefully) unbiased scientists.

## Ginkgo

*Ginkgo biloba* (hereafter just "ginkgo") is the formal name for the maidenhair tree, native to China, Korea, and Japan. *Ginkgo biloba* is thought to be the oldest living tree species, and besides the species itself being ancient, individual trees can live 1000 years and more (Lee & Birks, 2018). In ancient China tea made from ginkgo leaves was believed to strengthen the body and enhance cognition, perhaps because the longevity of individual trees seemed to be an indicator of its efficacy. Popular literature and aggressive marketing in the modern era suggest that ginkgo will lead to our cognitive salvation; thus, it is often placed near the top of lists of nutraceuticals that are potential cognitive enhancers. The ingredients thought to convey those great benefits include some nutrients found in many plants, such as the flavonoids mentioned in Chapter 6, and terpenoids (a class of organic compounds that seem to be everywhere). Quercetin, a flavonoid that is also derived from red wine, is a major active ingredient of ginkgo (see a bit more about quercetin in Chapter 14). Other active ingredients that are unique to ginkgo are the two terpene lactones: ginkgolides and bilobalise—terms you need not remember for the exam.

Now consider whether ginkgo merits the acclaim that it has received. Fortunately, we benefit from thorough reviews of relevant research by Liu et al. (2019) and by Cicero et al. (2018). In their review of research with animals Liu et al. noted that those pre-clinical studies showed positive impacts of ginkgo on Alzheimer's-disposed rodents, and that ginkgo inhibited the toxicity of the nasty form of β-amyloid protein. Others (Lee & Birks, 2018; Cicero et al., 2018) noted that ginkgo reduced reactive oxygen and enhanced neurotransmitter levels. Ginkgo also stimulates cerebral blood flow by dilating capillaries via the action of nitric oxide (NO). (Recall that cacao's circulation-enhancing capacity is also thought to occur by evoking nitric oxide.)

The review by Liu et al. of ginkgo's impacts included 28 randomized-control trials using both cognitively normal people and people with Alzheimer's. The studies chosen spanned publication dates from 1984 to 2018. A simple count of the main results of that review found 17 positive studies that affirmed that ginkgo effectively preserved or enhanced cognition, in contrast to 11 null studies showing no significant benefits from ginkgo extract. A superficial assessment of that 17 to 11 ratio could lead to doubts, but a closer look leads to different conclusions. First, of course, the 11 null studies do not establish that ginkgo had no effects, but rather that any effects were not large enough to reach statistical significance. But more importantly, much is learned from the differences between the null and the positive studies. The positive studies were generally longer in duration (most were over 22 weeks versus only two null studies that long), and the positive studies used higher ginkgo doses. Effectiveness occurred with daily doses of 240mg or more—a level more than twice as high as used in most of the null studies. And the null studies typically used healthy and younger participants, whereas the positive studies employed older participants who sometimes suffered from dementia. (Other reviewers have also concluded that ginkgo is more suitable for treatment of the elderly.) Thus Liu et al. concluded that at appropriate doses of over 240mg/day, that a long course of treatment with ginkgo extract would effectively aid cognitive preservation in the elderly. However, as is usually the case with such nutraceuticals and nootropics, the research to date does not give information about how the impacts of such treatment may change over time, nor does it inform how ginkgo treatment may have different impacts on people carrying different alleles of the Alzheimer's-relevant *APOE* gene.

Ginkgo extract is already widely used. Liu et al. reported that nine countries had jointly published guidelines for the treatment of dementia with ginkgo extract, and Lee and Birks noted that although it is available as a non-prescribed supplement in most countries, it is available by prescription in France and Germany for the treatment of "cerebral insufficiency" and dementia.

Although many billions are spent each year in the US on ginkgo products, ginkgo extracts are relatively inexpensive, with internet supplies costing in the range of $.15/day for 240mg doses. However, despite the positive impacts that it apparently has on elderly cognition, decisions about taking ginkgo must be tempered with awareness of its not-often-studied limitations and complications. For example, ginkgo can exacerbate the impacts of anticoagulant medications and interfere with SSRIs—(selective serotonin reuptake inhibitors) the often-effective anti-depressants. For most people, ginkgo appears to be reasonably safe and effective, but be careful.

### Bacopa

*Bacopa monnieri* (hereafter simply bacopa) is the formal name of a succulent plant that grows easily in tropical climates. In India's Ayurvedic tradition bacopa extracts have been used in traditional medicine for centuries. It is called "brahmi" in Hindi and in some research papers. Compared to ginkgo, in the US bacopa is not yet as well known or esteemed, but besides being used by practitioners of Ayurvedic medicine for its positive impacts on cognition, it is touted in the US as an effective ingredient in at least one widely advertised brain elixir. And the advertising for that elixir notwithstanding ("...or your money back"), an extensive body of research really does suggest promise.

Some of the active components of bacopa that readers need not memorize are polyphenols that come in the form of twelve variations of bacopacides (a term that seems to imply killers of bacopas—but perhaps not). Besides the lethal-sounding bacopacides there are several other bacopa components called bacosides (dangerous for bacos?) and the ever-popular bacopasaponins. Although different studies of bacopa use different mixes of those many components, outcome measures show positive consistency.

Here I present a single excellent randomized-control trial that shows the impacts of long-term administration of bacopa on the cognitive processes of older people. Then I will discuss the conclusions from several recent reviews that summarize both animal and human research.

Peth-Nui et al. (2012) conducted a randomized, double-blind, placebo-controlled trial of 60 healthy older people (mean age 63) who were given a placebo or a bacopa extract of either 300mg or 600mg per day for 12 weeks. Attention was assessed by differences in event-related potentials (EEG measures of N-100 and P-300 waves) that were evoked by "oddball" signals. As noted for the "oddball" paradigm mentioned in Chapter 11, in response to a unique signal, spikes of those waves emerge more quickly and are stronger when attention is better. Working memory was assessed using various tests of memory, accuracy, and reaction time. Availabilities of the neurotransmitters acetylcholine, dopamine, and noradrenaline were assessed by enzyme assays. A finding that has been frequently replicated in other research was that bacopa enhanced acetylcholine. Bacopa also improved working memory and attention focus (as indicated by the EEG measures). Peth-Nui et al. concluded that the cognitive and attention improvements followed from bacopa enhancing acetylcholine levels.

An early review of human randomized-control trials of bacopa by Pase et al. (2012) characterized bacopa research as in its infancy. The six studies that fit their criteria administered placebos or bacopa extracts ranging from 300mg to 450mg per day for at least 12 weeks. In those six studies bacopa improved performance on nine of the 17 tests of free recall memory with little evidence of improvement in other cognitive domains.

Two years later, Kongkeaw et al. (2014) did a thorough search of major scholar indices for randomized-control trials of bacopa impacts on human participants. The nine studies that met their criteria provided 437 people for their meta-analysis. The reviewers judged the quality of those studies to be high and concluded that bacopa improved performance substantially and statistically significantly on a choice reaction time task and on the trail-making test—a measure of processing speed and cognitive flexibility (both significant at $p < .001$).

Several years later, Chaudhari et al. (2017) noted from the animal studies they reviewed that bacopa extracts reduced damage from reactive oxygen species and protected cells of the prefrontal cortex and the hippocampi from toxicity and from the DNA damage that accompanies Alzheimer's dementia. Chaudhari et al. concluded that bacopa also protected neurons that depend upon acetylcholine (supporting the conclusions of Peth-Nui et al. reviewed above), and that bacopa reduced both the amyloid precursor protein responsible for the β-amyloid plaque formation and reduced the plaques themselves. Bacopa also reduced stress-caused damage in the hippocampi.

As noted above for ginkgo, one of bacopa's means for protecting the brain and aiding cognition is by increasing cerebral circulation. An important study using rats by Kamkaew et al. (2013) compared bacopa's capacity to increase cerebral circulation with similar impacts from ginkgo and from donepezil—a drug used to treat Alzheimer's. After eight weeks of dietary supplementation, compared to placebo, both bacopa and ginkgo increased cerebral blood flow in the rats' brains (by 25% and 29%, respectively, $p < .05$) with no similar positive effect from the Alzheimer's drug.

With no serious complications, the reviewed research with humans showed positive bacopa impacts on memory including "logical memory" and paired-associate learning. Chaudhari et al. concluded that those cognitive benefits from bacopa depended largely upon its antioxidant and anti-inflammatory actions. They noted additional benefits to health from its action as an anticonvulsant, a "cardiotonic," a bronchodilator, and by offering protection from peptic ulcers.

Finally, Manap et al. (2019) provided an even later review of bacopa impacts from research with both animals and humans. Echoing the conclusions from the previous reviews, the animal research showed that bacopa protected the brain from oxidative damage, especially in the hippocampi and prefrontal cortex, prevented β-amyloid plaque formation, and protected neurons from the toxicity caused by plaques. As noted in the human study reviewed above by Peth-Nui et al., long-term exposure of the animals to bacopa extracts also enhanced the synthesis of acetylcholine, regulated other neurotransmitters (including serotonin), and increased cerebral blood flow. In turn, those impacts prevented or delayed age-related cognitive deterioration in the animals. Finally, bacopa actively inhibits inflammation in the brain by inhibiting inflammation-promoting enzymes and preventing the release of inflammatory cytokines from the brain's immune cells—the microglia (Nemetchek et al., 2017).

Randomized-control trials of young, middle-aged, and older human participants summarized in the Manap et al. review found improved cognition in young medical students from bacopa administered for 42 days

(Kumar et al., 2016). In middle-aged people, a 3-month regime of bacopa enhanced retention (Roodenrys et al., 2002). Older Italian participants (mean age 73) without dementia received a placebo or 300mg per day of bacopa for 84 days. Those receiving bacopa showed substantial and significant improvement in a recall task and in the famous Stroop Task—a measure of attention. A relatively unique result from that study was that bacopa improved measures of both anxiety and depression (Calabrese et al., 2008).

**A bacopa summary.** The practitioners of India's Ayurvedic tradition considered bacopa to be a "medhya rasayana"—an herb to sharpen mind. They were correct, and modern research has shown us the means for bacopa's stellar accomplishments. The physiological issues we associate with Alzheimer's are all attenuated by bacopa. That is, bacopa reduces inflammation by downregulating the microglia, keeps β-amyloid plaques from forming and from damaging neurons, keeps acetylcholine levels appropriately high, regulates other essential neurotransmitters, reduces damage from reactive oxygen species, and improves cerebral blood circulation. That is a very large basket of benefits at a supplement cost that can be as low as around US $.25/day. But even with that large basket, perhaps this should be said after noting strong impacts from any of the nutraceuticals: impactful ingredients may have substantial side effects. Check such substances carefully before taking them, and beware of interactions with other drugs.

## Choline

Choline is one of the really important nutrients we should know about. It is a water-soluble nutrient in the B-vitamin family that is plentiful in eggs and meat. Choline is a component of the memory-vital neurotransmitter acetylcholine. Several compounds are available that affect the brain's choline levels (Colucci et al., 2012). Phosphatidyl choline is a variant of choline that is a component of lecithin, and that (naturally) contains choline. Hereafter I shall use the term choline to subsume its various forms unless researchers designate a specific variant (such as in the study below by Ylilauri et al., 2019).

As noted in Chapter 11, benefits accrue to brain and cognition when nutrients such as ginger enhance acetylcholine levels. Choline itself should then be similarly effective. To address that issue, Ylilauri et al. assessed levels of the dietary choline and phosphatidyl choline consumed by almost 2500 Finnish men for 22 years. Note that phosphatidyl choline is a form that especially affects neural membranes. Cognitive capacity was assessed on a good selection of tests and the researchers accounted for a host of potential confounds including age, energy intake, education, smoking, BMI, diabetes, physical activity, heart disease, medications, and consumption of alcohol, fiber, fruits, berries, vegetables, and dietary fats.

During the 22-year period of the study 337 men (13.5% of the total group) were diagnosed with dementia. Total dietary choline did not correspond with dementia risks at a statistically significant level; that is, after taking account of the potential confounds listed above, the risk ratio calculated from the multivariate equation for the 624 men in the highest choline quartile was (a suggestive-but-non-significant) RR = .88 ($p$ = .18). Phosphatidyl choline consumption had a stronger relationship with dementia. After taking those same potential confounds into account, the multivariate calculation of risk ratio for the men in the top quartile of only phosphatidyl choline was RR = .72 ($p$ = .03; i.e., for every 100 men with Alzheimer's in the bottom quartile there were only 72 in the top quartile).

Examining cognition rather than only dementia, in the subset of 482 men for whom cognitive data were available, both total choline and phosphatidyl choline corresponded positively with cognitive scores. Specifically, total choline intake correlated positively with tests of verbal fluency, verbal memory, and visual memory. Phosphatidyl choline intake correlated positively with cognitive processing speed, verbal fluency, and visual memory. Those relationships of both choline and phosphatidyl choline with the cognitive tests were not affected by which of the alleles of the Alzheimer's-relevant *APOE* gene were carried by the participants.

Those correlational findings were significant and substantial, but the randomized-control trials that explain the likely causes of those relationships were done with smaller creatures. With both normal mice and Alzheimer's transgenic mice, Velazquez et al. (2019) tested choline supplements across their "lifetimes" from age 2.5 months until their enforced demise at 10 months. The control animals received choline levels in their diets that were essentially normal, but the choline-supplemented mice were given doses at around five times that normal level. The research design featured four groups, the Alzheimer's-disposed mice with and without choline supplementation, and the normal mice with and without the extra choline.

Instead of tests of vocabulary or reciting numbers backwards, the main test of cognitive capacity of the mice was learning to navigate the Morris water maze, a test of spatial memory. As expected, maze learning was quite slow in the Alzheimer's mice without choline supplements. However, for the Alzheimer's mice given the extra choline, learning the maze was as quick as for both groups of cognitively-normal mice—both the normal mice with and those without extra choline. (Actually, it appeared that the extra choline provided a small benefit for the normal mice too.)

The authors assessed a number of physiological indicators that were all enhanced by the supplemental choline and that could explain the superior maze performance by the lucky critters receiving those supplements. Specifically, in the choline supplement group of transgenic Alzheimer's mice, the β-amyloid plaques were substantially reduced in the hippocampi, certainly in part because the amyloid precursor protein was better controlled in those supplemented animals. Fortunately, the Alzheimer's mice with choline supplementation also had less microglia activation than the other Alzheimer's mice, reducing the potential for damaging inflammation from overly-active microglia. Because choline lowers nasty homocysteine levels, and because lower homocysteine levels lead to lower β-amyloid levels (as noted in Chapter 5), Velazquez et al. speculated that the reduced plaques in the Alzheimer's animals receiving the choline supplements may have been due to the choline reducing homocysteine.

Applying their observations to humans, Velazquez et al. suggested that the high levels of dementia seen in the UK may stem from the lack of national standards for choline. But they added that for preventing dementia and cognitive decline, the current US RDA of 425mg of choline for women and 500mg for men may be much too low.

In support of that conclusion, consider that in the research by Velazquez et al. the choline-supplemented mice received 4.5 times the RDA for mice. (Yes, I realize this leads to interesting questions about mouse RDAs, but ... ?). They noted that the tolerable upper limit of choline for humans is seven to eight times higher than the RDA amounts. In other words, we people too could take rather large choline supplements with large potential benefits with little danger of unwanted side effects. However, because choline supplementation has not proven to benefit people with advanced Alzheimer's, Velazquez et al. suggest that their lifetime approach should be used to slow age-related cognitive decline.

Where should our choline come from? We can get some from normal diets. For example, one egg yolk has around ¼ of our RDA at 147mg, but if we sacrificed the egg producer, three ounces of chicken liver would provide 247mg. Not for me though. An equal amount of *grass-fed* beef has only 55mg, but with those numbers in mind, consider some tempting exchanges: Instead of eating the three ounces of not-too-appetizing chicken liver, for the same choline benefit, you could eat a 15-ounce steak from a grass-fed bovine. Other grass-fed animals like sheep are similarly generous with their choline, but we must be cautious around those red meats.

Instead, should additional choline come from supplements? Given that we make some choline in our livers but depend upon animal sources to top off levels to RDAs, some nutritionists emphasize that although plant-based diets are good for the environment, the resultant choline deficiencies risk brain health (Derbyshire, 2019). Thus choline supplements probably benefit especially those favoring vegetarian and vegan diets. The pros and cons of such supplementation are described in a National Institutes of Health website at https://ods.od.nih.gov/factsheets/Choline-HealthProfessional/. That article spells out risks (some speculate cardiovascular) and benefits (based on some of the research described here).

The Covid-19 outbreak reminded the US Center for Disease Control and Prevention to recommend that pregnant women take choline supplements in order to prevent the deficient fetal brain development (frequently seen with viral epidemics) that can result if pregnant women become infected (Freedman et al., 2020). Even in normal times, extra choline is recommended for pregnant women.

**Dangers from anticholinergics.** Anticholinergic drugs block the action of the neurotransmitter acetylcholine. However, anticholinergic drugs are sometimes prescribed to people with Parkinson's disease to reduce tremors, and some anti-depressant drugs are anticholinergics, with different ones having different degrees of acetylcholine suppression. Anticholinergics are also sometimes prescribed for COPD, asthma, bladder control and motion sickness. Benadryl is an anticholinergic too and so are over-the-counter sleeping pills that contain Diphenhydramine.

If supplemental choline prevents cognitive decline and dementia, as suggested above, then perhaps anticholinergic drugs increase the potential for dementia. Fortunately, the tests of that hypothesis are in. Several recent studies with thousands of participants found that indeed the anticholinergics lead to more cases of dementia. Another side of that relationship is that people already suffering from dementia more frequently have a history of using anticholinergics (in contrast to people without dementia; Campbell et al., 2010; Coupland et al., 2019). Perhaps we should not be overly concerned; some reviewers suggest that anticholinergics foster dementia only after years of exposure. Still, some caution is appropriate.

Judging from the multivitamin used in my house, choline supplements are not usually included in multis, but they are easily available online. Supplements with choline bitartrate, choline chloride, and phosphatidyl choline are widely available, and affordable, but determining which forms are more bio-available is not easy. We use one with phosphatidyl that costs around $.10/day; it has not yet made me a stable genius, but hope lingers.

Besides the research reviewed above affirming the value of choline and phosphatidyl choline, other reviewers defend the cognitive benefits from citicholine. For example, the review by Colucci et al. (2012) of only nootropic drugs that boost cholinergic activity discusses the positive impacts of citicholine and other alternatives to the choline-boosting forms that I review here. Supplements of any of those may eventually prove to be very important for brain and cognition but, as noted above, some reviewers suspect too much may have negative cardiovascular implications.

### Spermidine

Spermidine is a vital polyamine that influences a host of vital biological functions. Like other mammals, we make spermidine in our bodies, but all of us mammals also derive it from dietary sources. Thus some of the following assesses impacts of spermidine levels that have been experimentally enhanced by benevolent researchers.

The recent review by Madeo et al. (2020) concluded that spermidine extends lifespan and healthspan. Those impacts were seen in research ranging from *in vitro* tissue samples to studies of a variety of species, including yeasts, fruit flies (*drosophila*), roundworms (*C. elegans*), and, of course, mice (*M. mouse*— just guessing). In the mouse studies reviewed by Madeo et al., it was noted that the life-extension effect resulted even if spermidine supplementation began late in life. With impacts on such a wide array of species, it is apparent that something important at the cellular level results from spermidine.

Clearly, spermidine declines as people age, but there have been few randomized-control trials using intact humans. However, although spermidine tends to be quite low in most elderly people, spermidine levels in the serum of people who live very long lives tend to be as high as spermidine levels in middle-aged people. Such correlations support the animal research that shows spermidine's causal role in prolonging lifespan and (hopefully) healthspan. Other correlational research by Schwarz et al. (2020) found that older people with higher spermidine intake had greater hippocampal volume and cortical thickness. At this writing, those researchers are beginning to undertake randomized-control trials to determine causal relationships.

The animal research shows the means for those positive impacts: Spermidine reduces chronic inflammation and reduces blood pressure. Most importantly, it assists the removal of damaged mitochondria, reducing the oxidative damage that "sick" mitochondria cause, and allowing new replacement mitochondria to develop and assume their energy-generating duties (perhaps after completing apprenticeships (?)). Those antioxidant and anti-inflammatory functions are especially important in tissues with high-energy demands, such as in the cardiovascular system and the brain. Some of the animal research showed enhanced synaptic functions as well. Madeo et al. cited research showing that rats exposed to pesticides that enhance Parkinson's disease were protected from the expected loss of dopamine neurons if they had been given supplemental spermidine.

With that array of important impacts on animals (and even yeast) it is natural to expect that enhanced spermidine would reduce cardiovascular disease and reduce age-related cognitive decline and dementia in people. Testing that expectation in correlational research, Kiechl et al. (2018) studied diets assessed by repeated dietitian-administered and validated food-frequency questionnaires from 829 participants in a 20-year span from 1995 to 2015. The people were divided into thirds based on spermidine intake. After taking into account various potential confounds (age, sex, calories consumed, and lifestyle factors) mortality risk was substantially lower for those in the third consuming the most spermidine, with a hazard ratio of HR = .76 (meaning only 76 deaths in the high spermidine third for every 100 deaths in the low third; $p < .001$). Kiechl et al. estimated that those in that top spermidine group would live 5.7 years longer than those in the lowest third. (Longevity is not our main concern here, but as noted previously, death invariably causes cognitive decline.) I think that eating a few extra mushrooms (see below) is a small price to pay for the possibility of more years above ground.

In another somewhat-preliminary correlational study, Pekar et al. (2020) recruited 80 elderly participants (mean age of 83) from nursing homes. Instead of assessing spermidine from food logs, spermidine measured from blood serum was correlated with mental performance. The results showed a modest by statistically significant Kendall rank correlation between spermidine concentration and mental acuity assessed with the Mini-Mental State Examination (tau-b = .153, $p = .025$).

In one of the few randomized-control trials with people Wirth et al. (2018) compared a 1.2mg daily dose of spermidine (in spermidine-rich wheat germ extract) with a placebo condition in only 30 randomly assigned adults (age 60 to 80). Those adults had all reported a subjective cognitive decline. The participants were tested pre- and post-treatment on standard measures of memory, executive functions (digit symbol substitution), and "mnemonic discrimination"—the ability to differentiate highly similar previously seen objects from an array of seen and not-seen objects.

With only 15 participants per condition, Wirth et al. assessed effect sizes rather than statistical significance from the 3-month spermidine treatment. The spermidine group showed very substantially enhanced mnemonic discrimination compared to controls (effect size Cohen's d = .77) and, unlike the controls, showed improvement from pre- to post-measures (d = .79). Similar improvements were not found on standardized tests on memory and executive functions. Those suggestive results will be affirmed (or not) when

Wirth and colleagues publish their on-going follow-up study of appropriate length and size.

Although research on spermidine's impacts on brain and cognition is not yet conclusive, it is tantalizing. Given the studies currently ongoing, more firm conclusions are (perhaps) only a year or two away. Even with the current limitations, I believe we should consider the inclusion of spermidine-rich foods in our own normal diets. The lists of those foods consistently begin with mushrooms and wheat germ, but (happily) the lists include pears, green peas, and aged and fermented cheese (including the blue cheese that we can put on our phytonutrient-rich salad). (From Chapter 6 you may recall other benefits from not-necessarily-magic mushrooms.) My quick web search for spermidine supplements found some availability for spermidine extracts—mostly derived from wheat germ. Some were expensive at well over a US $1.00 per day. Most had been rated by a few people, indicating that despite hints of delivering genius and (relative) immortality, spermidine supplements are not yet widely used.

**A questionable summary.** Some of the researchers and reviewers contributing perspectives have cited randomized-control trials where some of the nutraceuticals have been combined. I have not reviewed those combined-therapy approaches here because it is difficult enough to determine effectiveness levels of individual supplements. But an obvious issue relates to the combined impacts of (say) ginkgo, bacopa, choline, and spermidine. Hypothetically, if 10 years of taking a choline supplement led to a risk ratio of RR = .80 for Alzheimer's (versus placebo, but remember, I am just guessing here), and if similar risk ratios were achieved from bacopa, from ginkgo, and perhaps even from spermidine supplements, would their impacts be additive, yielding absolutely wonderful ratios from the combination? Perhaps—just perhaps—one day we shall know the answer. (Remember, as noted in Chapter 7, the impacts of tea and coffee did seem to be additive.)

# Chapter 13

# Alcohol I: controversies

One of the studies that nudged me toward writing this book was the research by Topiwala et al. (2017), mentioned in Chapter 3 and reviewed more thoroughly below. Their well-designed and through study concluded that drinking any amount of alcohol was definitely harmful to brains and, because of the nature of the brain harm, probably harmful to cognition. I was sufficiently concerned that I taped the study abstract to the door of the small refrigerator that cools the household beer. That abstract asked me to keep the door closed—a request I often ignored—but the warning was worrisome.

Yet, in the last couple of decades, the popular media have reported on research showing various benefits from low to moderate alcohol use, especially benefits for cardiovascular health and longevity. Often those reports mentioned blessings from red wine, but some smiled upon moderate amounts of alcohol from any source. But with that ominous summary taped to my refrigerator, I dove into the alcohol research literature, finding other well-constructed studies and a major review. Several of the recent studies challenged the positive belief that moderate drinking could benefit general health, or specifically the cardiovascular system, or brain integrity, or cognition. But several others came to opposite conclusions. I craved a resolution.

When most other nutrients are studied, the research goal is usually to decide whether some increase above normal dietary levels might be helpful. That is not the usual research question with alcohol, because there really is no normal background level of consumption. The question for alcohol is whether any at all is harmful or beneficial for brain and/or cognition.

To share some of the consternation spawned by the contradictions in the research, I begin this chapter by reviewing the disappointing findings that even small amounts of alcohol are harmful to brain and cognition, and then I examine the best of the studies showing the opposite—that moderate alcohol consumption may benefit brain and cognition. Some of the positive studies suggest that red wine especially should be celebrated; I explore that possibility thoroughly in Chapter 14. After the arguments of this Chapter 13, with some assistance from Pollyanna I conclude Chapter 14 with conciliatory words that resolve all apparent dietary contradictions, and (with time, space, and the tolerance of editors) address other possible concerns such as finding purpose in life, securing true love, etc.

**The brain on booze.** It is not absurd to expect cognitive and brain benefits from consuming alcohol. Consider this recent study by Lundgaard et al. (2018) of mice enjoying a daily happy hour: The lucky "moderate" drinkers were given the equivalent of 2 ½ human drinks per day, whereas the not-so-lucky heavy boozers consumed three times that amount (appropriately characterized by the researchers as a "binge" level); controls had to settle for water. As expected, the heavy drinkers had poor outcomes. They suffered brain inflammation, especially in the astrocyte cells that regulate the brain-cleaning glymphatic system. Combined with other negative brain impacts, the alcohol-soaked astrocytes of the heavy drinkers failed to remove β-amyloid protein and plaques from those little brains.

On the other hand, the moderate imbibing mice benefited from their daily cocktail. Immediately after their daily boozing and after a month of those hazy days, compared to the non-alcohol-drinking controls they had reduced brain inflammation and increased efficiency of their brain-cleaning glymphatic systems. Perhaps we humans should expect similar benefit from moderate drinking. But will the research cooperate?

### Negative impacts on brain and cognition

**Reviews.** Wood et al. (2018) provided a major review of prospective studies collected from 19 countries with a total of over six hundred thousand people participating in the various studies. A review of that scope should lead to irrefutable conclusions, and the authors did not hesitate to announce that our brief human lifespans are shortened even more by consuming over five drinks a week. (Obviously, that is less than a single drink per day!) While their review was not specifically about brain impacts, as noted throughout, death discourages cognitive preservation. Together the reviewed studies showed various negative impacts from alcohol consumption including strokes, aneurysms, and other heart failure, although on the positive side alcohol seemed to reduce heart attacks. In general, however, no benefit to health or longevity was found from modest drinking. The researchers concluded that the upper safe limit is five units of alcohol per week. Note, however, that a unit is defined as eight grams of alcohol—considerably less than a more-typical 12-gram "drink."

Although that review was vast, direct causality from alcohol to health problems was impossible to establish because the studies were essentially correlational, with many being cross-sectional studies relating health at some point to drinking over various prior intervals. Besides the usual limitations of correlational research, that meta-analysis combined studies that assessed alcohol consumed in various ways (e.g., drinking beer with friends after work, or having rum for breakfast, or perhaps wine with dinner); nor were the sources of the alcohol differentiated (e.g., beer versus vodka). With those limitations, and with the conclusions not being about brain or cognition, we might be tempted to discount that vast review. But it was not alone.

Before assessing other reviews and some individual studies, consider that the differences between people who consume different amounts of alcohol are likely to be more important and substantial than (say) differences between people who use different amounts of olive oil or who take (or not) vitamin B supplements. The many possibly-confounding variables that may be different between people who drink a little or a lot may account for differences in cognitive abilities and brain structure. Advancing that idea, Nurk et al. (2009) noted that moderate wine consumption is likely to portend other favorable social and lifestyle factors that resist cognitive decline. Whether focused on wine only or on other forms of alcohol, consider an extension of that observation: It may be that the association of heavy drinking with cognitive deterioration is due to *un*favorable social and lifestyle factors besides alcohol—factors such as depression, or just being dumb. Those features do indeed accelerate age-associated cognitive decline. Those concerns are not unique to the alcohol research, but they are likely to be more important in interpreting the alcohol research than for most other nutrients. Fortunately, as the researchers of the studies reviewed below drew their conclusions, in each case, they took into account either a moderate amount or an exhaustive amount of those potentially-confounding factors.

**Brain impacts.** Supporting the conclusions from the massive Wood et al. review that any alcohol is detrimental to lifespan and healthspan, as mentioned in the introduction above, Topiwala et al. (2017) extended those negative conclusions to our concerns with brain and cognition. Published in the prestigious *British Medical Journal* their study was titled: "Moderate alcohol consumption as a risk factor for adverse brain outcomes and cognitive decline ..." That well-conducted study of the Whitehall II cohort (middle-class English folks who have been studied for decades) took into account a vast array of potentially confounding factors. I listed that entire array in Chapter 3; it took 10 lines. I note in summary here that the array accounted for factors ranging from initial IQ, socioeconomic factors, age, sex, education, exercise levels, cardiovascular health, and even personality variables such as impulsivity. For 30 years, the study tracked the drinking amounts and cognitive performance of the 527 middle-aged British men and women who completed the study and who were 73 (mean age) at the study's end. Because the researchers assessed cognitive capacities from start to finish, they could assess changes across that 30-year span. Happily for those of us who consume alcohol, there were no significant correlations between drinking and reduced performance on most of the cognitive tests, even though there were enough people in the study to allow detection of even small effects. However, drinking did lead to a decline across the 30-year span in lexical fluency—the vital skill of assembling words in meaningful ways.

But Topiwala and her colleagues also contributed some really bad news: Keep in mind that the MRI brain scans of those Whitehall participants were not done at the study's beginning, but provided only end-of-study data. Nevertheless, the scans led to correlational relationships that were completely negative. They showed that the amount of alcohol regularly consumed over the 30 years correlated with lower hippocampal volume in a dose-response relationship (i.e., more drinking corresponded with smaller hippocampi). When the people were divided into two groups defined by having either above-average or below-average hippocampal volume (a rather unrefined approach), the correlation with drinking was huge and statistically significant. That is, compared to abstainers, "moderate" drinkers of 14-21 alcohol units per week (up to around two typical drinks/day) were three times more likely to show hippocampal atrophy ($p$ = .007). But also compared to abstainers, participants who drank over 30 alcohol units per week (i.e., over three typical drinks/day) were 5.8 times more likely to show hippocampal atrophy ($p$ = .001). It is not trivial to lose hippocampal volume and the episodic memory capacity it supports.

Other bad news from Topiwala and colleagues was that alcohol consumption was associated with reduced grey matter density, especially in hippocampi, although fortunately frontal brain regions were not affected (a modicum of at-least-neutral news). Drinking more also correlated with reduced white matter integrity for those Whitehall participants, meaning that communication between brain structures was less efficient—especially the between-hemisphere communication through the 200 million axons of the corpus callosum.

Overall, drinking correlated with greater negative features in the Whitehall men than the women, but the men drank twice as much as the women (as in many populations). In summary, in this very well-constructed study, even while taking into account almost all the potentially-confounding factors that could reasonably account for brain degradation, there was substantially less brain volume in really important structures in the drinkers—even the drinkers of small amounts.

When another study of brain shrinkage from even small amounts of drinking appeared recently, it splashed into local news outlets (as is often the case) as if it were a new revelation. The half-page coverage in my city's newspaper included in its title that alcohol was linked to "smaller brains." It frightened some of my friends, who asked me about the study. The study used yet another cohort of (over 36 thousand) British people, but unfortunately took into account fewer potentially-confounding variables than the Topiwala et al. research. The authors concluded in their abstract (Daviet et al., 2022, p. 1) that:

> *alcohol intake is negatively associated with global brain volume measures, regional gray matter volumes, and white matter microstructure. Here, we show that the negative associations between alcohol intake and brain macrostructure and microstructure are already apparent in individuals consuming an average of only one to two daily alcohol units, and become stronger as alcohol intake increases.*

Like the review described above by Wood et al. of overall health impacts, no protection for cognition or brain structure result from even light drinking in the studies by Topiwala et al. and by Daviet et al. For those who drink any alcoholic beverages, those correlational relationships are clearly bad news.

But there may be causes for that bad news that open other paths for understanding relationships between alcohol and brain, or alcohol and cognition. For example, although beverage choices were not described in either if those large negative studies, it seems likely that for those English participants, that the tradition of post-work meetings in pubs (often owned by breweries) could lead to relatively more beer consumed than other alcoholic beverages. Beer drinking may be a part of the problem. Another potentially important factor is that those after-work beverages are more likely to be consumed with minimal food—at least minimal in contrast to cultures where alcohol is more traditionally consumed with meals. As discussed in Chapter 14, those two factors of beverage choice and timing are likely to be important.

### Positive impacts on brain and cognition

Like those negative studies, these positive studies were selected because they were well constructed, had large numbers of participants, and accounted for reams of potentially-confounding variables.

In a detailed and well-constructed longitudinal study that spanned 25 years, Richard et al. (2017) studied 1,344 community-dwelling older adults in an American community. Alcohol consumption was first assessed by questionnaire between 1984 and 1987, and again at the study's end, in 2009. Cognitive function was assessed at 4-year intervals between 1988 and 2009. The conclusions from their *Journal of Alzheimer's Disease* research paper were dramatic (Richard et al., 2017, p. 803):

> *Relative to nondrinkers, moderate and heavy drinkers (up to 3 drinks/day for women and for men 65 years and older, up to 4 drinks/day for men*

*under 65 years) had significantly higher adjusted odds of survival to age
85 without cognitive impairment (p <0.05). Near daily drinkers had 2-3
fold higher adjusted odds of cognitively healthy longevity versus living to
at least age 85 with cognitive impairment (odds ratio (OR) = 2.06; 95%
confidence interval (CI): 1.21 – 3.49) or death before 85 (OR=3.24; 95% CI:
1.92-5.46). Although excessive drinking has negative health consequences,
these results suggest that regular, moderate drinking may play a role in
cognitively healthy longevity.*

Wow! In real words, elderly drinkers were over three times more likely to just survive to 85, and when they did so, they were two to three times more likely to do so with intact cognitive abilities. At first glance, those results for elderly Americans are completely opposed to the findings from the much-younger participants in the British studies. And whereas the studies of the British drinkers mainly assessed brain tissue impacts from alcohol (with the cognitive assessments in the Topiwala et al. study showing little), that American study was about longevity and cognition. Perhaps those things are keys to the differences. Perhaps.

In another study of Americans, Zhang et al. (2020) compared their self-reported alcohol consumption with measures of cognition obtained over an average of nine years for almost 20 thousand middle-aged adults. Participants' average age was 62—close in age to the Brits in the Topiwala study and much younger than participants in the Richard et al. study of Americans. The participants were part of the Health and Retirement Study—a representative sample of the US population (thus with more women than men, and more white than black people, etc.). Cognitive tests were administered every two years, so that each participant was tested at least three times. The possibly-confounding factors of age, sex, race/ethnicity, years of education, marital status, smoking, and body mass index were taken into account.

Participants were categorized as Never Drinkers, Former Drinkers, Light-to-Moderate Drinkers (hereafter L-M Drinkers), or Heavy Drinkers. L-M Drinkers were women who consumed fewer than eight drinks per week and men consuming less than 15. (Note that "drink" here reflects a typical description of alcohol consumption, with more alcohol than the "alcohol unit" used in the Topiwala study; the Glossary has more precision.) The large number of 20 thousand participants lends stability of the findings. (E.g., whereas only 10% of the participants were Heavy Drinkers, the actual number in that category was around 2,000).

Total cognitive functioning was defined by combining scores from tests of word recall (immediate and delayed), mental status (tests of knowledge, language, and orientation), and vocabulary (essentially word definitions). There were two methods of assessing cognitive differences between the alcohol consumption categories. For the first method, participants were divided into the two cognitive categories of Smart or Slow (my terms), based on whether their overall cognitive scores across time were above or below the mean.

Supporting results of the Richard study, being an L-M Drinker kept participants out of the Slow group with an Odds Ratio of OR = 0.66 ($p < .001$; see Glossary if in need of interpretation of the odds ratio). One of the surprising results was that the three categories of drinkers (Former, L-M, and Heavy Drinkers) all were better in cognitive performance than the Never Drinkers, although the L-M Drinkers were best.

The second method of assessing cognitive differences between the categories of drinkers examined the rate of decline in cognitive performance across the nine years of the study. Those results were consistent with the former analysis. That is, in contrast to the relatively rapid cognitive decline across that 9-year period for the Never Drinkers, consumption of any alcohol correlated with more stabile cognitive scores ($p < .002$). But the best consumption pattern for cognitive preservation was consuming 10 to 14 drinks per week—the moderate drinking.

So far the really positive studies have involved US participants. Perhaps that is important. Probably not. Instead, consider people of the Netherlands. In the best study I reviewed for this chapter (in my view), 2613 middle-aged men and women in a small town in the Netherlands participated in a longitudinal study (Nooyens et al., 2013). The study spanned five years, with cognitive measures taken at the beginning and end of that interval, and with drinking monitored throughout. At the study's conclusion, those respondents were all between 48 and 75 years old. The features that cause me to celebrated this study include (a) that the sources of alcohol were taken into account (e.g., red wine versus beer, etc.), (b) the comparison group for moderate and heavy drinkers was more thoughtfully selected than in most other studies, and (c) most importantly the researchers were much more thorough than usual in accounting for the many potentially-confounding factors that could impact cognitive changes across the 5-year span of the study.

The comparison group for the drinkers consisted of people who consumed very little alcohol rather than (as in most studies, like the Zhang et al. study above) people who abstained. That little-consumption comparison group is preferable because the usual selection of abstainers often includes former drinkers—sometimes former heavy drinkers—making comparisons with (say) moderate drinkers less meaningful. (Some reviewers, such as Dhir (2018), assert that using abstainers as the comparison group is a major flaw.)

Global cognitive decline over the 5-year span for the participants in the Nooyens et al. study was based on comparing performance at the end with initial cognitive measures. Thus as in the two studies reviewed immediately above, assessing cognitive decline over time allowed much stronger inferences of causality between alcohol and cognition. The global cognitive measure resulted from combining the measures of memory function, information processing speed, and cognitive flexibility.

Adjustments were made for the potentially-confounding variables of age, education, and initial cognitive function. Among the many other factors taken into account were smoking, physical activity, and diet (including consumption of tea and coffee, fruit and vegetables, and total fat and total calories). Assessments were also made on vitality, mental health, past depression, and marital status. Health variables taken into account were cardiovascular factors such as blood pressure, cholesterol levels, heart disease, diabetes, waist circumference, etc. Because so many variables were taken into account, some compound scores were calculated by combining measures of similar variables. Better than placing participants into only two or three consumption categories, men and women were placed separately into five categories (quintiles) determined by the amounts of alcohol regularly consumed.

The results for women provided the most striking results. For the women the *smallest cognitive decline* over the five years of the study corresponded with being in the group with the *highest* alcohol consumption (corresponding to two to three drinks per day; $p < .02$). Compared to women who drank very little alcohol, those women in the top quintile showed less than half of the cognitive decline. That is an amazing result.

The results for men were weaker but somewhat similar, up to a point. On average, the men consumed much more alcohol than the women. Research shows consistently that heavy drinking is bad for brain and cognition, so it is not surprising that a substantial amount of cognitive decline was found for men in the quintile with the highest consumption. Thus instead of a straight-line relationship between increasing alcohol amount and positive cognitive scores, the curvilinear results showed the greatest *cognitive flexibility* to be in the men who drink a moderate amount—in the middle quintiles. However, the correspondence of consumption with cognition was not statistically significant for men, and the measure that seemed to be most affected by drinking—the cognitive flexibility measure—was only one of the measured components of cognitive decline. With those limitations in mind, these data for men cannot be interpreted as showing general cognitive protection from moderate drinking.

At this point, this series of well-constructed studies leads to the apparent contradictions that even moderate amounts of alcohol lead to brain pathology, but (from other studies) that similar amounts seem to protect cognition. However, recall from Chapter 2 that sometimes even obvious and substantial Alzheimer's-related brain pathology can exist in people who show no apparent cognitive decline. Perhaps the "apparent contradictions" in the alcohol literature show a similar weak relationship between (at least some) brain pathology and cognition. The next chapter features other possible explanations for those apparent contradictions and to vastly revised conclusions about the impact of alcohol on brain and cognition. I have said often that nutrition is complex, and now confront the reality that alcohol impacts are too. In fact, to clarify that complexity, a new chapter is required.

Chapter 14

# Alcohol II: Red resolutions

With 2613 participants in the Nooyens et al. (2013) study that ended Chapter 13, it was possible to do meaningful analyses separately for the different alcoholic beverages (e.g., wine versus beer and other spirits). As noted above, the initial findings were that higher consumption of alcohol by those Dutch women corresponded with better cognitive preservation across the five years of the study. However, wine was reported to be the principal alcoholic beverage of those women, and when the impacts from only the red wine were separated from the impacts of all their other alcoholic beverages, an entirely different interpretation was required. For beverage categories other than red wine, there were *no consistent relationships* between maintaining cognitive acuity and amount of alcohol regularly consumed. Neither small nor moderate amounts of non-wine alcohol provided any slowing of cognitive decline.

## Different beverages have different impacts

However, the results for red wine alone were spectacular. A strong linear relationship was found between red wine consumption and cognitive preservation. That is, after adjusting for the lifestyle factors mentioned above, during the five years of the study the women who consumed the most red wine declined the least in global cognitive function ($p < .01$), declined the least on the memory measures ($p < .01$) and declined the least in cognitive flexibility ($p = .03$). Those who drank 1.5 glasses of red wine per day had the best cognitive results. In fact, for women, the entire positive dose-response relationship between alcohol and cognitive preservation was due to the strong relationship of red wine to cognitive measures. (Here the "dose-response" term implies that for each increased amount of wine consumed, the cognitive scores were proportionally higher.)

But we must not forget the men. Although the men of the Nooyens et al. study preferred beer, by drinking twice as much as the women they managed to consume as much red wine as the women did. Thus it seems likely that the moderate (and non-significant) cognitive boost that men received from moderate alcohol was, as with the women, due to their red wine consumption. It seems clear that without red wine in the mix, moderate alcohol consumption was *not* protective of cognition or brain structure. That is certainly true for the women, and probably true for the men.

**Wine or beer.** Somewhat similar findings were noted in a longitudinal study conducted across two years of over 2500 people in China. Deng et al. (2006) adjusted for potentially-confounding factors of age, sex, education level, blood pressure, smoking, stroke history, and Mini Mental State Exam (MMSE) score. (Thus, there was a smaller set of potential confounds taken into account than in most studies, with variables like income and other health and social indicators left out.) Even moderate beer drinking was found to increase dementia probabilities, whereas moderate wine consumption reduced dementia risks. Although the study was far from perfect, the finding of cognitive benefits from the wine support the Nooyens et al. results, and the cognitive problems from beer consumption could be interpreted as supporting the bad outcomes from drinking noted for the British participants in the studies by Topiwala et al. (2017) and by Daviet et al. (2022).

On to Norway and a study I mentioned in Chapter 7 for positive impacts of tea on cognition. Recall (probably not) that Nurk et al. (2009) looked at the joint and separate correspondence of chocolate, tea, and wine on cognition in a sample of over two thousand Norwegians between the ages of 70 and 74. Interpreting causal relationships from these results is not as obvious as in the longitudinal studies reviewed above because cognition was assessed only once, and then compared with the self-report of habitual consumption of chocolate, tea, and wine. However, the cognitive test battery was an excellent selection composed of both general and specific measures, and the potentially-confounding array of nutrition, health, and education factors that were accounted for was comprehensive and thus similar to the best of the studies described immediately above. Consumption of either chocolate, or tea, or wine improved cognitive performance, but consumption of all three was best. Recall from Chapter 7 that the more tea consumed, the better were the cognitive scores in a dose-response relationship. Positive chocolate impacts on the cognitive measures peaked at 10 grams per day and then leveled off (10 grams is roughly equivalent to a chocolate bar). The best impacts from the wine on cognition were when consuming between 75 and 100mL per day. (Note that a typical bottle of wine is 750mL.) The researchers noted that of the three foods, the positive effect on cognition was the most for wine.

### Perhaps some other resolutions

Recall from Chapter 13 the spectacular results from the positive study by Richard et al. (2017) of elderly Americans. Even alcohol consumption on the high side of moderate seemed to extend longevity and preserve cognitive capacity. Perhaps those positive relationships were at least partially due to red wine consumption. Unfortunately, we have no direct data on the beverages those 80-year-olds consumed, but we do know about general beverage preferences: From 1992 to 2013, preference for wine rose from 37% to 46% for Americans over 50, and according to Rivas (2013), wine was the most preferred among all alcoholic beverages. A more recent 2019 Gallup survey of consumption found wine to be the most preferred (versus beer and spirits) alcoholic drink for Americans over 55, but not for younger people. Indeed the older Americans with whom I associate usually prefer red wine as their beverage of choice, at least until the hot weather arrives when some gravitate toward chilled white. Certainly, some red wine was consumed by those older folks in the Richard et al. study.

**Age?** For a moment, let us return to considering alcohol rather than red wine. Independent of beverage choices, perhaps being elderly is sufficient to enhance the positive alcohol-cognition relationship noted in some of the studies reviewed in both Chapter 13 and this one. The 62-year-old people in the positive Zhang et al. (2020) study seemed to benefit cognitively from alcohol consumption, although the even-older 85-year-olds of the Richard et al. (2017) study seemed to derive astonishing (to me) cognitive benefits from their drinking. Other cross-sectional research by Beydoun et al. (2014) using the cohort drawn from the Baltimore Longitudinal Study of Aging found positive correlations of alcohol consumption with cognitive preservation (women only in this case) but only for participants over age 70. In contrast, there were negative correlations between alcohol and cognition for those under 70. Does it make sense (i.e., is there supportive data or logic) that age could affect the relationship of alcohol consumption with cognition?

Recall from Chapter 2 that among the many discouraging features of aging brains are substantial reductions of both neurotransmitters and neurotropins. But one of many impacts of *moderate* alcohol in the brain is the increase of neurotransmitters—a feature that leads to its addictive appeal for some. To be specific, moderate amounts of alcohol enhance the neurotransmitters dopamine (in the nucleus accumbens, eliciting pleasure), noradrenaline (activating), and GABA (controlling anxiety; McIntosh & Chick, 2004).

It is sheer speculation on my part, but it seems likely that enhancing neurotransmitters in an older brain where they are in short supply could make more of a positive difference than enhancing them in a younger brain that is probably not deficient. And given age-inspired neurotropin decline, it is noteworthy that Zhang et al. (2020) cite research showing alcohol stimulation of brain neurotropins. Those facts support the supposition that modest levels of alcohol might indeed benefit aged brains more than younger ones.

**Timing and culture.** Besides people in different cultures and age groups choosing different alcoholic beverages, another factor that probably contributes to differences between alcohol-cognition studies may be the timing of consumption—a factor related to culture. The binge drinking of college-aged Americans is legendary. If one of those youngsters consumed their "weekly allotment" (say of 12 drinks) in only one evening each week, the short-term and the long-term impacts of that pattern on brain and cognition could be awful.

On the other hand, red wine is typically consumed with meals by Mediterranean people and those of us following the Med or MIND diet (e.g., Panza et al., 2018). The wine is therefore likely to remain longer in the stomach where the metabolizing of alcohol begins, literally changing the nutrients absorbed. Slower consumption and consumption with food also reduces spikes of blood-alcohol levels, certainly to the benefit of brains. And with a slower passage through our gut, wine nutrients can interact with other nutrients from the food, or with meal-related fluctuations in the gut's microbes (see more about that below and in Chapter 16.)

**Wine-supplied nutrients.** Based on the strong evidence of cognitive benefits from red wine, in combination with the inconsistent evidence of similar benefits (and sometimes harm) from other garden-variety alcohol, we can certainly suspect that benefits from the red wine come from nutrients other than alcohol, or perhaps elements in combination with alcohol. With that in mind, consider the likelihood that other alcoholic beverages may similarly contain extraneous substances that are either beneficial or actually harmful. The benefits from red wine tell us little about the benefits of alcohol, just as the benefits derived from coffee inform us little about the benefits of caffeine. Thus when researchers fail to differentiate between different alcoholic beverages, but instead combine them all together, we should expect a great variety of sometimes-contradictory research results. And that does indeed reflect the current state of the research literature on alcohol impacts on brain and cognition.

### Atrial fibrillation—a digression

A similar observation of different impacts from different forms of alcoholic beverages and different patterns of drinking is found in the research literature on alcohol impacts on the atrial fibrillation of the heart (hereafter just a-fib). Because cardiovascular issues are not our major concern, I will avoid lacing this brief digression with citations, but we know that a major share of the alcohol-cardiovascular research asserts that low-to-moderate alcohol consumption benefits some aspects of cardiovascular health.

However, the relationship of alcohol with a-fib appears to be entirely negative. That research shows a direct dose-response relationship between the amount of alcohol consumed and the development of a-fib; in short, even moderate alcohol conveys no benefits at all for a-fib—only harm from even small or moderate amounts. I add a really big "however" here. However, there is one excellent-but-contrary study with almost 23 thousand participants. That study by Di Castelnuovo et al. (2017) accounted for a large and appropriate selection of potential confounds. Over the 8-year period of the study, more than 500 of the participants developed a-fib. However, the amount of alcohol regularly consumed by the participants did *not* correspond at all with its development. The researchers noted that their null results were unique, but that the studies mentioned above were from the US and northern European countries. Di Castelnuovo et al. hypothesized that whereas their Italian population preferred wine that was consumed with meals, that the European and American pattern of drinking more and at irregular times explains the contrasting results.

In short, the researchers believe that, like the contradictory findings concerning alcohol and cognitive impacts, that the contradictions in the a-fib research can be explained by the same factors. That is, for the reasons mentioned above and elaborated below, red wine consumed with meals results in different outcomes than those from other beverages consumed in different patterns, especially different outcomes for brain and cognition.

## Nutrition that interacts with alcohol

As noted above, other elements of nutrition may interact with wine and other alcoholic beverages, perhaps accounting for beneficial impacts in some research and detrimental impacts in others. Specifically, consider that as mentioned in Chapter 8, alcohol interferes with the absorption of five of the eight vitally important B vitamins (i.e., B-1, B-2, B-3, B-7, and B-9). Evidence is solid that insufficient levels of those Bs are really bad for brains and cognition. Thus it is likely that in cultures where B-laden foods are in short supply (e.g., in countries like Ireland and the UK where B-vitamin enrichment of flour is not mandated by law) that alcohol may have a more negative impact on brain and cognition by further limiting those scarce vitamins. In fact, in an article with the interesting title "Does thiamin [vitamin B-1] protect the brain from iron overload and alcohol-related dementia?" Listabarth et al. (2020) suggest that deficits of Vitamin B-1 weaken the blood-brain barrier's capacity to block the passage of iron into the brain. Iron accumulation in the brain then damages the structure and can cause the cognitive deficits frequently seen with alcoholism and Alzheimer's.

However, in cultures where B-laden foods are more available, perhaps moderate drinking of alcoholic beverages may be less detrimental to B-vitamin levels and thus less detrimental to brain and cognition. (E.g., The US mandates enrichment of flour with four of the B vitamins.) Having said that, a caveat is required: Whereas some research in UK has found negative impacts on brains from even moderate drinking (i.e.,Topiwala et al., 2017; Daviet et al., 2022) and some research in the US has found beneficial impacts from moderate drinking (i.e., Richard et al., 2017; Zhang et al., 2020) my suggestion that those differences may be influenced by dietary B-vitamin levels is purely speculative. But personally, as a moderate consumer of alcohol, if I were not already taking a multi-vitamin supplement loaded with Bs, I would certainly consider some B supplementation.

**Paths for red impacts.** Now consider a more fine-grained analysis of *how* red wine promotes brain health and cognitive capacities (This section may provide more information than required for the exam, but it is interesting...) In his chapter "Red wine retards abeta [β-amyloid] deposition and neuroinflammation in Alzheimer's disease" Dhir (2018) reviewed a vast array of research from a variety of sources that established first that red wine does indeed promote cognitive capacities and slow the progress of Alzheimer's, and secondly he explored the research that determines many (but undoubtedly not all) of the causal paths from enjoyment of red wine to brain health. The important characters in this saga are resveratrol and the many other polyphenols found in red wine, and quercetin—a polyphenol (and flavonoid) mentioned in Chapter 6 that is also a major active component in ginkgo (Chapter 12), and frequently studied in animal models. (It is interesting that resveratrol is an antifungal substance synthesized by plants in response to various stressors; it is extracted into red wine from grape skins during fermentation and it is plentiful on raw grapes too. Thus as a moderate consumer of both grapes and red wine, I feel only minimal threat from fungi.) I begin with Dhir's (2018, p. 296) conclusions:

> *Some of the important mechanisms [for red wine's impacts] include its antioxidant and anti-inflammatory activity besides acting on abeta [β-amyloid] clearance in multiple ways. Resveratrol is the main ingredient present in red wine that has been studied extensively for its protective effect in AD [Alzheimer's dementia]. Quercetin is another polyphenol that is also beneficial for neurodegenerative disorders, including AD.*

Cicero et al. (2018) reviewed several randomized-control trials using people—studies that showed the administration of resveratrol (versus placebo) dramatically enhanced cerebral blood flow and benefited various cognitive measures. (Enhanced cerebral blood flow generally fosters spectacular cognition.) Another of the major activities of resveratrol is to reduce the destruction caused by reactive oxygen species. Resveratrol manages its repair functions in multiple places and in multiple ways, including by improving levels of the indigenous "master" antioxidant that we all depend on—glutathione. One of the studies reviewed by Cicero et al. even showed improved connectivity from resveratrol—connectivity through the white matter between hippocampi and frontal, parietal, and occipital lobes.

Note, however, that another recent review and meta-analysis of resveratrol's impacts that was published earlier (but in the same journal) found no evidence of cognitive enhancement. Farzaei et al. (2018) attributed those null findings to resveratrol supplements being very poorly absorbed and thus having low bioavailability, in the range of less than 1%. Those observations reinforce the suggestion that positive impacts from resveratrol in red wine may depend upon either interactions with other nutrients consumed with meals and/or the processing of resveratrol by gut bacteria into other nutrients.

Reconsider four of the major elements of Alzheimer's, outlined in Chapter 1: Accumulation of clumped β-amyloid protein between neurons, tangles of misshaped tau proteins within neurons, brain inflammation from over-eager astrocytes, and mitochondria damage from oxygen radicals. Cicero et al. noted that resveratrol has its positive impacts by affecting all four of those elements—by directly reducing β-amyloid plaques and tau tangles, and by having powerful antioxidation effects, inhibiting free-radical damage and by reducing inflammation. Resveratrol also has positive impacts on Parkinson's and Huntington's disease. (Some research also shows that combining the hormones melatonin and vitamin D with resveratrol boosts its positive impacts on the brain.)

But resveratrol and quercetin are not the only molecules sequestered within red wine that maintain brain health. There are various polyphenols contained in red wine, and red wine has around five times as much of those beneficial substances as does white wine. Secondly, even different reds differ from each other in the combinations of their various polyphenols. Those differences in turn lead to different brain effects, some of which have been studied. For example, all the transgenic mice in the study by Wang et al. (2006) were genetically programmed to develop Alzheimer's. Compared to control mice who were regularly given either water or water laced with plain alcohol, those who were in the lucky group given cabernet sauvignon for their candle-lit dinners improved in measures of neuropathology and in spatial memory. But those brain impacts from the Cabernet were different than the improvements that were obtained in another study of Alzheimer's mice who consumed red muscadine wine (Ho et al., 2009; I know nothing about muscadine, nor does my Glossary).

**Help from the biome.** Another approach to understanding the neuroprotective benefits from red wine was undertaken by Esteban-Fernández et al. (2017). Those researchers identified the metabolites of red wine that are formed by bacterial action in the human gut. They exposed neurons (*in vitro*) to those metabolites and then subjected those neurons to stressors. The pre-exposure of the neurons to the wine-derived metabolites protected the neurons from the stress, enhancing their survival.

González-Domínguez et al. (2021; described more completely in Chapter 16) provided more direct support for positive impacts of the metabolites of red wine on cognition. Red wine metabolites in plasma correlated positively with cognitive preservation across a 12-year span. However, reinforcing the distinctions emphasized in this chapter, a marker for total alcohol (ethyl sulfate) correlated with cognitive decline.

Another factor to consider: nutritionists often note that physical condition may have substantial impacts on tolerance for and benefit from consuming alcohol. Those of us in good physical condition may benefit from moderate amounts that could be excessive and harmful for people in poor physical condition.

### An alcohol summary

Several sometimes-excellent studies have shown that moderate amounts of red wine appear to benefit cognition and brain. Even though red wine confers cognitive protection, we certainly do not know everything about the contribution to those benefits from the specific nutrients in the wine, or even everything that could be important about gut microbiome interactions.

However, the mixed results for alcohol from other beverages should dampen our confidence that even modest levels of alcohol from other sources promote cognition and brain integrity. That should remind us that González-Domínguez et al. noted somewhat parallel relationships between coffee and caffeine. As described more fully in Chapter 16, although they found some metabolites of coffee to protect cognition, caffeine itself apparently was not protective.

Another potentially-important issue is that studies of physiological impacts from alcohol may have different implications than studies of cognitive impacts. They are certainly related, but recent research on Alzheimer's dementia shows clearly that it may take years for physiological deficits to foster cognitive decline. That issue would be better informed if more studies, like the one by Topiwala et al. (2017), assessed both physiological and cognitive impacts.

Thus general conclusions about alcohol impacts are difficult to make. Perhaps some differences in impacts by different beverages result because different beverages have different nutrients, but also because those different beverages are typically preferred by different people at different ages and in different cultures, and because they are consumed in different patterns. (E.g., who drinks Scotch with dinner?) Life is complex. So, it turns out, is nutrition.

An admonition directed toward non-drinkers that usually concludes a typical paper about possible health benefits from alcohol is that if one does not drink to not begin a habit of alcohol consumption based on the potential advantages to (usually) cardiovascular or general health. Even with our focus on brain and cognition, that seems good advice, especially in light of the research showing that in some circumstances even moderate drinking can be harmful, and in most circumstances heavy drinking will certainly "dumb us down." (But keep in mind that moderate and heavy are likely to be different amounts for different people.)

My admonition is a variant of the warning to not begin drinking in response to the positive research: If you drink, consider red wine in moderation, but with any alcohol consumption, make sure to have adequate amounts of the B vitamins, whether from food or supplements. Those Bs are crucial because alcohol reduces the effectiveness of the Bs, and the Bs are certainly vital for brain and cognition. Keep vitamin D levels up too.

# Chapter 15

# Contented mitochondria

Our mitochondria are much like the mitochondria in all creatures, even those of us who are not mammals. Thousands of mitochondria can inhabit each of our cells, occupying themselves with supplying the physical and mental energy we need for … well … for everything. It is their central importance in our lives that led to this chapter being organized about the various nutrients that boost mitochondria function, rather than being organized around a class of nutrients.

Because their function is so fundamental, some researchers believe that the mitochondria are the key to understanding how and why there are well-documented correlations between dimensions as diverse as intelligence, health, resistance to cognitive decline, and even to longevity itself. Consider the title of Geary's (2019) review describing the mitochondria as "The spark of life and the unification of intelligence, health, and aging." In a variety of fields, modern science is beginning to recognize the central importance of the mitochondria. If our mitochondria are in good shape, so (usually) are we, both mentally and physically.

On the other hand, in Chapter 2, I mentioned that mitochondria decline with aging and with stress, and that the decline of mitochondria in turn has the potential to degrade our responses to future stressors and to damage brain and thus accelerate cognitive decline. The declining health of our mitochondria is therefore both a result of our aging and a likely cause of age-associated deficits (Piccard et al., 2015; Sun et al., 2016). And indeed deteriorating mitochondria in the brain are one of the hallmarks of Alzheimer's and other neurodegenerative diseases such as Parkinson's (Zhang et al., 2018).

**Evolutionary origins.** Mitochondria have an intriguing origin story: Modern theories that cannot be verified with new research suggest that mitochondria originated as bacteria, eventually evolving into their current form, much like modern birds evolving from dinosaurs, but much earlier. At some point, they somehow became fully integrated into living cells, developing symbiotic relationships with the cells. Today those "residual bacteria" are present in all us "eukaryotes." (Eukaryotes are all plants and animals that are built of cells—cells that have nuclei, DNA, and the other adornments of normal cells.) The mitochondria celebrate their separate existence by maintaining their own genes—genes that are distinct from those that comprise the 46 chromosomes that hang out in the nuclei of our human cells.

**More recent origins.** Our mitochondria are a gift from our mothers. With no assistance from our fathers, like other mammalian females with motherly concern our mothers packed tens of thousands of mitochondria into each oocyte—the cells that became eggs. Our fathers did not bother tucking any into their sperm. The lack of thoughtful advanced packing by fathers is a topic sometimes broached by wives (e.g., mine) and mothers.

**Generating energy.** The many mitochondria that reside within each of our cells generate energy by combining glucose, fatty acids, or ketones (the metabolites of fatty acids) with oxygen. Brain mitochondria have different preferences; they rely primarily on glucose and manage largely to avoid processing fatty acids. The initial result of mitochondrial processing is an energy-packed molecule called adenosine triphosphate, usually written simply as ATP. But there is a dark side to the production of ATP. Byproducts of ATP manufacturing are the highly reactive forms of oxygen introduced in Chapters 1 and 2 as reactive oxygen species. As mentioned at various points in the preceding chapters, their high reactivity leads them to combine with other molecules that are then unable to fulfill their usual obligations. We can think of that process as a form of rusting. On the plus side, however, the reactive oxygen species are required for some cell functions and for the adequate response of the immune system against pathogens (Pagano et al., 2020). Nevertheless, they must be controlled.

### Damage and antioxidants

Oxidative stress occurs when the quantity of those highly reactive oxygen molecules exceeds the level of control provided by other available molecules that serve as antioxidants. Oxidative stress can take many forms, including causing mutations in the DNA and damage to our RNA. Those and other injuries in turn interfere with protein synthesis and cause the progressive decline of our cells' abilities to perform their assigned tasks (Tadokoro et al., 2020). Like patricidal children, the reactive oxygen molecules can even damage the mitochondria that produced them, especially when antioxidants are in short supply. For example, animal research shows that low levels of the antioxidant vitamin B-9 (folate) result in damaged mitochondrial DNA. Because our brains require voracious amounts energy, the cells of our brains (and our cardiovascular system) are especially vulnerable to injury from reactive oxygen and thus especially in need of antioxidants.

But irrespective of whether our diets include normal amounts of antioxidants, with aging and stress, damage to our DNA occurs in all of us, especially to the DNA of our mitochondria. Because of the brain's special vulnerability, it is not surprising that the neurodegeneration in both

Alzheimer's and Parkinson's diseases is caused at least in part by oxidative stress and the resulting mitochondrial malfunctions and energy deficits.

## Effective nutrients

To determine what nutrients might be most therapeutic for resisting dementia, one approach is to identify those antioxidant nutrients that most effectively control those pesky reactive oxygen species. Another is to determine nutrients that boost mitochondrial performance, and a third approach involves assessing metabolic differences in the brains of cognitively normal people versus those suffering from neurodegenerative diseases such as Alzheimer's. Those various research traditions led Fenech (2017) to conclude that the production of the energy-packed ATP molecules in aging brains could be enhanced by various vitamins. The Fenech list of mitochondria-maintaining vitamins includes seven of the eight B vitamins (with only B-7 somehow missing the list), but perhaps to make up for that omission, vitamin H (biotin)—often considered to be one of the B vitamins—was included.

**Mushrooms (again) and avocados.** But as with the search for effective antioxidants, the search for the nutrients that enhance mitochondrial nutrition has led well beyond our favorite vitamins, and on to foods such as mushrooms, avocados, and eventually, to pomegranates. Mushrooms were celebrated in Chapter 6 for their provision of phytonutrients, including the important antioxidants ergothioneine and glutathione, and in Chapter 12 for their contribution of spermidine. Avocados are also notorious for increasing glutathione levels and, as noted in the next chapter, for maintaining proper balances of gut bacteria. Some of the lesser antioxidants, such as vitamin C, serve to preserve glutathione levels by eliminating some of the reactive oxygen molecules that glutathione would otherwise have to bother with.

**Pomegranates and urolithin A.** Pomegranate juice is one of those foods celebrated lately in the popular nutrition media as an answer to just about everything. Fad or not, the research indicates that pomegranates may deserve their pop-media notoriety. In fact, there is evidence that pomegranate juice may delay the aging of mitochondria as effectively as any other food, and given the central importance of the mitochondria to almost everything, perhaps it is appropriate to see pomegranates as a kind of universal elixir.

First, consider the animal research. That research consistently shows surprisingly large impacts on the mitochondria from long-term consumption of either pomegranate or the most prevalent pomegranate metabolite in humans—urolithin A. One of the directly observable positive effects of both pomegranate and urolithin A is the removal of old and dysfunctional mitochondria, facilitating the subsequent biogenesis of new ones (Tan et al., 2019). Pomegranate and urolithin A achieve that cleansing and renewal by transcribing (activating) specific genes responsible for mitochondrial quality control. Those processes negate the negative impacts of the reactive oxygen molecules that would otherwise overpopulate and damage their host cells, and they attenuate inflammatory responses, and the damage to cells that can be caused by mutated mitochondrial DNA. In summary, Tan et al. concluded that pomegranate extract could "alleviate mitochondrial dysfunction in aging and mitochondrial-related diseases."

The ultimate impacts of the molecular processes fostered by the presence of pomegranate and urolithin A are to improve energy generation, physical strength, endurance, healthspan and lifespan. Those impacts are shown in species ranging from roundworms (*C. elegans*) to fruit flies (*Drosophila*) and rodents (Ryu et al., 2016). (Remember that when a nutrient impacts organisms from widely different phyla, the evidence that basic cellular processes are affected means we should certainly expect similar benefits for us human mammals.)

Another avenue for benefits from pomegranate and urolithin A was demonstrated in research on transgenic mice disposed to suffer Alzheimer's. Urolithin A imparted cognitive protection in those unfortunate rodents, probably by triggering neurogenesis—the creation of new neurons from neural stem cells. Gong et al. (2019) concluded that urolithin A showed promise as a treatment for Alzheimer's. We can better assess that promise for people by looking at these first human randomized-control trials addressing those issues.

In a double-blind randomized-control trial Andreaux et al. (2019) assessed the impact on mitochondria-related biomarkers that resulted from daily doses of urolithin A given across four weeks. The participants were 36 healthy but sedentary and elderly people. Very unfortunately, there were no assessments of brain or cognition. After four weeks of treatment, the urolithin A improved mitochondrial fatty acid oxidation at a level that was similar to improvements from a 10-week aerobic exercise program. And the increasing ratio of mitochondrial DNA to cellular DNA indicated accelerated mitochondrial reproduction. That enhanced mitochondria generation was undoubtedly due to the observed transcription of mitochondrial genes— transcription that occurred at a level that was also similar to that observed following multi-week aerobic exercise training. Keep in mind that, as is often the case, this type of research adds the studied nutrient to a normal human diet, rather than to a diet that restricted the key nutrient. Thus it suggests that in general we would benefit by increased intake of urolithin A.

As is the case for various other essential nutrients, urolithin A production from pomegranate depends upon the bacterial denizens of our gut microbiome. But unfortunately, not all of us have the proper gut microbes for that conversion. And even with the proper microbes, the efficiency of that process declines as we age. Thus it seems likely that as we age, pomegranates (and nuts and berries that are also rich in the precursors to urolithin A) may become increasingly important. One day (but not today, and not even in the next chapter on the microbiome) we may know exactly how to arrange our gut microbial balance to optimize the production of Urolithin A.

Pomegranate juice is expensive, selling for almost $5/quart in my local groceries. But although that seems expensive, that cost is comparable to what I might spend for some quite-basic but health-giving red wine. But the pomegranate juice provides an entirely different mix of nutrients, and in my case, will probably last longer. If your mitochondria are aging (and they are!), perhaps give it a try. Your mitochondria may be grateful.

**CoQ10.** Coenzyme Q10, known as CoQ10, plays a viral role in the mitochondria of all our body's cells, and it is a potent antioxidant. Even though our bodies may make sufficient CoQ10, it is reduced by the statin drugs that many people use to control cholesterol. Thus CoQ10 supplements are often recommended for people who take statins, but the research suggests that CoQ10 may be good for everyone. Much of the following owes a debt to a thorough but highly technical review by Pagano et al. (2020). Pagano et al. described how several supplements, including CoQ10, affect the mitochondria and all of the major functions assigned to the mitochondria.

For example, Pagano et al. reviewed several *in vitro* studies of human cells treated with CoQ10. CoQ10 reduced the production of reactive oxygen, reduced inflammation, and increased the energy production of the mitochondria. Animal research with transgenic Alzheimer's mice showed CoQ10 to improve learning and, perhaps accounting for that, to reduce β-amyloid plaque. Other research with Alzheimer's rats found CoQ10 to enhance hippocampal synaptic plasticity.

On the other hand, research with humans has produced equivocal results. While CoQ10 appears to be generally neuroprotective, with some positive impacts on Parkinson's patients, randomized-control trials with Alzheimer's patients have not shown CoQ10 to delay the progression of their dementia. The potential reasons for the lack of positive impacts on Alzheimer's people are complex. Pagano et al. suggested, for example, that CoQ10 may be maximally effective only when combined with other pro-mitochondria nutrients. Furthermore, there is ample evidence that some effective metabolites of CoQ10 are produced by our gut's microbiome, and of course that means that variations in our gut microbes probably portend variations in the impact of CoQ10 and other mitochondrial nutrients.

Primary natural dietary sources of CoQ10 include oily fish such as salmon and tuna, and liver and whole grains. Some nutritionists assert the level found in normal diets is often sufficient. Even if that is the case, if on statin drugs, supplemental CoQ10 is widely recommended. CoQ10 supplements are readily available, but moderately expensive (although MitoQ, a related compound described below, is considerably more expensive).

### Antioxidants in our futures

The nutrients described below may all effectively extend the time that aging people maintain cognitive proficiency. Levels of proof of their efficacy for human cognition vary from strong evidence for MitoQ to less substantial evidence for the others. Keep watch for future developments.

**MitoQ.** Mitochondria-targeted ubiquinone, known as MitoQ, is a CoQ10 molecule that has an added electronic charge that induces it to cling to mitochondria. That modification supposedly makes it more available to mitochondria than naked CoQ10 molecules. Like CoQ10, MitoQ has powerful antioxidant characteristics, but unlike CoQ10, MitoQ is not a component of normal diets.

Braakhuis et al. (2018) provided a systematic review and meta-analysis of animal research with MitoQ. After initially identifying over 10,000 potentially-relevant articles, 19 randomized-control trials met their criteria. They examined the biomarkers of age-associated oxidative stress. MitoQ intervention produced a statistically significant reduction in nitrotyrosine—an important indicator of cell damage and inflammation. Those reviewers concluded that MitoQ may promote general cellular efficiency and decrease concentrations of reactive oxygen species, potentially reducing age-related oxidative stress.

That promising finding was supported by research with mice that showed positive brain/cognition impacts from MitoQ. Specifically, the MitoQ-treated mice experienced slowing of the progression of Alzheimer's, and even reversal of cognitive deficits, with added longevity in the bargain. MitoQ seemed to have its most beneficial impacts on older mice. Unfortunately, preliminary studies on human Parkinson's patients did not show similar positive results, perhaps because neurodegeneration had already progressed too far (Zhang et al., 2018).

Rossman et al. (2018) conducted a randomized control trial with people that featured a powerful cross-over design in which each person served as their own control. Prior to the study, the participants had experienced some cardiovascular impairment. Half of the group of 20 otherwise-healthy men and women ages 60 to 79 took 20mg/day of MitoQ for six weeks; the other half took placebo. After that initial 6-week treatment and a subsequent 2-week washout period, the two groups switched conditions. The flexibility of blood vessel linings was assessed by measuring arterial dilation with increased blood flow. When taking the supplement, dilation of subjects' arteries improved by 42%, appearing to be younger by 15 to 20 years. Such an improvement was thought to provide a 13% reduction in heart disease. That research showed reduced oxidative stress (the main cause of arterial stiffness with age) and reductions in low-density lipoprotein (bad cholesterol). Rossman et al. concluded that MitoQ and other therapies that reduced reactive oxygen species may be effective in preventing age-related vascular dysfunction. Although the data seemed strong, that conclusion seems equivocal. Furthermore, Rossman et al. noted that the level of improvement of 42% in arterial stiffness from only six weeks of MitoQ supplementation was equivalent to that produced by other longer-duration interventions such as caloric restriction-based weight loss (around 30% improvement) and aerobic exercise (around 50% improvement). They suggested that because most of us do not meet current healthy-lifestyle guidelines, that MitoQ could serve as an alternative or complementary strategy for maintaining cardiovascular health.

Whereas that study was not about cognition or Alzheimer's, remember that cardiovascular health is clearly and consistently related to cognition. And the same levels of oxidative stress that harm the epithelial cells of the circulatory system also produce observable damage to neural tissue. Redressing that damage in the circulatory system certainly redresses it in the brain as well.

The recommended dosage of MitoQ can be purchased for about $2/day, but it is new, and at $700/year perhaps we should await further research.

**NAD+.** Nicotinamide adenine dinucleotide, mercifully written simply as NAD+, is another potentially-spectacular remedy for tired mitochondria. Fortunately, NAD+ is produced in all the cells of our bodies, but unfortunately, it declines dramatically with aging, apparently contributing to both metabolic diseases and to neurodegeneration. NAD+ itself is enhanced by the precursors (that you need not memorize) nicotinamide mononucleotide (usually just NMN) and nicotinamide riboside (NR in the research literature). Those two NAD+ enhancing nutrients can be consumed by people, apparently without obvious side effects. Tryptophan is also a precursor of NAD+. And a substantial amount of research shows that NAD+ levels are enhanced by flavonoids (Ruan et al., 2018)—another reason to emphasize the fruits and veggies of diets like the Med and the MIND.

As a rate-limiting precursor of a family of proteins known as "the seven sirtuins," NAD+ levels in the body determine the rate that those seven proteins are produced. Like the seven samurai of late-night movie fame, the seven sirtuins are vital, and protective. But unlike the samurai, the sirtuins prevent age-associated accumulations of mutations by repairing DNA damage. And because the sirtuins and their impacts are vital, wise and sometimes entrepreneurial researchers suppose that restoring NAD+ to youthful levels may restore our aging metabolism and our aging brains. Indeed the title of one recent research article asked whether NAD+ might be a "silver bullet" for metabolic health. Perhaps, because research shows that increasing sirtuin levels by NAD+ supplements extends lifespans in critters from nematodes (*C. elegans*) to rodents.

Researchers have detailed knowledge of how NAD+ achieves its vast positive impacts including skin repair, cardiovascular benefits, neural repair after various forms of research-induced brain damage, and longevity itself. For example, Grabowska et al. (2017) noted that damaged DNA can decrease levels of NAD+ and then decrease the positive activities of the sirtuins. In turn those sirtuin deficits can disrupt DNA repair, resulting in even more NAD+ deficits and associated problems for our mitochondria, our bodies, and our brains. Those problems result largely from oxidative damage from the reactive oxygen species that get too frisky when our mitochondria age and become dysfunctional. The reactive oxygen molecules then cause even more damage to the mitochondria etc. etc.

The evidence that enhanced NAD+ levels extend lifespans in various animals has inspired hundreds of research papers. The recent review by Braidy and Liu (2020) culled 147 articles from an initial pool of 1545, finding 113 "preclinical" and 34 clinical studies (i.e., randomized-control trials with real people) that met their criteria. Their review concluded that the great benefits to an array of critters resulting from various methods for boosting NAD+ have not yet been proven in us humans.

That tepid conclusion has not stopped pharmaceutical entrepreneurs from rushing to discover and patent drugs that boost NAD+ and (hopefully, in the future) to do the research that establishes effectiveness with authentic humans. In the meantime, in their review, Braidy and Liu noted that although 15 clinical trials with humans were ongoing at the time of their 2020 review, none published to date provided assurances that at this time, we should be taking supplements to boost our NAD+. If a flood of positive papers do not sprout like my front-yard mushrooms by 2023 or so, perhaps we can assume that the promise of the animal research has not born fruit for us humans. But at this time, to me, the potential from boosting NAD+ is enticing.

**Two amino acids: Glycine and N-acetylcysteine.** It is thought by some that deficiencies in older people of our beloved and vital antioxidant glutathione may be caused by deficiencies of two of its three amino acid precursors—glycine and n-acetylcysteine (often referred to as NAC). My search for relevant supporting research focused first on Glycine impacts on cognition. The published studies were mainly of impacts on schizophrenia; for our interests on delaying cognitive decline, there was insufficient information. On the other hand, following some animal research there were reasons to believe that NAC supplementation might be effective in preserving cognitive capacities. Although the studies that Skvarc et al. (2017) found for their review were methodologically inconsistent, Skvarc and colleagues concluded that NAC improved cognition, but they were uncertain whether that improvement was sufficient to be considered meaningful.

Weak support notwithstanding, several formulations—some patented— have combined those two precursors of glutathione and marketed them as anti-aging elixirs. That potential path to boosting mitochondrial function was tested in a *human* pilot study by Kumar et al. (2021). Their very limited study featured only eight older adults taking one of the available formulations for 24 weeks. That patented formulation combined glycine and NAC and was given the trade name "GlyNAC." Physiological changes were assessed across those 24 weeks and during a subsequent wash-out period. The title of the Kumar et al. study serves as a brief summary. "Glycine and N-acetylcysteine (GlyNAC) supplementation in older adults improves glutathione deficiency, oxidative stress, mitochondrial dysfunction, inflammation, insulin resistance, endothelial dysfunction, genotoxicity, muscle strength, and cognition." To this point, I have usually resisted citing research on nutrient combinations. However, the improvement in health indicators and in cognition from the GlyNAC combination in the Kumar pilot was (if real, and replicated, etc.) astonishing. Various indicators, including especially that the cognitive improvement corresponded with increases in the beloved neurotropin BDNF, suggested that the substantial cognitive improvements were not practice effects.

Hopefully, my astonishment will be justified when that research team completes and publishes their larger randomized-control trial. But until then, you can be the proud owner of a month's supply of the formulation they studied at the annual rate of around US $700. Yikes! Although I found no convincing evidence that either Glycine or NAC alone substantially boosted elderly cognition, remember that sometimes the magic lies in such nutrient combinations.

**Summary.** Unfortunately, reactive oxygen species are produced as a byproduct of energy production by our mitochondria, but some limited amounts are useful—even necessary. As the decades pass, the various evils caused by those frisky oxygen molecules include damage to our genes, our cardiovascular system, and ultimately, our brains. Both aging and stress exacerbate the problem of unwelcome oxidation and the resulting mitochondrial inefficiencies. And unfortunately, however effective we might be in mitigating stress in our lives, aging continues inexorably. Thus for lifespan, healthspan, or effective cognitive preservation, the weather-resistant fountain of youth remains elusive, at least for now. But even though randomized-control trials with people are still preliminary, anything (like MitoQ) that delays Alzheimer's in genetically predisposed mice is promising, and the impacts of MitoQ on the circulation systems of aged and vulnerable people are quite spectacular.

Beyond the nutrients discussed in this chapter, we can support our mitochondrial health and preserve our brains and cognitive capacities by engaging in the toughening activities discussed in Chapter 19, and by maximizing antioxidant nutrients from foods and common supplements such as multivitamins. Beyond those obvious and effective measures, consider too the benefits of urolithin A from pomegranates and the benefits from supplements of CoQ10 (especially if taking statins). And consider any of the activities and additives that enhance the impacts of the "master" antioxidant glutathione; those include adequate sleep and exercise and (especially) mushrooms, pomegranate, and avocados.

Remain vigilant for published research in reviewed journals (with actual human beings) on MitoQ, NAD+, and combinations like GlyNAC because in some future time, those new mitochondrial nutrients may prove to be exceptionally effective in defending brain and cognition. But remain skeptical of the "research" (and especially the testimonials) cited in the advertisements for (usually expensive) patented combinations containing those substances. Even beyond those three nutrients, with researchers aware of the central role of the mitochondria for everything in our bodies requiring energy, intense searches continue for nutrients and supplements to boost mitochondrial function. The future may hold some pleasant surprises.

Chapter 16

# The microbiome: Denizens of our gut

Some of the small residents of our bodies have horrified us for decades, such as the worm-like mites that hide in our eyelash follicles and come out to play at night. But only recently have we come to fully appreciate our resident intestinal "gut" bacteria. The sophisticated term for that vast and varied collection is the "microbiome" or simply the "biome." Thanks to whoever counted in that dark and dank interior, we can be assured that each of us harbors more bacteria than human cells within out body. The actual number is estimated to be from 10 trillion to 10 times that many; 95% of them live, work, and (presumably) play in our gut.

**The many kinds we entertain.** If there is to be a theme for Chapter 15 on mitochondria and this Chapter 16 on the microbiome, perhaps it should be about the vital need to care for the little ones that we depend upon and that depend upon us. In Chapter 15, the little ones were mitochondria that probably evolved from bacteria, but now we consider impacts on brain and cognition from real live bacteria, not some ancient transformed anomaly.

Even newer than the study of the microbiome is the study of the viruses that also thrive in our gut—the "virome." Recent analyses of worldwide samples from people identified 140 thousand different gut viruses. But viruses are not cells, and so do not add to the count of trillions of non-human cells that comprise our biome. Studied by researchers at Ohio State University, the majority of the players in the human virome are phages—viruses that invade bacteria, though often in symbiotic relationships. Perhaps a research paper I came upon recently is a harbinger of things to come. Mayneris-Perxachs et al. (2022) titled their paper "*Caudovirales* bacteriophages are associated with improved executive function and memory in flies, mice, and humans." We know so little about the relevance of the virome to cognition, mental states, and brain processes that they will receive no further mention here, but for readers aspiring to become viral scholars, see Gregory et al. (2020) and the Mayneris-Perxachs paper mentioned above.

Fungi too lurk in some of the dark places within us. They form communities of molds and yeasts collectively known as the "mycobiome." As with the viruses, we know little about our gut fungi except that their presence activates our immune system when other unwelcome fungi appear in other parts or our bodies. I shall write no more about fungi; I have already told more than I know.

**Good and bad in the microbiome.** Although Hippocrates believed most of our ills originated in the gut, he was not an accomplished gut scientist. Thus most biome research is recent (and, as evident from this chapter, somewhat scattered). The research informs us that some members of our microbiome are very beneficial—close to essential—whereas others are troublemakers. The new appreciation of the impact of our microbiome on brain and mind has contributed to some neuroscientists referring to our gut as our "second brain." That attention has led to positive article titles such as "Microbes may hold the key for treating neurological disorders," and "Gut microbes could unlock the secret to healthy aging," and even "Clues to brain health may lie in the gut;" on the dark side though, "Scientists identify gut-derived metabolites that play a role in neurodegeneration." (If insufficiently fulfilled, Google those real titles for their sources). Perhaps there is truth in those titles, but generalizations about the impact of gut bacteria are complicated by the vast differences between us in the composition of our biomes—much greater differences than the differences between us in our genes.

**Sophisticated terms.** Naturally, a new science needs new terms. Besides more familiar ones like "probiotics" (foods that contain live bacteria destined for our gut) and "prebiotics" (foods that feed our resident gut bacteria) a new vocabulary has developed that could be used to impress your friends, but that you need not master for understanding this chapter. Postbiotic is the term for bioactive elements secreted by some of the bacteria of our biome; many are nutrients of some form or other. You might imagine that with "pre, pro, and post" that we might be done, but just for fun … an imbalance of good and bad gut bacteria is "dysbiosis;" an "operational taxonomic unit" is a grouping of gut bacteria based on their genetic resemblance; and both the "gut-brain axis" and the "microbiota-gut-brain axis" describe the two-way communication between the gut and the brain. Perhaps we should explore "psychobiotics"— nutrients that impact the residents of the biome that in turn influence our gut-brain axis. Then there is the "food metabolome"—the metabolites created by our resident bacteria from our food, and (naturally) the study of the metabolome, called "metabolomics."

## The smart gut

The enteric nervous system (enteric NS) is composed of the collection of neurons and glia that regulate our gut processes. Although the enteric NS anchors the lower end of the gut-brain axis, even without oversight from the brain, it is sufficiently sophisticated on its own to coordinate the gut activities needed for digestion. But having said that, a stream of information flows in both directions between gut and brain, traveling largely via the vagus nerve, with research showing that the information flow is essentially stopped when the vagus is cut (Forsythe et al., 2014). Although the vagus conveys information from the gut wall to the brain (and from brain to gut), other impacts of the microbiome on our brains and bodies depend on the various metabolites created by the microbiome. Those substances can affect the gut wall directly or pass through that vast interface between gut interior and exterior. Although the intestines are just under 10 meters in length, the many projections (villi) and nooks and crannies on the intestinal walls yield a surface area of around 200 square meters—approximately the size of a tennis court. Somehow that seems excessive for processing breakfast.

**Research approaches and causal paths.** Most research on the microbiome assesses the bacteria already present in our gut. The results are correlations of mental or physiological conditions with assessments of bacteria types and quantities—types often identified from bacterial RNA or DNA extracted from fecal material. As always, such correlational relationships lead to questions of causal directions to be resolved (hopefully) by randomized-control trials.

In the randomized-control trials, bacteria are typically infused in probiotics, or nourished via prebiotics, or, when animals are the participants, transferred from another animal. Although most randomized-control trials are done with animals, some exceptions are described below and in Chapter 18. Fortunately, the creatures who volunteer—usually mice or rats who like us humans tend to be omnivores—entertain many of the same gut bacteria that we do. And besides having a similar microbiome, those animals often have many of the same neurochemicals and neural structures that we humans cherish. Thus we should usually take that research seriously. As said before, at the biological level we humans are really not that unique.

**Metabolites that affect cognition.** As an example of typical research progression from human correlations to animal randomized-control trials, Razazan et al. (2021) noted that some of our colon-based bacteria produce metabolites known as short-chain fatty acids; those short-chain fatty acids can then enter the bloodstream and affect important free-fatty acid receptors (FFAR2s) in brain neurons. (Razazan et al. introduced those FFAR2s to us in Chapter 11 because the FFAR2s were also activated by basil—yet another reason to seek out pesto.) Levels of FFAR2-stimulating short-chain fatty acids are lower in older people with cognitive impairment, and in people with Alzheimer's. (Although you need not remember them, those short-chain fatty acids are acetate, propionate, and butyrate.) Those relationships within people are correlational, but Razazan et al. (2021) noted that stimulation of the FFAR2s in animal brains by those metabolites can protect brains against accumulation of the toxic β-amyloid proteins that we dread.

Besides the path for impacts from gut to brain and cognition described in the previous paragraph, various other causal paths are available. For example, some denizens of our metabalome can harm the brain and cognition by producing toxins such as those found at high levels in the cerebrospinal fluid of people suffering from multiple sclerosis (Ntranos et al., 2021). Others aid us by assisting the digestion of nutrients, and some modify nutrients into other brain-useful metabolites. Some of those metabolites are neurotransmitters, like serotonin, that leave the gut, cross the blood-brain barrier, affect brain neurons, and ultimately affect mood and cognition. For other examples, recall the Chapter 14 discussion of cognitive benefits derived from the biome-produced metabolites of red wine, and similar benefits noted in Chapter 15 from the urolithin A produced by gut bacteria from pomegranate.

**Biome impacts on critter cognition.** With aging, the microbiome of mice changes, potentially having a large brain/cognition impact. To assess those impacts, Boehme et al. (2021) transplanted microbiota from the fecal material of young mice into mice old enough to show cognitive deterioration (forgetting names, misplacing keys, etc.). Besides the probable trepidation experienced by the recipients, the new fecal material in the oldsters improved brain and immune function to "youthful" levels. (We were not told how smart they were when young, but perhaps that is not really important.)

Rodrigues et al. (2021) focused on diabetes. Keep in mind that poorly-controlled blood glucose levels can damage the brain, degrade cognition, and substantially enhance dementia risk (Crane et al., 2013). Using mice, Rodrigues et al. studied two bacterial species of the *Lactobacillus* genus (i.e., *gasseri* and *johnsonii)*. (As discussed in Chapter 18 some *Lactobacillus* bacteria also foster resistance to depression.) Some of the mice in the Rodrigues et al. study were made susceptible to type-2 diabetes by being fed an unhealthy Western-style diet. However, half of those unfortunate mice were given daily doses of the two *Lactobacillus* strains, and those bacteria allowed the recipient mice to resist developing the glucose intolerance and insulin resistance that characterize diabetes. Detailed analyses showed the avenues for that impact to be via positive effects on the liver and on lipid metabolism. Those positive impacts resulted in turn from those two *Lactobacillus* strains improving the functioning of the liver mitochondria by somehow transcribing mitochondrial genes. And those *Lactobacilli* also increased levels of our favorite endogenous and exogenous antioxidant—glutathione. (Remember glutathione levels are also enhanced by mushrooms, avocados, and by red wine's resveratrol.) The enhanced glutathione levels then protected the mitochondria from damage caused by reactive oxygen species. The causal direction from gut bacteria types to positive physiological outcomes was well established by that study.

**Gut bacteria and their metabolites affect human cognition.** Correlational relationships of specific gut bacteria with dementia were assessed by Vincigurra et al. (2020). They noted several studies showing that the Med diet correlated with higher levels of beneficial bacteria of the genus *Bifidobacteria* (double dog?)—bacteria associated with control of inflammation and reduction of cholesterol. Other reviewed research showed that people suffering from Alzheimer's had low levels of several anti-inflammatory gut bacteria (e.g., *Bacteroides fragilis*) and high levels of pro-inflammatory bacteria (e.g., *Escherichia coli*). Although those studies resulted in correlations, there are a few randomized-control trials with people that show direct impacts from specific foods on concentrations of beneficial or worrisome gut bacteria. For example, Thompson et al. (2021) found that avocados enhance positive balances of gut bacteria and their metabolites.

For a brilliant recent example—perhaps the most convincing research in this series—in a comprehensive prospective study González-Domínguez et al. (2021) assessed cognitive decline across the 12 years of their longitudinal research, ending when the participants averaged 76 years old. They assessed correlations of cognitive decline with metabolites assessed from plasma at the study's beginning. The (almost 900) French participants were free of dementia at baseline, when they contributed their serum samples. The mental tests to assess cognitive change were both varied and comprehensive.

The researchers concluded that very strong protection from cognitive decline was correlated with metabolites derived from polyphenol-rich foods such as were described in Chapter 6—mostly the vegetables and fruits that we associate with the Med and the other diets recommended in Chapter 4. González-Domínguez et al. noted similar powerful protection against cognitive decline correlated with a cacao metabolite (i.e., 3-methylxanthine; OR = .75). And reinforcing my frequent celebration of mushrooms, the mushroom metabolite ergothioneine was similarly correlated with cognitive preservation (OR = 0.90) undoubtedly in part by protecting hippocampal neurons against oxidative stress.

On the other hand, González-Domínguez et al. noted that artificial sweeteners apparently cause damage from reactive oxygen species by dysregulating energy metabolism. (For example, they noted that the odds ratio for negative cognitive impacts from saccharin was OR = 1.26.)

Confirming the complexities discussed in Chapter 14 of different cognitive impacts from alcohol versus red wine, González-Domínguez et al. found that some metabolites of red wine appeared to protect cognition, with a substantial odds ratio of OR = 0.70. On the other hand, reflecting the conclusion that all alcoholic beverages do not convey cognitive benefits, ethyl sulfate, a marker of total alcohol intake, strongly correlated with subsequent cognitive decline (OR = 1.82).

And similarly reflecting the complexities of cognitive impacts from coffee versus caffeine, on the one hand, González-Domínguez et al. found that various metabolites of coffee appeared to protect against cognitive decline (OR = .57). But on the other hand, biomarkers of caffeine had inconsistent relationships with cognitive decline, reflecting the uncertainty of caffeine impacts described in Chapter 7. That relationship of positive coffee impacts with null or even negative effects from caffeine is appropriately termed the "caffeine paradox." Another seeming paradox was that whereas some of the metabolites of fruit and citrus correlated with higher cognition, markers of commercial fruit juice indicated no cognitive benefits from the juice alone.

## Other impacts of the microbiome

Some paths lead from the microbiome to impacts on psychological states such as our level of optimism, stress tolerance, anxiety, and depression; those later paths are discussed in Chapter 18. Some denizens of our biome even affect us when they are dead (as illustrated by the "zombie" research of Nisheda et al., 2017, also described in Chapter 18).

**Effects at all ages.** In all the stages of life, proper microbiotic balances benefit the development and/or the maintenance of the immune system and both the central- and the autonomic-nervous systems in all of us mammals. Those physiological developments are, in turn, essential for the normal behavioral and mental development of the young. Thus animals born with artificially sterile guts do not develop normally, at least until appropriate microbes are introduced into their diets. But even then, normal development occurs only if that bacterial introduction is done while the critters are still young; long-term neurological damage results if biome restoration is begun too late. (Those observations have stimulated concerns for the biome of human infants, and for impacts on them from the biome of their mothers, especially when infants are premature or born without exposure to the bacteria that are present with vaginal delivery. But that is not our topic here.)

**Microbiome impacts on psychopathology.** To appreciate the relevance of the next research, note that irritable bowel syndrome corresponds with an imbalance in the gut microbiome. Zhang, Wang et al. (2021) hypothesized that imbalances in the gut microbiome might also contribute to dementia. If so, there would probably be a positive correlation between an indicator of that biome imbalance—irritable bowel syndrome—and dementia. Zhang, Wang et al. studied over 1700 people who had been diagnosed with irritable bowel syndrome; all were at least 45 years old. During the 16-year follow-up period, compared with a matched control group, those with irritable bowel syndrome were almost three times more likely to develop any dementia and six times more likely to develop Alzheimer's. Those are some serious numbers! For those who developed Alzheimer's, the irritable bowel people developed dementia seven years earlier than the control-condition people. Being a correlational study, the causal relationship from poorly balanced gut microbes to dementia is not firmly established, but clearly, a substantially disrupted microbiome *might* enhance prospects for Alzheimer's and other dementias. The possible paths for that biome-dementia relationship could be the positive causal impact of a well-balanced microbiome on the neurotransmitters serotonin and GABA, and on our favorite neurotropin— BDNF (de J.R. De-Paula et al., 2018).

Another possibly-related relationship is that of unhealthy gut bacteria (or lack of healthy bacteria) as a potential cause of autism spectrum—a possibility supported by autistic people showing frequent digestive problems. That possibility has led to experimental therapies for autism that are based on restoring healthy gut bacteria. For example, transgenic mice created to experience autism-like behaviors that were given a course of *Lactobacillus reuteri* experienced relief from their dysfunctional social behavior, but no relief from hyperactivity, suggesting a different cause for the social and hyperactivity components of autism (Buffington et al., 2021). The association of abnormal levels of the inhibitory neurotransmitter GABA seen in some people with autism, and the role of the gut in GABA production, suggest some theoretical support for that approach.

### Summary and recommendations

**Fiber.** Fiber is especially important for the well-being of our microbiome, because many of our beneficial microbiome denizens depend upon otherwise-indigestible fiber for their sustenance. And of course we benefit doubly from consuming high-fiber foods because those that give us fiber are often the same plants that provide the terrific phytonutrients reviewed in Chapter 6. In fact, Oliver et al. (2021) suggest that replacing low-fiber foods with those that are high would result in major positive health gains for people who consume Western diets. An increase in fiber beyond the average daily consumption for a typical American (15 grams) to the RDA of 20 grams for women and 30 for men would lead, according to Oliver et al., to lower risks of a wide array of discouraging health effects including diabetes, heart disease, some cancers, and deaths from all causes. Some recent longitudinal research even shows an association of years of fiber consumption with reduced dementia (Yamagishi et al., 2022).

**Balancing bacteria.** Research shows clearly that some specific metabolites correspond with various benefits to the brain and cognition, but on the other hand that various deficiencies and imbalances correlate with cognitive decline, dementia, and metabolic conditions that ultimately cause cognitive decline, such as obesity and diabetes. Other negative impacts on health from deficits in the microbiome, such as suppressed immune functions, are beyond the scope of this coverage. Overall the research literature reviewed above and in Chapter 18 shows that it is important to maintain a proper balance of different kinds of gut microbes, keeping the nice ones productive while discouraging the grumps. (de J.R. De-Paula et al., 2018). But how?

**Sources and kinds.** Even with new and scant research, we can entertain some recommendations for maintaining the health of our microbiome. Note that healthful probiotics reside in fermented milk products such as yogurt and kefir, and in fermented vegetables such as un-pasteurized sauerkraut, pickles, and kimchi. To be sure that live bacterial strains inhabit those products, they must be refrigerated; otherwise fully-sealed-but-not-refrigerated products probably contain only deceased organisms. (However, as noted in the study by Nisheda et al. (2017) to be reviewed in Chapter 18, even "zombie bacteria" may make a contribution to health.)

When specific strains are listed on labels, look for some species of *Lactobacillus.* Many grocery-store probiotics include those delightful organisms, including the store-brand yogurt in my refrigerator (with three of the five bacteria strains in that yogurt being species of *Lactobacillus*). A label indicating that a food is a probiotic without identification of specifics is not enough to allow confidence of vast benefits. For example, a jar of probiotic spicy kimchi previously hiding deep in our refrigerator indicated that the kimchi was a product of "wild fermentation" so that the mix of bacteria depended on "Mother Nature's mood at the time." Thus the kimchi could be great, but maybe not.

Beyond possibly nurturing the live bacteria we host, be conscious that some medications, especially antibiotics, can kill them in terrifying numbers. Take seriously the admonition from various nutritionists that for overall health, and for brain health in particular, it is as important to consume gut-healthy meals as meals that are heart-healthy. Tell your doc.

Finally, a focus on metabolites that support cognition should lead us to select foods shown to lead to those beneficial metabolites. Pay attention to those foods specifically noted by González-Domínguez et al., especially those rich in polyphenols (including fruit, but not necessarily fruit juice), cacao, coffee (but not necessarily caffeine), mushrooms, and red wine (but probably not alcohol). And as the paleo-dieters would advise (Chapter 17) avoid the artificial sweeteners.

Chapter 17

# Intriguing dietary options

If tempted to snack while digesting this chapter, consider this option: Forego the fruit, the carrots, the leafy greens, and especially the chocolate and red wine, and consider instead frying some bacon with a well-marbled t-bone swimming in the fat. Your snack could be in sync with some of the dietary advice mentioned below.

It would kill too many bytes to write about every dietary plan (or fad) that has achieved some popularity or notoriety in the last couple of decades. Some new ones, like the "climatarian" and the "flexitarian," are essentially less restrictive vegetarian diets or modifications of the Med or similar diets. Those seem reasonable and healthy, but because they are only modest modifications of diets celebrated in Chapter 4, I shall not bother them here. Some others have been designed to benefit people with special conditions such as gluten intolerance. They too shall be neglected here. Others may be temporarily effective for weight loss, but possibly hazardous in the long term, like the bacon-fried steak suggested above. Because some curious dietary recommendations have arrived only recently and may be departing soon, there is often insufficient research to comment on or review. And because few of them, fad or otherwise, make cognitive sharpening a priority, many will not receive even a mention here.

**The spectrum of advice.** Some modern dietary approaches make recommendations about macro-nutrients—proteins, fats, and carbohydrates. But some are more narrowly crafted, asking us to avoid foods that may actually provide important or even essential nutrients, and some of those are hyped with impressive web advertising. Often we receive heartfelt warnings that our neurons or other body parts are turning to tapioca because we continue to eat rice, or lentils, or meat, or beans containing the "notoriously unhealthy" lectins, or cholesterol, or fructose, or just too much or the wrong kind of protein. Salvation is sometimes provided in a book that offers dietary remedies, occasionally with meal plans and recipes. Others offer a month's supply of capsules at a substantial saving for the introductory offer, of course with a "satisfaction or money-back" guarantee.

As an example of one of the narrowly-crafted approaches, I encountered recently the infomercials of an entrepreneurial cardiologist who warned we must avoid beans and other foods containing "dangerous lectins." Those "nasty" lectins spawn "endotoxins that will cause a leaky gut" followed by all kinds of problems for brain and body. As with almost all such stories, there is an element of truth. Indeed it is true that major health problems can be caused by "leaky" intestines that allow bacteria and other unwelcome intruders to escape through our intestine wall and into our blood stream. And lectins in some form may indeed cause leaks, but attributing leaky guts to lectins derived from normally-prepared food is striding far away from real facts.

You do not really need to know all this, but lectins are actually a type of sugar-binding protein that keeps some nutrients from being absorbed. Nevertheless, in small quantities lectins are beneficial. And small quantities are what we consume, even from high-lectin foods, because those foods are almost always washed and cooked—processes that essentially reduce the lectins to negligible levels. There is no evidence that normal dietary levels of lectin-containing foods (actually most beans, and many fruits, veggies, nuts, and grains) are harmful. In contrast, those foods are usually rich in well-studied and obviously-beneficial vitamins, minerals, and phytonutrients, and thus known to be good for cognition and brains too. For example, Ganesan and Xu (2017) note that lentils—although high in lectins in their pre-cooked form—correspond with reduced degenerative diseases such as cancer and other conditions that degrade cognition, including diabetes, obesity, and (yes, even) cardiovascular disease. Note too that the really-old-but-bean-consuming people who seem to live forever in the blue zones of the world seem to avoid the health problems of bean-induced leaky guts. Apparently, the entrepreneurial cardiologist missed some of that.

Surely you can live a healthy life without learning more about lectins. In fact, although there are important ideas and findings in this chapter, for diets as a whole, I believe the best evidence for healthspan, and for brain health and cognition was offered in Chapter 4. The evidence presented there was solid in showing that the Med, the MIND, and closely related diets keep our brains healthy and sharpen our cognition. Still, some of the dietary approaches outlined below offer tantalizing suggestions. An examination of some of those with promise follows. But be cautious.

### Ketogenic and related diets

**Keto diets.** To foster carbohydrate restrictions, some ketogenic diets (hereafter usually just keto diets) substitute fats for the required calories, with fats accounting for 70% to 90% of total calories, and with carbohydrates kept to less than 50 grams per day. As explained below, limiting carbohydrates in favor of fats essentially results in the creation of ketones. Other diets minimize carbohydrates by substituting more protein than is included in the typical keto diet.

Another approach to limiting digestion of (complex) carbohydrates depends on chemicals called carb blockers, more formally described as α-amylase inhibitors. I offer nothing more than this brief mention because impacts on brain and cognition have not been widely studied.

Those recommending more protein include the older Atkins diet and the South Beach diet. Both are somewhat ketogenic, as described below. The South Beach makes a clear distinction between good carbohydrates from natural sources such as fruits, veggies, whole grains, beans and legumes versus unhealthy carbohydrates from foods with added sugar, and baked goods. Certainly, that orientation is sensible, but because data on the impacts of Atkins and South Beach on brain and cognition range from unavailable to skimpy, I focus on the modern ketogenic diets.

To achieve the high-fat and low carbohydrate percentages required for aggressive keto diets, one avoids many veggies, most fruits, beans, grains including bread, and even milk. Thus many nutrients are eliminated that have been recommended by scientifically-oriented nutritionists—sometimes nutrients that are the primary components of the MIND and the Med diets. All that sounds downright dangerous, especially when the permitted (and sometimes encouraged) fats include the saturated fats in the bacon-fried t-bone that I considered above. Established nutrition research clearly shows that those saturated fats cause problems—at least when they are part of a normal diet. Some research with critters even shows how cognitive problems can result from high-fat diets that negatively prime the hippocampi to respond to stressors with inflammation (Sobesky et al., 2014).

Expectations for benefits from keto diets are expressed in titles such as "Eat fat, live longer?" (a *Science Daily* title in the 5/9/17 issue, but notice the "?"). In fact, early research with rodents showed that when high-fat diets were contrasted with diets high in carbohydrates, the high-fat critters really did live longer; some research even showed that the high-fat diets increased cognitive capacities, along with reduced inflammation and suppressed tumors. With such counter-intuitive findings, researchers focused on how high-fat regimes could possibly be healthy.

**Benefits of ketones.** The flow of logic begins with ketones. When the body is deprived of dietary carbohydrates, leading to low levels of blood glucose, our helpful liver transforms stored and circulating fats into ketone molecules that circulate throughout body and brain. Then our resourceful and adaptable mitochondria substitute (for the missing glucose) two of the three kinds of ketones that are circulating (those two ketones are β-hydroxybutyrate and acetoacetate, but you need not remember them). That substitution process is especially important for our brains because, as you know, brains require a constant high level of energy merely to survive, let alone to function well. But even beyond enhancing the brain's contentment and survival, there are other benefits to substituting ketones when carbohydrates are in short supply.

Salomón et al. (2017) noted that one of the highly toxic byproducts of glucose conversion to energy is the evil molecule methylglyoxal. High levels of methylglyoxal contribute to Alzheimer's and to other age-related diseases, including cancer, diabetes, and cardiovascular diseases. Of course, our lives would be mostly unhealthy and short if the story ended there. But very fortunately, methylglyoxal can be controlled. Even with a more normally balanced diet than the keto, some conversion of fats into ketones occurs in the liver. Salomón et al. demonstrated that one of those ketones detoxifies evil methylglyoxal, reducing methylglyoxal's contribution to degenerative diseases. That analysis concluded that either (or both) of the two main components of the keto diet—increasing fats or severely limiting carbohydrates—should limit methylglyoxal and should therefore be a major benefit to brain and body, and thus to cognition.

Another possible means for the keto diet to control Alzheimer's is by countering the brain's loss of energy. That is, as Alzheimer's develops, although the brain's energy supply from ketones remains constant, there is a reduction in the brain's processing of carbohydrates into energy. Thus Cunnane et al. (2016) suggested that diets that enhance ketones may mitigate dementia by preventing the brain's energy deficits from developing as quickly as they would without the ketones.

**Keto diets and cognition.** Confirming those positive expectations, a recent and thorough review of long-term studies showed cognitive benefits from ketogenic-style diets. Grammatikopoulou et al. (2020) assed the randomized-control trials published through 2019 that used actual people to assess the impacts of keto diets on age-related cognitive decline and on Alzheimer's. Ten randomized-control trials met the stringent inclusion criteria for the review. Those studies compared keto diets against placebos, or normal diets, or meals that lacked ketogenic agents. The keto diets assessed in those 10 studies lasted between 45 and 180 days and improved cognition irrespective of the length of time on the diet. The longer keto-diet periods also improved memory. The conclusion that keto diets enhance cognition was supported by the positive correlation between higher plasma levels of ketones and cognitive performance. Grammatikopoulou et al. concluded that ketogenic diets hold both short-term and long-term promise for improving cognition in people suffering both Alzheimer's dementia and mild cognitive impairment.

Nevertheless, following a different but thorough recent review, Vinciguerra et al. (2020) reached a different conclusion—that the case for positive impacts of ketones on cognition is not yet proven. Furthermore, they noted the possible risks of keto diets when used for long periods, and they recommend that time-limited keto diets be used in only specific cases; they noted that risks could be especially high in elderly people.

For delaying age-associated cognitive decline, Vinciguerra et al. clearly favored reliance on the Med and on variations of the Med that are culturally appropriate, rather than on keto diets. With that in mind, but also with some positive results from the keto research, consider the potential benefits of carbohydrate-restricted diets that are less focused on fats.

**Carbohydrates and cognition.** Lots of past research shows that administering carbohydrates—often in glucose drinks—produces short-term benefits in both physical endurance and cognition. However, a recent review specifically of carbohydrate impacts on cognition by Hawkins et al. (2018) noted that the immediate impacts of carbohydrates are mixed, with positive impacts when base-rate levels of blood glucose are low, but not always when they are higher.

However, in contrast to the usual short-term benefits from added glucose, research shows consistently that cognitive problems result from long-term high-carbohydrate consumption, with cognitive deficits developing even when the high consumption does not lead to weight gain. Most importantly for our interests, Hawkins et al. asserted that cognitive impairment follows from long-term (or lifetime) exposure to high levels of especially refined carbohydrates.

Supporting that assessment, Momtaz et al. (2018) noted the correspondence of dysregulated blood glucose with Alzheimer's. They cited research showing that 81% of Alzheimer's people have either type-2 diabetes or other imbalances of glucose metabolism. That often-seen co-occurrence of diabetes with Alzheimer's is sometimes referred to as "type-3 diabetes." Furthermore, Vinciguerra et al. noted that 30% of patients with type-2 diabetes have mild cognitive impairment, with diabetes being the causal element in that correlation, clearly increasing neurodegenerative disease risk.

Krikorian et al. (2012) had noted that excessive insulin (known formally as hyperinsulinemia) promoted brain inflammation and neurodegeneration. Thus they suggested that a diet low in carbohydrates might retard neurodegeneration in people by downregulating insulin, even in people already experiencing mild cognitive impairment. To test that hypothesis, Krikorian et al. randomly assigned only 23 older adults already experiencing mild cognitive impairment to a control condition of diet-as-usual or to a very low carbohydrate condition. Those two dietary conditions continued for only six weeks. Even with the low experimental power associated with the few participants and short duration, the low carbohydrate diet did indeed result in improved verbal memory performance ($p = .01$) as well as benefits to a remarkable series of physiological indicators including weight reduction ($p =$ .0001), waist size shrinkage ($p = .0001$), lower fasting glucose ($p = .009$), and lower fasting insulin as well ($p = .005$). In further support of their hypothesis, plasma ketone levels correlated positively with improvements in memory ($p = .04$). However, Krikorian et al. noted that the control of insulin rather than the extra ketone molecules could have been the direct cause of improved memory from the carbohydrate restriction.

At this point, we have multiple explanations for how high carbohydrate diets can harm the brain and degrade cognition. The high insulin levels suggested by Krikorian et al. could be a direct cause, as could the reduced ketone levels that follow from deriving energy largely from carbohydrates. Other aspects of carbohydrate metabolism within the mitochondria seem implicated as well. Recall that carbohydrate metabolism produces the evil methylglyoxal described above, enhances inflammation, and produces the various reactive oxygen species that cause mutations of both mitochondrial DNA and cellular DNA. Those mutations in turn damage both the mitochondria and the cells that host them, degrading cognition as one of the many unwelcome byproducts.

For our purposes, it is not essential that we know the relative potency of those various routes that intervene between sustained high carbohydrates and cognitive decline. We know the moral of the story, that moderating carbohydrate intake will almost invariably reduce insulin levels, increase ketones, and reduce the need for our mitochondria to produce energy from only carbohydrates. Irrespective of the underlying causal paths, research shows that carbohydrate restriction has positive impacts on cognitive processes, and on the various physiological parameters that we know to influence cognition. Undoubtedly our genes play a role as well.

**Carbohydrate interactions.** Hawkins et al. suggested that both the short-term and long-term relationships of carbohydrates with cognition are probably moderated by our genes, gut microbiome composition, age, and other factors, including when and how we consume carbohydrates (as noted for alcohol in Chapter 14). That suggestion reinforces a theme noted in other chapters: Nutrition is not simple; nutrients interact with each other, with the environment, with our genes, and certainly with the microbiome.

### Caloric restriction

Reducing caloric consumption to around 75% of normal usually benefits the lifespan, healthspan, and cognitive functions of several species of experimental animals, including the usual assortment of mammals. One of the keys to those benefits may be the "anti-aging" hormone klotho. Klotho is produced in the kidneys. It activates vitamin D receptors and, according to Haussler et al. (2016,

p. 166), klotho "modulates the 'fountain of youth' array of genes, with the klotho target emerging as a major player in the facilitation of healthspan by delaying the chronic diseases of aging." Unfortunately, like (it seems) almost every similar physiological element that extends healthspan and is neuroprotective in us humans, klotho declines substantially with aging.

To assess dietary impacts on klotho, Shafie et al. (2020) placed rats on various diets, including caloric restriction, extra protein, extra fats, and combinations of extra protein with caloric restriction. Their title summarized the findings: "High protein and low-calorie diets improved the anti-aging klotho protein in the rats' brain…" The extra protein and the caloric restriction diets also led to improved maze performance. Other research supports the impact of caloric restriction (and physical exercise) in enhancing klotho levels.

But those beneficial impacts from caloric restriction can be different for lifespan versus healthspan, and they can vary by sex, they can be different for different individuals, and even within an individual there can be tissue-specific impacts with some positive and others not so much (Wilson et al., 2021). For details concerning the many physiological paths that may be taken with dietary or caloric restrictions, readers well versed in biochemistry are referred to that extensive analysis by Wilson and colleagues. Wilson et al. even propose a new title for a new field: "nutrigeroscience" to indicate the science of how the management and restriction of nutrition can affect longevity.

However, because people usually find any caloric restriction to vary from difficult to awful, most randomized-control trials have been undertaken with overweight people seeking weight loss. But even then, positive associations of caloric restriction with enhanced cognition are not consistent. The occurrence of the negative or null findings with people are very possibly due to caloric restriction leading to the experience of hunger and then preoccupation with food (as suggested by Leclerc et al., 2020). Another possible explanation, discussed below, is that the positive impacts seen in animal studies of caloric restriction may be due to the rhythm of eating rather than the amount eaten—in short, due to intermittent fasting rather than to total calories consumed. Wait for more about that.

**Caloric restriction in humans.** The two studies reviewed below examined reductions in daily calories rather than periodic fasting. The researchers avoided mentioning death threats to persuade participants to persevere, but Witte et al. (2009) randomly assigned 50 moderately-older participants (mean age of 60) to one of three dietary conditions for three months. Although the caloric restriction condition asked participants to reduce their caloric intake by 30%, adherence to that restriction was only approximate. The two control conditions were a regular-diet condition and one with increased unsaturated fats. A significant increase in verbal memory scores (20%, $p < .001$) was achieved only by the few participants in the calorie-restricted condition; that improvement correlated with adherence to the diet. Reductions in the inflammation-indicator C-reactive protein and reduced plasma insulin levels also resulted from the caloric restriction and also correlated with memory improvements ($p < .05$). Levels of our favorite neurotropin, BDNF, were not affected by the dietary restriction.

A much longer randomized-control trial called CALORIE lasted for two years. After some attrition, 53 participants remained at the end (Leclerc et al., 2020). To motivate cooperation for that long time span, (and in lieu of kidnapping) monetary payments were given. A 25% caloric reduction was prescribed for the 34 healthy and non-obese participants between ages 21 and 50 who were in the caloric restriction condition. However, those restricted participants actually subsisted for the two years on 85% of their normal caloric intake. That is still a substantial reduction, but the shift from the planned 25% to the actual 15% reduction shows the difficulty of maintaining such restrictions. Even though the participants were not originally obese, the calorie-restricted participants lost an average of 9kg (20 pounds–mostly fat, but including some lean tissue) while the 19 people in the control condition had little weight change.

Potential confounding factors taken into account were sleep quality, moods, stress, and energy expended. The main result was that compared to the control condition, caloric restriction resulted in greater improvements in spatial working memory (assessed by the Cambridge Neuropsychological Battery). That relationship was a trend at the end of the first year, but statistically significant after the second year ($p < .01$). However, Leclerc et al. acknowledged that those effects were mediated by improvements in sleep quality, and energy expenditure from physical activity. Furthermore, Leclerc et al. noted that other research showed that mild cognitive impairment and negative hippocampal changes can follow from weight gain, clearly suggesting that weight loss (rather than calorie restriction per se) could benefit hippocampi and thus memory capacity.

Thus on balance, the results of the two studies on calorie restriction with humans showed some cognitive benefits. They were not spectacular, but one possible response is that irrespective of the mediating impact of weight loss, sleep quality, and physical activity, that the bottom line is important—that for whatever reason, caloric restriction ultimately resulted in some cognitive sharpening.

**Paths from caloric restriction to brilliance.** Another consideration supporting that conclusion is that all of the animal research contributing to the reviews shows physiological changes (to say nothing of increased lifespans) that themselves underlay cognitive brilliance. In fact, other analyses of the data from other people participating in the CALORIE studies showed reduced damage from reactive oxygen species following the caloric restriction (Redman et al., 2018). Those physiological effects clearly protect neurons and cognition.

One final noteworthy feature of the Leclerc et al. (2020) research was that the reduction in protein intake (not carbohydrates or fats) was the dietary element that correlated with improved memory performance. Leclerc et al. asserted that despite popular sentiment to the contrary, research has not shown consistent positive relationships between protein intake and cognition. That observation is interesting, but certainly not conclusive, and very probably depends on the base-rate protein intake of the study participants.

### Fasting instead

Because real people obviously have great difficulty adhering to a diet of 75% or even 85% of their normal caloric intake, with the meager exceptions noted above we are not overwhelmed with randomized-control trials testing caloric restriction with human subjects. Thus most of the related research done with people has pivoted to assess whether similar benefits could be obtained from intermittent fasting rather than continuous caloric restriction.

**Un-confounding restriction and fasting.** Perhaps fasting is a better choice than calorie restriction anyway, as strongly suggested by this study of mice who tried various dietary regimes (Pak et al., 2021). Previous research with animals achieved caloric control usually by restricting feeding times—by intermittent fasting. Typical results were improved blood glucose control, and, corresponding with that, a higher ratio of fat to glucose utilized for energy production. That combination of fasting with caloric restriction also led to reduced frailty and greater longevity. However, Pak et al. noted that calorie restriction and fasting were almost invariably confounded in those studies. To assess fasting with and without caloric restriction, in a thoughtful design, Pak et al. created four dietary regimes. The dependent measures were not about brain and cognition, but did include the important health measures mentioned just above—measures that have major impacts on brain and cognition.

One group of mice ate all they wanted whenever they wished (no restriction). Another group was given 70% of a normal mouse diet, dispensed to them over the day to avoid actual fasting (caloric restriction only). A third group ate a full amount but in a limited time period each day (fasting only), and the most unfortunate of the volunteers were asked to consume 70% of normal calories, but only during a limited interval each day (caloric restriction plus fasting).

The surprising result in this research by Pak et al. was that the great benefits to health and lifespan only materialized if some fasting occurred. Caloric restriction alone resulted in some positive control of blood glucose, but in contrast to prior research, the caloric restriction alone actually reduced the mouse lifespans. That is a poor exchange, but those calorie-restricted beasts may not have been relishing life anyway. On balance, the results clearly supported the hypothesis that fasting, even without restricting calories, is better than caloric restriction alone for healthspan, lifespan, and undoubtedly for brain and cognition as well. At least at this point, that seems to be the case if one is a mouse. (It is interesting, isn't it, that sometimes a single study can cause re-evaluation of decades of prior research.)

**Fasting styles and reviews.** For a review and analysis of research on intermittent fasting we benefit from a recent *New England Journal of Medicine* paper on the "Effects of intermittent fasting on health, aging, and disease" by de Cabo & Mattson, 2020). Directly relevant to our interests in brain and cognition, de Cabo and Mattson noted that studies of animal cognition have shown gains from caloric restriction (though often confounded with fasting)—gains in the form of improved spatial memory, associative memory, and working memory. Furthermore, they cited research showing that alternative-day fasting slowed disease progression in transgenic animals disposed to suffer both Alzheimer's and Parkinson's diseases. Naturally, those studies led to similar studies of fasting with people.

For us humans, two different rhythms of fasting are usually chosen. The first method features eating normally (with no restrictions at all) five days per week, but restricting eating on the other (fasting) two days per week. Some approaches allow up to 1000 calories per day on the fasting days, but some suggest lower levels, and some are initially generous but gradually reduce fasting-day calories in subsequent weeks. The second of the two fasting approaches limits the hours for eating each day, with the time allowed for eating as short as one hour per day. More humane approaches allow more normal intervals for eating—intervals that may last as long as 10 hours (e.g., breakfast at 9am and no food after dinner ending at 7pm). Both fasting approaches seem to help in weight loss with no obvious health problems resulting.

According to the analysis by de Cabo and Mattson, intermittent fasting is effective because as little as 10 to 14 hours of fasting depletes glycogen levels and stimulates the metabolic conversion of fats to ketones. As noted above, the mitochondria then substitute those ketones for glucose in energy production, resulting in reduced stored fat, reduced appetite, less threat from methylglyoxal, and fewer pesky and destructive reactive oxygen species. Increased ketones also result from the 5-2 style of fasting. Even if 500 to 700 calories are consumed on each of the two fasting days, ketone levels are elevated on those days.

Thus the approaches to intermittent fasting reviewed above achieve their benefits through the same means as the more mainstream keto diets. In addition to the means described above for the keto diets, other paths for benefits from both keto-style diets and intermittent fasting were noted by de Cabo and Mattson. Those included improved cardiovascular function, improved insulin and glucose levels, suppressed inflammation, mitochondrial rejuvenation and creation, cell repair and the recycling of molecules from expired cells, healthful weight loss, and general stress resistance and cell survival. Every one of those physiological enhancements leads to brain maintenance and inhibits or delays age-associated cognitive decline.

But even more central to our interests, de Cabo and Mattson noted that the ketones resulting from either keto diets or fasting affect both neurotransmitters and neurotropins. Elevated ketone levels activate the wonderful neurotropin BDNF (and other neurochemicals that can also act as transcription factors, activating various genes). Those genetic impacts in turn enhance neurogenesis and synaptic plasticity. As noted previously, BDNF expression in turn fosters brain maintenance and development—providing the essential physiological elements for cognitive enhancement and for resistance to neurodegenerative diseases. Intermittent fasting also increases the neurotransmitter GABA, with its calming impacts reducing the potential for neural damage when neurons become over-activated. All of the foregoing, but especially ketones encouraging the neurotropin BDNF and the neurotransmitter GABA, suggest that intermittent fasting and caloric restriction should indeed have mighty impacts on the brain, cognition, and moods.

### Paleo diets

An issue to ponder concerns the logic of paleo diets—diets based on the idea that we humans were shaped by evolution to flourish in the natural environments of our pre-agriculture ancestors. That pre-agriculture period lasted hundreds of thousands of years, and most evidence would suggest that the following short agriculture period of a few thousand years has not substantially changed us. A basic tenet is then that we modern humans would benefit from a diet that duplicates that early diet—whatever it was.

But of course there were and are many different "paleo" diets. Some current-but-pre-industrial cultures, and some that are even pre-agricultural, still consume foods much as their ancestors did for millennia. Some of those diets, like that of the Inuit, are largely based on animal proteins and fats, whereas others are based on vegetables and grains, and still others on root vegetables.

Some of the facts supporting a paleo diet are that our modern diets often have many elements that range from not nutritious to downright harmful. Remember that the notorious Western is often contrasted with the Med and the MIND, with the Western found to be wanting, even when fed to rodents.

It might be sensible to avoid definitions based on specific cultures—fictional or real—and instead to define a paleo diet by the modern foods that we should avoid—foods that were certainly unavailable to people in any paleo culture. That list of banned foods would include dairy (with a few exceptions), added sugars, and most any other kind of food additives. Processed foods from crackers to hot dogs would be condemned too because of losing the nutrients blessed in previous chapters (and because of often adding junk). Some paleo adherents eat lots of meat, but perhaps given the underlying logic of the approach, they should resist meats contributed by overly-fat creatures that have been eating their own unnatural diet of corn, various grains, and other products of monoculture farming.

What then should paleo fans eat? Paleo adherents advocate the consumption of a large variety of (locally sourced if possible) organic and non-genetically modified foods that are neither highly processed nor derived from monoculture agriculture. Probably adding large white grubs to lunch is not necessary, but we should await final word on that.

The logic of paleo also affirms that we should not consume supplements. Knowing that our ancestors were shaped by evolution to thrive on the balance of nutrients available nearby and from the natural environment, those natural nutrients should be sufficient for us. But having read this far, you are aware of the problems with that approach, especially given that some nutrients are not absorbed well in elderly folks.

Another concern related to the previous point is that Mother Nature does not care about the health and length of survival of elderly folks like me—at least she does not care once we are past our age of reproduction and of raising our kids (perhaps caring for our grandkids too). Once we are done passing our genes to the next generation and nurturing those genes while they reside in our immediate descendents, Mother N. considers the fate of the genes left in our elderly bodies to be irrelevant. Thus even if some form of paleo is great for the young, nature provides no assurance that the nutritional content will be adequate for elderly people whose nutritive needs may be vastly changed from their youth, and whose ability to absorb and process nutrients may be fading.

We can end this rather quickly because, although a hot topic, I see no substantial research suggesting that paleo diets will be good for brains or cognition, and it seems the paleo receives almost as much criticism from mainline nutritionists as does the poor disparaged Western. Even the "Proceedings of the 2nd annual symposium of the German Society for Paleo Nutrition held in 2014" published in the *Journal of Evolution and Health*, yielded nothing that I could find connecting paleo with cognition.

## Summary of intriguing diets

Taken together, research on the ketogenic and other caloric restriction/fasting diets leads to the conclusion that we could surely harvest some health and cognitive benefits by at least occasionally urging our livers to release a few ketone molecules from their captivity. I suspect with some training, I could refrain from eating for 14 hours or so—at least occasionally. Taking a break from continuous noshing could be healthful for the brain and body too. (Perhaps a long sleep could suffice.)

But as for the paleo, we should of course adhere to the aspects of that approach that follow established research, such as minimizing food additives, avoiding excess sugar and salt, and serving highly processed foods only to people we dislike. But none of that requires any knowledge of paleo, at least as paleo has been presented. The basic premise of paleo that we will be healthier if we eat like our pre-agriculture ancestors is…well…inaccurate, often impossible, and (I believe) somewhat preposterous.

Remember too that insofar as the ketogenic diets substitute animal proteins and fats for carbohydrates, that for the human population as a whole those dietary approaches are absolutely unsustainable. The climate and most of us denizens of the earth simply cannot absorb even more costly production of calories from animals; there are simply too many of us.

Chapter 18

# Resilience: Resistance to stress, anxiety, and depression

In Chapters 4 through 17 I did not emphasize impacts of nutrition on resilience. Now that changes. Resilience is defined here as stress tolerance, and resistance to the moods of depression and anxiety (collectively hereafter just "moods"). This chapter will have nothing to do with whether those moods entice us to munch chocolate, other comfort food, worms, or even the (baked, not fried) 17-year cicadas that were plentiful in the American North East during the summer of 2021.

Because inflammation and oxidative stress are both linked with stress intolerance and the unwholesome states of depression and anxiety, to resist those states we benefit from all of the previously-reviewed nutrients with anti-inflammatory and antioxidant characteristics. Similarly, because low energy can accompany negative moods, the mitochondria are often implicated, so nutrients that protect the mitochondria and boost their function are relevant as well.

In fact, any of the nutrients that keep our brains healthy and that sustain our cognitive abilities are indirectly or directly relevant to these topics. However, I focus mostly on the specific nutrients shown to *directly* restrain those unpleasant states, and to a lesser extent, the nutrients affecting mitochondria, and those affecting the neurotransmitters that are directly linked with stress tolerance, depression, or anxiety. Thus the neurotransmitters serotonin, noradrenaline, and dopamine receive attention because their deficits often correspond with depression, and boosting their levels often relieves depression. For controlling anxiety the inhibitory neurotransmitter GABA and the endocannabinoid system are involved, and both are affected by nutrition. (The endocannabinoid molecules and their receptors are distributed throughout the brain; they influence mood, cognition, and immune functions. See Glossary for slightly more.)

### Stress

As in Chapter 2, stress is defined here as our internal response to stressors. Stressors vary from threats—especially social threats—to the experience of harm or loss. Stress, depression, and anxiety are not separated by clear boundaries. That is, anxiety is often a component of a stress response, and chronic depression itself is both a stressor and a frequent result of sustained stress. For clarity, note that although the term "oxidative stress" has been mentioned throughout, oxidative stress—when reactive oxygen species are too plentiful for effective control by antioxidants—is one of many components of the stress response.

Stress requires extra nutrients. Those nutrients should subdue inflammation, tame reactive oxygen species, and reduce the C-reactive protein and excessive homocysteine that both result from stress and contribute to the symptoms of stress. (Recall that elevated homocysteine levels can damage arterial walls and kidney function, and can contribute to cognitive decline and even Alzheimer's.) Vitamins C, D, and the B vitamins combat those physiological components of stress responses, but those vitamins are not always successful, because the body's stress responses reduce levels of vitamin C, and inhibit absorption of the B-vitamins. Thus supplements may be required and are often recommended. For example, the study by de Jager et al. (2012), reviewed in Chapter 8, showed that homocysteine levels were reduced by 30% in the randomly assigned elderly people receiving a supplement of three B-vitamins (B-6, B-9, and B-12). That B-vitamin treatment also had significant positive impacts on cognition and brain volume. Dietary zinc and a healthy microbiome are also major contributors to stress tolerance, but are discussed more fully below in the section on depression.

**Stress and mitochondria.** Our mitochondria are pressed into extraordinary service to restore the energy that is drained as we experience chronic stress. As you know, mitochondrial hyper-activity produces high levels of reactive oxygen species that then cause damage to DNA and other cellular components. In Chapter 15, I described the nutrients that increase our potential stress tolerance by repairing the self-inflicted damage caused by overly-excited mitochondria. Those restorative nutrients included the B vitamins, urolithin-A (with our gut bacteria creating it from foods like pomegranate), and CoQ10. (Other unproven supplements with potential for boosting the mitochondria that were mentioned briefly in Chapter 15 include MitoQ and NAD+.)

**Stress tolerance and toughness.** Because physiological toughness and psychological resilience reduce the negative impacts of stressors on lifespan, healthspan, and general well-being, I provide a brief description of physiological toughness and psychological resilience here. Await Chapter 19 for a chapter-length presentation of toughness and resilience. My previous book (Dienstbier 2015) describes how physical exercise, cognitive stimulation, confronting manageable stressors, practicing self-control, meditation, and affectionate activities can lead to physiological toughness. Physiological toughness is reflected in well-bulked-up brain structures, especially the prefrontal cortex and hippocampi. And it is reflected in the enhancement of neurochemicals, especially the neurotransmitters and neurotropins. Those physiological modifications lead, in turn, to resilience, as defined in the opening paragraph of this chapter.

**Stress and the major diets.** Given the mix of valued nutrients in diets like the Med and MIND, and the potential that those nutrients may be even more effective in combination than they are in isolation, as anticipated, those major diets have been shown to repair stress-induced damage. For example, in an excellent study using primates Shively et al. (2020) randomly assigned 38 female monkeys (macaques) to enjoy either 31 months of a diet based on the Mediterranean diet or on one equivalent to the sad Western diet. The two diets were formulated with equal amounts of protein, fats, and carbohydrates, but except for some lean protein from fish and dairy the Med sourced protein and fats mainly from plants, and it was rich in monounsaturated fats. Shively et al. based their version of the Western on the consumption patterns of middle-aged Western women; it featured animal-sourced protein and fat, high levels of saturated fats and sodium, and low levels of mono fats and omega 3s.

Across the 31 months of that study, stress was induced by social isolation from other monkeys, and by having blood drawn and other tests administered. Those stressful procedures were administered first during a baseline phase and later at 12 and 29 months into the diet phase of the study. As described in Chapter 19, activities that result in physiological toughness change the pattern of arousal to stressors, and it is that changed arousal pattern that leads to stress tolerance. Specifically, toughened people and animals show higher initial sympathetic NS responses to *intense* stressors (but not to modest stressors); thus, they have the energy required to cope effectively. But toughened people also have quicker recovery to base-rate levels when arousal-demanding emergencies are over. In the research by Shively et al. the Med diet animals showed that tough arousal pattern in response to the periodic stressors they experienced, in contrast to the Western diet animals. The greater toughness of the Med animals was also reflected in their pituitary-adrenal-cortical arousal responses being less than those of the Western group ($p = .01$).

Other arousal pattern issues result from aging. Aging in both humans and monkeys leads to gradual increases in base rates of sympathetic NS arousal, and declines in base rates of the parasympathetic nervous system (parasympathetic NS). But those age-associated changes were less in the Med diet monkeys. Thus their arousal patterns in response to both stressors and to aging showed the Med diet animals to be physiologically tougher in ways that control both stress responses and anxiety.

In a study with even larger primates Baynham et al. (2021) gave cacao laden with flavanols, or a low-flavanol control chocolate drink to young men. The design was a powerful crossover design with each person participating in both conditions. The drinks were consumed 90 minutes before an 8-minute mental stress test. The study title summarized the findings that "Cocoa flavanols improve vascular responses to acute mental stress." Even though enhanced cognition was not assessed directly, attenuated cardiovascular responses to acute stressors lead ultimately to a healthier cardiovascular system, with positive implications for brain and cognition.

## Anxiety

Because anxiety disorders are common, anxiety control has been a central focus of therapeutic research. For example, there have been legions of studies on the impacts of omega 3 fatty acids on both short-term and long-term anxiety. Indeed there are good reasons to expect anxiety suppression from omega 3s. Diets rich in those fatty acids attenuate the anxiety-driven behavioral responses of animals. For example, in "open field" tests where anxiety motivates critters to scoot to the walls and poop, with omega 3s there is less scooting and pooping. And animals favored with omega 3 supplements in randomized-control trials show corresponding suppression of stressor-stimulated pituitary-adrenal-cortical (PAC) arousal. (PAC arousal is described in Chapter 2 and in Glossary.) Furthermore, omega three deficiencies in young animals result in reductions of our favorite neurotropin BDNF, particularly in the hippocampi, potentially downgrading the ability of the hippocampi to control anxiety and to control PAC arousal to future stressors. Thus omega 3s may provide anxiety control for us humans too, but at this point, the research is not compelling.

**Anxiety and the nutraceuticals.** Because both bacopa and ginkgo (reviewed in Chapter 12) enhance cerebral blood flow into the brain and increase supplies of neurotransmitters, particularly acetylcholine (Chaudhari et al., 2017), it seems likely that they might aid in the control of depression and anxiety. And indeed research by Calabrese et al. (2008) found that 300mg per day of bacopa administered for 84 days to older Italians without dementia improved measures of both anxiety and depression.

Using a different research approach, Savage et al. (2018) concluded that ginkgo was similarly effective. Knowing that the neurotransmitter GABA suppresses anxiety, Savage and colleagues cast a wide net, reviewing research from a variety of research approaches including *in vitro* studies showing nutrient impacts on GABA, or animal studies of nutrients affecting anxiety, or similar human clinical trials. From that broad search, they concluded that some preclinical and clinical research does indeed suggest such positive impacts on anxiety from a variety of 10 "phytomedicines." Besides ginkgo, the other anti-anxiety nutrients snagged in their broad research net were kava, valerian, pennywort, hops, chamomile, passionflower, ashwagandha, skullcap, and lemon balm. But similar reports supporting control of anxiety from those phytomedicines are rare. In fact, the evidence is modest even for impacts on anxiety from bacopa and from ginkgo.

Even with modest reasons to expect control of stress responses and anxiety from various nutrients, and even with some encouraging research outcomes—albeit sometimes preliminary ones—other recent reviews have been tepid, at best.

**Anxiety and broad-brush reviews.** Firth et al. (2021) addressed this issue with an unusual but thorough approach. Their title accurately indicates that they searched for *any* "Effects of dietary improvements on symptoms of depression and anxiety." After sifting through all the randomized-control trials published through March, 2018, they identified 16 for inclusion in their meta-analysis. The reviewed diets lasted between 10 days and three years; impacts were assessed on mostly non-clinical levels of both anxiety and depression. The dietary interventions in their analysis included four that were designed to reduce weight, four crafted to reduce fat intake, and the others adding various nutrients. Despite that wide array of interventions, whereas the interventions reduced depression symptoms at moderate effect sizes (discussed below), there were no impacts from the dietary interventions on anxiety.

It is curious that despite their being substantial overlap between members of the research group conducting the review by Firth et al. and the research group of the Savage et al. 2018 review discussed above, that the Savage et al. results point toward positive impacts of some nutrients on anxiety, whereas the Firth et al. review does not. On balance, at this point, there is not much solid evidence of substantially-effective nutrients directly contributing to the control of anxiety. Perhaps nutrient control of depression is more effective.

## Depression

Depression corresponds with reduced cortical and hippocampal volume, and with reduced levels of neurotropins and important neurotransmitters, especially serotonin, but with reduced dopamine and noradrenaline often implicated as well. Depression often (but not always) correlates with enhanced base rates of cortisol, and it regularly corresponds with pituitary-adrenal-cortical (PAC) arousal cycles that are dysregulated from normal diurnal rhythms. Although those relationships with depression are correlational, the available evidence suggests that reductions in some neural structures, neurochemical depletion, and disruption of arousal cycles can cause or at least contribute to depression. Depression itself has crucial impacts on wellbeing and is a risk factor for a later diagnosis of dementia (Burton et al., 2013). The association of depression with deficits in major brain structures and neurochemicals suggests that the toughening activities that build brain structures and replenish neurochemicals (discussed much more in Chapter 19) should have anti-depressant impacts.

But many nutrients similarly enhance neurochemistry and grow and maintain neural structures. Therefore those nutrients should be similarly effective as antidepressants. Indeed that is exactly what the research literature shows. To illustrate, I begin with the larger dietary categories because diets similar to the Med and the MIND have been shown to enhance neural structures and neurochemicals. Thus adherence to such diets should mitigate depression.

**Healthful diets reduce or prevent depression.** Several reviews with meta-analyses support the importance of healthful diets in controlling depression. The first, by Lassale et al. (2019) was of 20 longitudinal and 21 cross-sectional studies that compared adherence to various diets including the Med, the DASH, etc. with depression. The most compelling evidence was from four longitudinal studies that assessed the Med, finding a risk ratio for depression of RR = .67 (i.e., for every 100 depressed people in the low-adherence group, there were only 67 in the group adhering most closely to the Med). Another four longitudinal studies found anti-depressant benefits from diets crafted to reduce inflammation (with RR = .65). Another contemporary review by Wu et al. (2020) of essentially-correlational studies of older adults over age 65 showed that healthy diets corresponded with reduced depression with an odds ratio of OR = .85.

The recent review by Firth et al. (2021) was introduced above in the anxiety section. Recall that they searched for randomized-control trials of literally any dietary manipulation having impacts on either anxiety or depression, and that they concluded that positive dietary impacts on anxiety were not proven. Despite the wide array of interventions assessed in their review, the interventions reduced depression symptoms (with an effect size assessed as Hedges g = .27). That is a moderate impact, but the dietary impacts on depression were greater for women than for men. Similar positive impacts on depression with null impacts on anxiety were noted in a review mentioned in Chapter 10 by Kirkland et al. (2018) of magnesium impacts. Kirkland et al. concluded that magnesium therapies were useful for depression.

**Depression and B vitamins.** Recent reviewers have emphasized the therapeutic role of some of the B vitamins (e.g., Fenech, 2017; Moore et al., 2018). The most recent of the reviews, by Yanjun Wu et al. (2022), conducted a meta-analysis of 18 correlational studies. Results indicated that lower incidences of depression were associated with a higher intake of vitamins B-2, B-6 and B-12, with stronger effects from each of those B-vitamins for women than men.

Following the writing of that review, a major study of impacts of folate (B-9) and B-12 on depression was conducted by Laird et al. (2021). The participants were almost 4000 Irish citizens over the age 50 who participated as part of the Irish Longitudinal Study on Aging; the chosen participants were all free of depression symptoms at the study's beginning. Recall that Ireland does not mandate B-vitamin flour fortification, but even where mandates exist, such as in the US, vitamin B-12 is not usually included. At the start of that 4-year longitudinal study by Laird et al. the folate and B-12 were assessed from plasma. Taking into account potential confounding factors such as physical activity, chronic disease burden, vitamin D status, cardiovascular disease and antidepressant use, B-9 (folate) levels did not correspond with later assessments of depression. On the other hand, B-12 levels did. The lowest third of the participants in plasma B-12 were 51% more likely to experience depression over the next four years, versus those in the top third in plasma B-12. B-12 seems prophylactic for depression.

**Depression and vitamin D.** Despite the null results for vitamin D in the study by Laird et al., above, the presence of receptors for vitamin D (remember, it is actually a hormone) in various brain structures, including the amygdala and hippocampi, suggests the likelihood of impacts on brain, and thus potentially on cognition and depression. Some research with animals shows positive behavioral impacts, but studies and reviews with human participants of impacts specifically of vitamin D on depression are (to say the least) inconsistent. Given that inconsistency, Alavi et al. (2019) conducted a carefully-done randomized-control trial that included only elderly depressed men and women with mean age over 65. At the study's beginning, vitamin D blood levels of all of the participants were below the recommended amount (as could be expected in the Spring, after the low sunlight of an Iranian winter).

Individuals in the vitamin D group then received a very large dose of 50,000 IU of vitamin D3 weekly for eight weeks, bringing their blood levels well above the recommended minimum and to around twice their starting levels. (That huge weekly dose translates to 350mcg/day or over 17 times the normal RDA and several times more than the normally acceptable upper limit.) Whereas the depression test scores of the placebo group remained unchanged from beginning to end, the 39 vitamin D participants experienced a remarkable and significant drop ($p = .0001$) in depression test scores. I estimate the effect size for that improvement to be approximately $d = .90$—a remarkable impact for an 8-week intervention. Some of the other research reviewed by Alavi et al. showed positive vitamin D impacts on depression only for people older than

40. Conclusions from the broader literature and from this study support the usefulness of vitamin D treatments for elderly and depressed individuals, especially if they are somewhat deficient (as is very common) in vitamin D levels.

**Depression and the omega 3s.** There is no clarity in this section. If you find that frustrating, skip through it lightly. An early review by Appleton et al. (2015) had concluded that omega 3s were not therapeutic for depression. A later update of that review (Appleton et al., 2021) examined 34 studies with a total of almost 2000 participants. That second review reached a similar conclusion, specifically (in the latter case) that omega 3s provided no meaningful benefits for participants with major depressive disorder.

In support of those conclusions, in a randomized-control trial described as the largest on this question to date, Okereke et al. (2021) assigned over 18 thousand adults over 50 years old to placebos or omega 3 supplements for a mean of 5.7 years. Okereke et al. described their findings as mixed, but concluded that omega 3 supplements were useless for preventing depression. Note, however, that the participants were initially free from either depression or any depressive symptoms.

Between that initial negative review and the following negative randomized-control trial, a review by Bae and Kim (2018) came to mixed conclusions. From the six randomized-control trials in their review, including over 4600 elderly people (mean age 77), Bae and Kim noted first that the studies of participants without depression affirmed the previous conclusions—that no protection from depression was achieved by taking omega 3s. However, an entirely different result was found for those initially with depression. For those elderly and depressed people, omega 3 supplements of 1.3g/day were highly therapeutic, with a huge effect size of Hedges $g = .94$.

The research by Yu et al. (2020) potentially explains how omega 3s could act as antidepressants. Remember that chronic depression often causes deficits of both neurotransmitters and neurotropins, and depression causes shrinkage in the hippocampi and various cortical areas. Yu et al. found that the omega 3s stimulated the brain's astrocytes to produce neurotropins, including the great BDNF, thereby providing the means to transcribe the genes that produce the proteins that rebuild deficient brain structures and that replenish neurochemicals.

Consider the conclusions above that vitamin D seems to have positive impacts on depression only for elderly and somewhat depressed individuals, especially if they were initially deficient (as is common) in vitamin D levels. Although similar answers for omega 3s are less clear, it does seem that the current differences in outcomes may result from such supplements being useful and effective only when prior deficiencies exist. And indeed, that conclusion may apply to may of the nutrients discussed throughout.

**Zinc.** As mentioned in Chapter 10, zinc is essential for everything important in the body. Zinc levels support epigenetic functions, immune-system processes, cell reproduction, and cell survival. For our concerns with depression and anxiety, zinc is essential for the production and regulation of neurotransmitters, including serotonin, noradrenalin, dopamine, glutamate, and GABA. Thus zinc insufficiency should be one of the usual suspects when neurotransmitter deficits cause cognitive impairment, depression, or anxiety. People who experience any of those conditions should be assessed for zinc levels.

Sure enough, there are reams of research papers that assess zinc deficiencies or supplementation to explain or treat depression, or hyperactive conditions, and even autism. From that large array of research, one consistent finding is the linkage of zinc deficiency with depression (especially, but not entirely, for women; see Maserejian et al., 2012). Li et al. (2017) provided a recent meta-analysis summarizing findings from nine studies that affirm the relationship of insufficient zinc with depression. Although each of those nine studies took into account different combinations of potentially-confounding variables, most of the nine accounted for age, sex, race, education, marital status, BMI, smoking, alcohol, and energy intake. Combining data from those nine studies, Li et al. calculated the risk ratio for highest versus lowest dietary zinc to be RR = .67, indicating that for every 100 people in the low zinc group who suffered depression, there were only 67 in the group consuming the most zinc.

Three other recent reviews mentioned in Chapter 10 support those relationships of zinc deficiencies and depression. Those reviews assessed randomized-control trials showing that supplements that restore zinc levels can act as antidepressants (Piao et al., 2017; Wang et al., 2018; Wessels et al., 2017). Piao et al. cited research showing that zinc-deprived animals were cognitively impaired and responded to stressors as if they were depressed. Piao et al. concluded their review by noting zinc treatments may be therapeutic for mood disorders and for neurodegenerative diseases.

**Saffron.** Despite the apparent difficulty of obtaining saffron in appreciable quantities, when Marx et al. (2019) searched for randomized-control trials of saffron impacts on depression and anxiety, they identified 23 studies that were worthy of inclusion in their review and meta-analysis. As mentioned in Chapter 11, their review of the animal research showed that saffron is a regulator of neurotransmitters, the immune system, inflammation, oxidative stress, pituitary-adrenal-cortical arousal, and neurotropins, including BDNF. Clearly, saffron does many good things for brains, and it is obvious that depression is associated with many bad brain things. Thus saffron should affect depression, even in people.

In their review, Marx et al. included studies of both depressed and non-depressed people and they even incorporated two prior meta-analyses that had shown positive impacts of saffron on depression. They also included research that compared saffron with antidepressant medications, and they assessed saffron's usefulness as an adjunct to established treatments for depression. Trials in their review lasted an average of six weeks, with 19 of the 23 studies administering 30 mg per day of saffron. Of those 23 studies, 21 were Iranian and two were Australian, perhaps accounting for the unusual standardization of the saffron dose used in the research. (Note that Iran produces more saffron than the next five producing countries, combined.)

Compared with placebos, saffron had amazing effect sizes for depression (Hedges' $g = 0.99$, $p < 0.001$) and even very strong impacts on anxiety ($g = 0.48$, $p < 0.001$). Saffron even showed effectiveness as an adjunct to established antidepressants. When saffron was compared with those antidepressants, saffron was equally effective, (i.e., there were no differences between the saffron and the standard medications; $g = -.17$, $p = 0.33$, NS). Unfortunately, saffron's future usefulness will be limited by being more expensive than most established antidepressants. Marx et al. noted that the reported effect sizes are larger than typically seen for standard antidepressant medications, and in combination with noting that the research is largely from one region and even from one research group, they suggest caution at this time before advising that saffron be used therapeutically.

**Other possible anti-depressants.** The research is thin to non-existent on the impacts of magnesium on the mood states of anxiety and depression, and there is no compelling reason to believe that SAMe (formally adenosylmethionine) is effective, especially for clinical depression. On the other hand, the clinical evidence for anti-depressant impacts from St John's wort is positive and substantial (Ng et al., 2017), but it is not superior to standard medications for depression. It is effective as an anti-inflammatory and by suppressing MAOIs, the enzyme that reduces levels of some of the major neurotransmitters, including serotonin, dopamine, and noradrenaline.

## Microbiome impacts on resilience

The levels and the kinds of gut bacteria that we host have impacts on our moods (de JR De-Paula et al., 2018). Certainly, part of the explanation for the impacts of the microbiome on depression and other states is that our gut bacteria manufacture over 90% of our body's total serotonin—serotonin that can enter general circulation and then cross the blood-brain barrier into the brain (Kaplan et al., 2015; Bravo et al., 2011). Remember that deficiencies of brain serotonin can cause depression, and that some effective antidepressant medications increase and normalize brain serotonin levels.

Recall that low levels of the neurotransmitter GABA are associated with anxiety. Like serotonin, GABA is produced by various known species of gut bacteria (in the genus *Bacteroides*). Those same bacteria were found (from human stool samples) to be deficient in depressed people (Strandwitz et al., 2019).

Another part of the answer to biome impacts on stress tolerance, anxiety, and depression comes from research with the usual lab denizens. Chevaliar et al. (2020) showed that transplanting fecal material from stressed rodents into contented ones downregulated the endocannabinoid systems in the recipients, nudging those formerly happy creatures toward depression (and not merely because they hated the fecal transplant idea). Exercise similarly increases endocannabinoids by changing the balance of gut bacteria in favor of those bacteria that produce the endocannabinoid molecules.

**Other microbiome impacts.** Research of that type with critters led Sawada et al. (2017) to study the impact of a strain of *Lactobacillus gasseri* on Japanese medical students who were taking a potentially-stressful course in cadaver dissection. The students participated in a double-blind randomized-control trial with a crossover design—a powerful design in which each of the men (yes, only men) served as his own control. The students were first randomly assigned to four weeks of receiving either a placebo or a probiotic containing the *Lactobacillus gasseri*. A three-week washout period followed with neither probiotics nor placebo consumed. Then for the next four weeks, the former probiotic-condition students received the placebo, and vice versa for the control students.

The results were spectacular. The probiotic treatment significantly reduced anxiety ($p < .05$) on both anxiety measures, and reduced depressive mood on one of the two measures ($p < .05$). Various dimensions of sleep quality were also assessed by questionnaire, with overall sleep quality significantly improved by the probiotic.

The physiological differences between conditions similarly supported the efficacy of the probiotic. Stool assessments showed that the probiotic treatment caused substantial changes in the microbiome, completely eliminating some bacteria known to increase inflammation. The probiotics even had impacts on genetic transcription. Specifically, the genes in blood leukocytes that are normally activated in stressful episodes were suppressed by the administration of *Lactobacillus gasseri*. Cortisol levels were also reduced ($p < .05$). Thus the probiotic had physiological toughening impacts identical to those from some nutrients and from some toughening activities.

That same research team tested whether "zombie" (i.e., dead) forms of the same strain of bacteria could improve stress-related behavior and relieve symptoms of irritable bowel syndrome. Nisheda et al. (2017) used heat to "inactivate" *Lactobacillus gasseri*. (To be clear, they killed the little buggers.) In the randomized-control trial, the 69 Japanese medical students (both females and males this time) received either the deceased bacteria or a placebo during the 12-week period of preparation for their national professional exam.

Besides having positive impact on the anxiety levels of (only) the women students in the study, the dead bacteria led to significantly improved sleep quality, as assessed both by questionnaires and by EEGs. The consumption of "zombie" bacteria also reduced basal cortisol levels and reduced expression of stress-responsive microRNAs in circulating leukocytes, improved functioning of the parasympathetic NS, and normalized bowel habits even during the stressful preparation for the exam. The impact of the dead *Lactobacillus gasseri* suggests that some components of those dead cells may have caused gut cells themselves to react in meaningful ways.

With such impressive individual studies, we should expect the reviews to be equally supportive. Indeed, in their summary of research on "Microbes and the mind ..." Smith and Wissel (2019) cited studies with humans showing that in general people with psychopathologies such as chronic anxiety, depression, or even autism have gut bacteria that are different from people without those pathologies. And they noted that several specific species of gut bacteria corresponded with anxiety and with depression. Even the total bacterial load proved to be important; a robust population of gut bacteria corresponds with positive moods and states of well-being, whereas low levels portend negative well-being. (Contemplate that when considering your next bacteria-destroying antibiotic.)

Noonan et al. (2020) provided a particularly thorough review of the impacts of the microbiome on anxiety and depression. They examined studies published in the last 15 years that focused on probiotic and prebiotic therapies for clinical levels of depression and anxiety—levels that go well beyond the mood shifts experienced by the Japanese medical students of the studies reviewed above. Noonan et al. found only seven randomized-control trials that fit their rigorous criteria, and even those studies were limited by short durations and limited numbers of participants. Nevertheless, Noonan et al. concluded that the reviewed studies showed that both probiotics and prebiotics (especially in combination) reduced depression; but as you might expect by now, similar impacts on anxiety were not as well established. Furthermore, they noted that individuals who had co-morbid gut conditions such as irritable bowel syndrome were most likely to benefit from probiotic and/or prebiotic treatments. Of the 12 bacteria strains tested in the seven reviewed studies, three strains seemed most effective for relieving depression. Two were in the genus

*Lactobacillus* (i.e., *acidophilus* and *casei*)—a genus obviously capable of heroic action. The third strain was *Bifidobacterium bifidium.*

All of the foregoing shows that the human microbiome functions like a kind of endocrine organ capable of producing important neurochemicals that can contribute to brain health, cognitive preservation, and even the physiological toughness described in Chapter 19. By making that contribution, the biome can reduce stress responses, reduce depression, and at least sometimes, and particularly in women, reduce anxiety as well.

**Summary.** Our nutrients and our microbiome indirectly and/or directly transcribe genes temporarily, and they methylate (and acetylate) genes more permanently, much as well-established toughening activities do. Those genetic modifications in turn impact neurotropins and neurotransmitters in ways that build brain structures, enhance cognition, and lead to stress tolerance and resistance to the moods we wish to keep at bay.

Chapter 19

# Nutrition toughens body, brain, and mind

A *National Geographic* magazine title (from November, 2005) asked "What if I said you could add up to ten years to your life?" A later title in *Newsweek* (July 24, 2013) asked "Is immortality plausible? Or is it quack science?" In my previous book on physiological toughness, I touched on those topics (Dienstbier, 2015, p. 121), but I said virtually nothing about nutrition, although I pretended to know something when I wrote that

> *gaining 10 more years from only dietary modifications is not going to happen. Instead, to get the full 10 years, we shall need to extract other implements from the scientific tool box. And besides settling for just the added years, let us include some adjectives like 'sharp,' or at least 'lucid,' keeping quality centrally in mind.*

It is often fun (but seldom graceful) to quote oneself, but that passage, perhaps in error, seemed to be an appropriate start for this chapter.

Before diving further into toughness, I note a recent paper that estimates the years that can be gained from wise choices of nutrition (Fadnes et al., 2022). Following a superbly extensive review of the relevant research, Fadnes et al. concluded that the actual lifespan gains from positive dietary modifications depend upon the age at which one either adopts better nutrition or removes the poor choices. Fadnes et al. even specify the potential gains in lifespan from the specific dietary elements that are increased (e.g., whole grains) or decreased (processed meats). Contradicting my uninformed introduction above, Fadnes et al. concluded that it may actually be possible to add a decade with wise food choices. But that was about lifespan, and one must begin healthy consumption while still young. Similar conclusions about cognitive brilliance must await further research.

Below I describe briefly how a couple of the "other implements from the scientific tool box" build the physiological toughness that leads to enhanced cognitive capacities and to resilience. Showing how toughness develops serves also to explain the nature of toughness beyond the brief paragraph offered in Chapter 18. The toughening activities I mentioned there were physical exercise, cognitive stimulation, confronting manageable stressors, practicing self control, meditation, and affectionate activities. Feeling concern for the wellbeing of readers who have ventured this far, I will limit my analysis here to the two activities we tend to think of first when considering activities that enhance lifespan, healthspan, and mental/psychological health—cognitive stimulation and physical exercise.

Below I first explain in general terms what physiological toughness means, and how it develops. Then I present research showing how enhanced cognitive capacities and resilience result from the long-term practice of physical exercise and cognitive challenge. Finally, I blend in information on how nutrition fits into that picture of toughness.

**Developing toughness.** Physiological toughness develops in response to systematically repeating cycles of toughening activities and rest. Performing the toughening activities requires neurological and endocrine processes that necessarily dispense neurochemicals and consume energy. Later, during rest, those previously depleted physiological systems are restored to their pre-activity levels. But the real magic happens when those cycles of activity and rest are repeated, and repeated. Just as repeating physical workouts results in greater and greater amounts of stored energy (especially with aerobic exercise), and larger and stronger muscles (especially with resistance exercise), the repeated use of almost any of the systems in our body, *including neural and endocrine systems*, leads to rebuilding the capacities of those systems to levels way higher than their original base rates.

Those processes of rebuilding depend, in turn, on our genes, because as we recover from any of those toughening activities, various genes are transcribed (activated), resulting in short-term protein production. But even long-term epigenetic modifications can result from toughening activities—modifications that cause the affected genes to become either more or less responsive to future transcription. Those epigenetic modifications may last for a month or two, or even for a lifetime, but they are individually tailored, depending upon our inherited genes. For example, cutting-edge research shows that people who have inherited different alleles of specific genes have different neural stem cell responses to both diet and to exercise (Klinedinst, 2020). Thus impacts on the brain from diets like the Med, or from exercise routines, are somewhat different for different people. Those differences in genetic makeup also affect the ways our brains respond to aging, so that aging-caused impacts on memory and cognition differ between individuals (de Lucia et al., 2020).

**Toughened arousal systems.** Whether from exercise, cognitive challenges, socializing, meditation, etc., toughening activities alternated with periods of rest eventually result in our hormones being balanced and well-regulated. As mentioned briefly in Chapter 18, toughening increases the capacity of the sympathetic NS, so that challenges or stressors requiring energy and arousal can be met with appropriately-intense responses. But being toughened also means that Sympathetic NS arousal more quickly returns to base-rate levels when high-arousal emergencies are over. Control of the Sympathetic NS also becomes more nuanced, with smaller responses to less important situations (compared to the larger arousal of un-toughened individuals). Toughness also leads to reduced pituitary-adrenal-cortical arousal (PAC) responses to many situations, and to lower PAC-system base rates, as indicated by lower cortisol levels, and to more stable diurnal shifts of PAC system arousal.

Because it is a central idea of this chapter, please note that those modifications to arousal systems from toughening activities are exactly the same modifications that resulted from the diet modifications offered to the monkeys participating in the study by Shively et al. (2020, reviewed in Chapter 18.) It was the monkeys benefiting from the Med-like diet (contrasted with those dissipating on the Western) whose sympathetic NS and PAC systems were obviously toughened. It is interesting, is it not, to see nutrition and toughening activities leading to the same physiological outcomes.

**Genetic responses.** Most importantly, genetic transcription and the subsequent epigenetic modifications that follow toughening activities result in enhanced supplies of essential neurochemicals and in bulking up the neural structures that were busily employed. Thus as toughness develops, supplies increase of great brain-building neurotropins such as BDNF; receptor densities for the neurotropins are enhanced as well. Toughness also implies adequate supplies and balanced levels of stimulating neurotransmitters such as glutamate, dopamine, and noradrenaline on the one hand, and inhibiting and calming neurotransmitters such as GABA and serotonin on the other. All of those modifications to body and brain are subsumed by the term physiological toughness.

Physiological toughness in turn leads to enhanced mental energy, sharpened cognitive capacities, and to psychological resilience. The cognitive capacities that are enhanced include the formation and retrieval of memories, fluid intelligence (i.e., problem-solving), and even the ability to maintain self control. Psychological resilience implies stress tolerance and emotional stability—especially appropriate control of anxiety and depression.

**Toughness influences future choices.** Once physiological toughness results in the experience of enhanced mental and physical energy, and of enhanced cognitive capacities, we are more likely to appraise life's various dilemmas as challenges rather than as threats, and thus we are more likely to approach them. Confronting new challenges toughens us even more. Thus as toughness develops we can enter an upward spiral where toughness leads to choices that in turn continue to toughen us.

## Toughness from cognitive challenges

With that abstract understanding of the development of toughness behind us, consider the specific case of how frequently engaging with cognitive challenge leads to physiological toughness and then to enhanced cognitive capacities and resilience.

"Use it or lose it" seems clearly to apply to the case of cognitively-challenging activities requiring mental energy and intensive mental processing, eventually leading to enhanced mental capacities. And indeed, a variety of correlational studies show that enhanced cognitive capacities do result from mentally challenging and stimulating activities such as learning a second language (e.g., Craik et al., 2010), or learning to play a musical instrument (Hanna-Pladdy & Gajewski, 2012), or from having more challenging occupations, or simply from leading more stimulating lives. (Hertzog et al., 2008, provide a thorough review indicating, for example, several times more Alzheimer's for the least cognitively active people). Reflecting the concept of cognitive reserve, early-life and mid-life cognitive activity also delays cognitive decline in the elderly years (Wilson et al., 2013). Even mice who benefit from cognitive enrichment in their puppyhoods show greater intelligence well into their dotage (Meany et al., 1990).

**Challenge reviews.** Except for the research with the smart mice, of course, those correlational studies are subject to the usual problems of interpretation of causality. Fortunately, Valenzuela and Sachdev (2009) conducted a meta-analysis of relevant randomized-control trials of cognitive enrichment training with people—training lasting from 10 to over 100 hours. Such training did enhance cognitive abilities, with an impressive effect size ($d = 1.00$; remember, effect size is explained in the Glossary). Unfortunately, most of the included studies assessed the same dimensions of cognitive capacity that were used in the training. Clearly, "training for the test" works, but it is hardly the holy grail we seek.

Fortunately, some positive exceptions exist where more general cognitive skills improved following unrelated training. For example, some video games have shown promise for improving fluid intelligence (Basak et al., 2008) and some individual studies (e.g., Park et al., 2014) and general reviewers have shown that such gains can accrue from training that employs a variety of stimulating activities (Tranter & Koutstaal, 2008). Although a few such studies show promise, the debate continues between those who believe we can get generally smarter from circumscribed training protocols, and those who do not. But positive interpretations are supported by studies showing physiological toughness resulting from cognitive training.

**Paths for challenge to enhance cognition.** Perhaps it is largely because most people eschew brain cannulas implanted for research purposes that it is mostly animal research that shows impacts of cognitive stimulation on neurochemistry (e.g., Meaney et al., 1990). During intense cognitive activity, the active neurons release transcription molecules that activate genes in neurons and glia. Those genes then (indirectly) create neurotropins such as the esteemed neurotropin BDNF. When the epigenetic modifications of methylation and acetylation also occur, some of those impacts can last a lifetime. The structural modifications from both the short-term and the long-term impacts on the genes can foster neural development. That development is most evident in the prefrontal cortex, the hippocampi, and the entorhinal cortex—a structure adjacent to the hippocampi that shows deterioration early in the development of Alzheimer's disease. In addition to aiding in neural maintenance and growth, other enrichment-stimulated neurotropins expand vascular networks in the brain. (All of these modifications are discussed more thoroughly in my earlier book—Dienstbier, 2015.)

The efficiency of neural transmission is enhanced by cognitive enrichment, especially in neurons that depend on the neurotransmitters glutamate and acetylcholine. Enrichment also results in greater sensitivity to cortisol due to increased receptor densities, especially in the hippocampi—sensitivity that enhances the control of cortisol during stress and the downregulation of cortisol when stress ends.

The most spectacular evidence for brain impacts from cognitive enrichment comes from MRI scans of people. For example, Draganski et al. (2006) scanned the brains of German medical students (and controls) three times. The first was at the start of the intensive study by the med students for a vital medical exam (the dreaded physikum). The second was three months later at the time of the exam, and the third was three months after the exam. Compared to the controls, during the intensive study before the exam, the hippocampi and nearby cortical areas grew remarkably and the hippocampi *continued to expand* during the 3-month post-examination period, apparently reflecting the development of new hippocampal neurons.

Similarly, Martensson et al. (2012) scanned the brains of Swedish military-language-school students before and after three months of intensive foreign-language study. Compared with university students, the intensive language study stimulated measurable growth in hippocampi and other language-related cortical structures. Thus the physiological research with both animals and people shows how mental enrichment can enhance the elements of physiological toughness that in turn underlay cognitive abilities and delay dementia.

## Toughness from physical exercise

With exercise, the "use it or lose it" expression does not seem to apply to cognitive preservation—at least not intuitively. It is not obvious why regularly taxing (say) leg muscles in daily workouts leads to brain development, or cognitive enhancement and emotional stability. But correlational studies show large and consistent positive impacts, sometimes in studies with thousands of participants. Those correlational studies suggest strongly that exercise sharpens cognitive capacities and leads to emotional stability. But it is the random-assignment studies we need.

**Randomized-control trial reviews.** Colcombe and Kramer (2003) reviewed the random-assignment studies published between 1965 and 2001 that assessed people who were at least 55 years old. Their review was subsequently updated with a meta-analysis by Hertzog et al. (2008). In those studies, aerobic exercise was contrasted with control conditions of (usually) either stretching and toning or non-exercise activities.

To fully appreciate these impacts of exercise on cognition, keep in mind that exercise training has no element of training for the test. Using cognitive tests before and after those months-long training periods, the impact of exercise programs on gains in measures of cognitive skills was very substantial (an effect size of $d = .48$). Heyn et al. (2004) did a similar meta-analysis of the impacts of exercise on delaying dementia, finding a similar effect size of $d = .57$. The largest impacts from exercise were noted for older participants and for women. Note that exercise, like various nutrients, has the most substantial positive impacts on people likely to be initially deficient.

**Paths for exercise to enhance cognition.** Some of the neurochemicals that support brain health and growth are first produced in the body in response to exercise, and then cross the blood-brain barrier to nurture the brain. Exercise also stimulates other neurochemical production directly in the brain. For example, a single bout of exercise releases the neurotropin BDNF, first in body and later in the brain, and a long-term exercise program increases the brain's BDNF base rates and receptor densities. Other brain-building neurotropins follow similar toughening-stimulated paths (Cotman et al., 2007; Zoladz et al., 2008; Erickson et al., 2013).

Like the benefits we gain from the phytonutrients discussed in Chapter 6 and the vitamins of Chapters 8 and 9, moderate exercise reduces oxidative stress by upregulating antioxidant enzymes and the "master" antioxidant glutathione, and by activating the DNA-repair functions of the seven sirtuins that were described in Chapter 15 (Grabowska et al., 2017). Exercise also removes arterial plaque, resulting (through several steps) in reduced inflammation, enhanced neurotropin levels, and attenuated stress responses (Chapman et al., 2010; Miller & Blackwell, 2006).

Another avenue for exercise mimicking various anti-inflammatory nutrients is through its impact on the microbiome. Vijay et al. (2021) randomly assigned 78 arthritic people to 15 minutes of strength-building exercise daily for six weeks. Compared with the non-exercising controls, the composition of gut bacteria changed. After the exercise, the gut denizens produced more of various anti-inflammatories, including some cytokines and the short-chain fatty acids discussed in Chapter 16. And the exercise resulted in higher levels of the endocannabinoids that were noted in Chapter 18 for their mood-stabilizing role.

Exercise also builds the brain's capacity to produce some essential neurotransmitters. Specifically, exercise increases noradrenaline (Brown et al., 1979) and serotonin (Greenwood et al., 2005) and controls cortisol during stress (e.g., Droste et al., 2007). Research with various critters shows that exercise programs enhance stores of brain glycogen, ultimately providing more mental energy (Matsui et al., 2012), and exercise builds the density of mitochondria within neurons (in mice, at least), also leading to enhanced mental energy (Steiner et al., 2011).

Brain scans reinforce those observations. Burdette et al. (2010) showed enhanced hippocampal blood circulation in randomly assigned elderly participants after four months of aerobic exercise training. With similar participants (and training) Colcombe et al. (2004) showed enhanced blood flow into prefrontal cortical and parietal areas of the brain structures. Such circulatory enhancements delay cognitive decline and dementia and protect against depression (Frasure-Smith & Lesperance, 2005; Jefferson et al., 2010). (Perhaps those observations remind you of similar impacts on enhanced brain blood flow from cacao, ginkgo, bacopa, and resveratrol.)

Colcombe et al. (2006) showed increases in the volume of both gray and white matter in frontal and temporal brain regions of randomly-assigned aerobically trained elderly participants. And in an outstanding study, Erickson et al. (2011) randomly assigned 120 older adults (average age 66 years) to a full year of aerobic training or to a control condition of stretching and toning. In contrast to the expectation for the normal rate of hippocampal shrinkage for the elderly of 1% per year, the aerobically trained participants showed a 2% increase in hippocampal volume (while the control people had 1.4% shrinkage). Hippocampal increases corresponded with improvements in fitness levels and with measures of cognitive performance.

## Integrating nutrition with toughening activities

As shown throughout all the previous chapters, besides all those physiological modifications and cognitive gains that are affected by toughening activities, those modifications and gains are all similarly affected by various nutrients. Undoubtedly you recall many of those specific similarities, and many were reiterated above. For example, like toughening activities, many nutrients have antioxidant and anti-inflammatory affects, many enhance neurotransmitters and neurotropins, some increase cerebral blood flow, and some have been shown to build brain structures, especially the prefrontal cortex and hippocampi. And like the toughening activities, many nutrients enhance cognition or at least delay cognitive decline, and many have been shown to enhance resilience. After all, that is the very reason those nutrients starred in their various sections of the preceding chapters. To preserve your patience, I will not elaborate further on those many parallels between toughening activities and various nutrients.

Those similarities of impact lead to the question of whether toughening activities and great nutrition might substitute for each other, or whether they simply complement each other in building physiological toughness, brain integrity, cognitive capacity, and resilience. At a basic level, that question is whether we really need to exercise or remain cognitively active (etc.) to flourish. Instead, could we become stable geniuses merely by daily consumption of some chocolate, or tea, or even red wine? On the other hand, if we exercise daily, or study Arabic, or learn to meditate, do we really need to eat the berries and the leafy greens and avoid that bacon-fried steak?

Despite the obvious parallels of impacts between various nutrients and toughening activities, few studies attempt to directly address that issue by comparing and contrasting influences on brain and cognition from great nutrients on the one hand and effective toughening activities on the other. A few studies combine nutrition and toughening to show joint impacts, but while that approach is informative, it does not address the specific questions of identity of impacts, or the question of substituting one for the other. Nevertheless, consider a few of those studies of combinations.

**Combining toughening nutrition and toughening activities.** Using Air Force personnel who were all undergoing a rigorous physical training regime for 12 weeks, Zwilling et al. (2021) randomly assigned them to either a normal diet that included placebo capsules, or the same normal diet but with capsules that supplied the nutrients of the Med diet. (Of course the capsules allow participants and researchers to remain blind as to the participants' conditions.) The Med diet supplements significantly enhanced the effects of exercise alone on a few of the several cognitive and the physical measures.

Those results should not be surprising for enterprising bodybuilders, except that the supplements consisted of Med diet nutrients, rather than muscle-building protein.

Another approach was taken in the following two studies, both mentioned in Chapter 15 on mitochondria. Andreaux et al. (2019) assessed the impact on mitochondria from daily doses of urolithin A (usually derived from pomegranate). The physiological improvements in the mitochondria from four weeks of the supplement were judged by the researchers to be at a level that would be achieved from 10 weeks of aerobic exercise. Andreaux et al. could not make direct comparisons of the impacts from urolithin A versus those from exercise, but nevertheless concluded that while both were effective, the nutrient was more so.

To appreciate this next study, recall that MitoQ is an enhanced form of CoQ10—and thus that MitoQ supports mitochondria. In a well-designed randomized-control trial, Rossman et al. (2018) studied impacts on arterial stiffness from only six weeks of MitoQ supplementation. They judged that the 42% improvement in flexibility from the MitoQ was somewhat equivalent to improvements achieved by caloric restriction (from other studies, estimated to be 30%) and to improvements from aerobic exercise (estimated to be 50%). Remember, benefits to the cardiovascular system lead to benefits to the brain, and then to cognition. But as with the study by Andreaux et al., the research did not provide direct comparisons of impacts from the nutrient versus from the exercise or caloric restriction.

Similarly, in their review Grabowska et al. (2017) noted research showing benefits to longevity and physical performance in mice and rats from combinations of resveratrol and habitual exercise. Grabowska et al. noted that resveratrol has its impacts through effects on the *FOXO3* gene—a gene that is also transcribed by even a single bout of exercise. The *FOXO3* gene influences a variety of vital functions that contribute to healthspan and lifespan in mammals like us. (Lifespan extension from combinations of resveratrol with exercise suggests the possible benefits of post-exercise thirst quenching with red wine. That is probably not a good idea, but still ...)

Grabowska et al. (2017) also noted that supplements of curcumin (from turmeric) had similar impacts, enhancing the effects of exercise training on exercise capacity, fatigue resistance, and general stress tolerance. Those positive curcumin impacts resulted from enhancing activities of the sirtuins that in turn repair DNA, support the mitochondria, and otherwise positively impact genes that affect various processes associated with aging. Also without making direct comparisons, Grabowska et al. noted that both exercise and curcumin positively stimulate those many vital impacts of the seven sirtuins.

An interesting randomized-control trial by Fitzgerald et al. (2021) is reviewed to illustrate at greater physiological depth how combinations of nutrition and toughening activities extend toughness as well as healthspan and lifespan. Before I review that study, some background:

Remember that a major way that toughening activities and dietary elements (etc.) have long-term genetic impacts is by causing epigenetic modifications that result in genes becoming either more or less responsive to transcription. I noted in Chapter 1 and elsewhere that a gene becomes less responsive when a methyl-group molecule is attached to the gene at a specific place—a processes called methylation (Schumacher et al., 2021). It is remarkable that with only 23 thousand genes in our human genome that we have 20 million (or so) possible methylation sites. That seems excessive.

Of those many methylation sites, there are a few thousand places that become systematically methylated or un-methylated as we age. It is not that overall methylation increases or decreases at those sites, but rather a changing pattern of methylation develops, with some sites losing and others gaining methylation as we grow older. With such age-related changes, it is possible to determine our biological age by comparing our individual methylation pattern with the patterns that are typical for people of different ages.

One set of 353 such genes was selected for the Horvath DNAmAge clock (the middle "m" stands for methylation; see Fitzgerald et al., 2021, for more about the "clock"). The Horvath clock predicts both healthspan and lifespan better than our chronological age, and is one of the most widely used of the four DNA clocks that had been developed by early 2022. Like two of the other developed clocks, the Horvath clock is based on epigenetic modifications of the genes in blood cells, not the brain cells that would be more relevant to our interests (Moore et al., 2013; Grodstein et al., 2020). As an indicator of the important impact of stress on aging, almost a quarter of the genes chosen for the clock regulate stress-relevant processes. (See Harvanek et al., 2021, for impacts of stress on indicators of genetic aging.)

In the introduction to their study, Fitzgerald et al. (2021) first reviewed two studies by other researchers that manipulated diet alone (i.e., studies not including exercise or other toughening activities). Using the Horvath DNAmAge clock, one of those studies found a reduction of a year and a half in biological age from a one-year Mediterranean diet—one that added extra vitamin D to the Med. That study by Quach et al. (2017) concluded that analyses of blood using the epigenetic clock support the observation that healthspan and lifespan are enhanced by plant-based diets with lean meats, moderate alcohol, some physical activity and cognitive stimulation.

The other study cited by Fitzgerald et al. showed a reduction of almost two years in biological age resulting from a 16-week course of massive vitamin D supplementation in people who were originally deficient in vitamin D.

Fitzgerald et al. considered their own research to be a pilot study because it randomly assigned only 43 healthy adult males between the ages of 50-72 to the no-intervention control condition or to the 8-week healthy-lifestyle treatment program. The dependent measure was change in biological age, as determined by the pre- and post-treatment epigenetic indicators of the methylation clock.

The healthy-lifestyle treatment was designed to affect sleep, exercise, relaxation, and diet. The diet was specifically designed to be nutrient rich, especially with phytonutrients, and included supplemental vitamin A, vitamin B-9 (folate), vitamin C, curcumin (presumably from turmeric), EGCG (from tea), and quercetin (associated with grapes, red wine, and ginkgo). The diet was also structured to lower glycemic cycling by restricting carbohydrates and by including "mild intermittent fasting." The supplemental probiotics included one from our favorite genus *Lactobacillus* (specifically the species *plantarum*). The regime included 30 minutes of exercise at least five days per week at around 70% maximum exertion and twice-daily breathing exercises to induce relaxation. At least seven hours of sleep was recommended.

Although the treatment was only eight weeks long, compared with themselves at pre-treatment, according to the methylation clock those in the healthy-lifestyle treatment condition were substantially (and almost significantly) "younger" by 1.96 years ($p = .066$). However, compared with the control people, at the study's end the treatment people were significantly "younger" by over three years ($p = .018$). Various biomarkers were also improved by the treatment. Those folks were getting younger!

**But immortality?** At this chapter's beginning, I noted that *Newsweek* had asked "is immortality plausible?" A literal interpretation of the Fitzgerald et al. research seems to provide a positive answer. Considered together, the two studies they reviewed and the new pilot study offered just above suggest requirements for continuous survival. First, we must select our nutrition carefully, especially the Med diet, perhaps with additional vitamin D. From their pilot study, we realize too that beside those additional vitamins and nutrients that a balanced life should include life-style adaptations such as adequate sleep, systematic relaxation, and daily exercise. If we do all that, the research suggests that we can essentially unwind the over-eager methylation that corresponds with aging. Then, with each week of healthful living resulting in unwinding multiple weeks from our personal methylation clocks, immortality seems to be in reach. Maybe, but keep the will, just in case.

**Toughening and nutrition: Identity or mere similarity.** Recall the question raised above of whether great nutrition and effective toughening activities might be substituted for each other. The next two studies—one with mice and one with real people—provide at least partial answers to that question.

You may not recall the mouse study by Huang et al. (2018; mentioned in Chapter 10) that showed positive effects from magnesium supplements and environmental enrichment on the cognitive capacities of aging mice. The mice experienced either enrichment alone, or magnesium supplements alone, or a combination of magnesium plus enrichment. For both young and elderly mice, the combination of enrichment plus magnesium was superior to either treatment alone—superior both for the development of synapses in the hippocampi and for improved cognition and spatial memory. Even though the research was with mice rather than people, and about magnesium rather than (say) the Med diet, the results argue against toughening activities and nutrition substituting for each other as if they had identical impacts; rather, their impacts seemed additive and thus probably different.

But for our needs, this final study by Sánchez-Villegas et al. (2016) is more directly relevant, and fortunately was done with people. Although the main focus of the study was on joint impacts of nutrition and some toughening activities on depression, in this case, depression can stand in for other aspects of resilience, and perhaps also for cognitive preservation.

Sánchez-Villegas et al. followed a large cohort of 11,800 Spanish university graduates for an average of 8.5 years to determine the relative contributions of diet, exercise, and socializing on depression. Adherence to the Med diet, physical activity and socializing with friends were each assessed with validated questionnaires. The research took into account a vast array of potentially-confounding factors, including various indicators of health, demographic variables, and lifestyle factors.

In the third of the participants who adhered least to the Med diet, there were 298 confirmed cases of depression in contrast to 250 cases in the third who were most faithful to that diet (reflecting a hazard ratio of HR = .84; $p = .06$). The top third in exercise and top third in socializing with friends were also contrasted with the bottom third in each of those two categories. The hazard ratio for exercise was an identical HR = .84 ($p = .05$); for socialization it was, HR = .79 ($p = .02$). Thus diet, exercise, and socialization were almost equally effective in resisting depression.

But then Sánchez-Villegas et al. computed a *Mediterranean lifestyle index* including all three of those factors, and then compared people in the top, middle, and bottom thirds of the index, taking into account the usual possibly-confounding variables. The hazard ratio for depression was HR = .50, indicating only half as many people in the top third (compared with bottom third) suffered from depression, and furthermore indicating that diet, socializing, and exercise did not substitute for each other, but rather that each apparently contributed unique means for preventing depression.

**Impacts of nutrition versus toughening: A reprise.** (For this discussion "cognition" stands in for resisting cognitive decline and fostering psychological resilience; "toughness" is short for "brain enhancement and physiological toughness.")

I have presented two contrasting themes: The first is that toughening activities and some nutrients have very similar impacts on cognition and toughness by taking the same mediating paths to cognition or toughness. For example, both the nutrition and the toughening activities may increase BDNF or ergothioneine, or they both might inhibit evil methylglyoxal or distorted tau protein in the brain. With such common paths, adding the nutrition and toughening activities together would add very little to cognition or toughness. Either would suffice to create genius or stability, and it should even be possible to substitute the one for the other.

The second theme, illustrated especially by the research of Sánchez-Villegas et al., is that toughening activities and certain nutrients have non-overlapping impacts on cognition or toughness—implying that they take different paths to the same positive impacts on brain and cognition. For example, antioxidant efforts by an effective nutrient but inflammation reduction by the toughening activity may both enhance cognition and toughness. With each making unique contributions to cognition and to toughness, combining them would lead to greatly enhanced outcomes as it did in the study by Sánchez-Villegas et al.

Although appearing contradictory at first, certainly both those themes are true—at least somewhat. Just as certainly, if we considered only the toughening activities (leaving out the nutrients for a moment) certainly, those same conclusions would apply: that the various toughening activities make both unique and common contributions to our well-being (as noted in Dienstbier, 2015). Finally, it is also apparent that the same conclusion applies to both unique and common contributions from different nutrients, even when those different nutrients foster the same results of enhanced cognition, or toughness.

That analysis, and especially the final point, reminds us (doesn't it?) of the great study of tea and coffee by Zhang, Yang et al. (2021) that was reviewed in Chapter 7. Using 365 thousand British people of the Biobank cohort Zhang, Yang et al. looked at the prevention of dementia and stroke. It was noted that for people who consumed *both* tea and coffee, the joint benefits were greater than those from consuming even ideal amounts of *either* tea or coffee. However, although those results suggested different benefits from tea than from coffee, there were undoubtedly some other benefits common to both beverages.

**Summary.** In the long-term, toughening activities toughen us through a variety of avenues that ultimately affect the functioning of our genes, largely through epigenetic processes. In their detailed analysis of impacts from nutrition and toughening activities, Grabowska et al. made similar observations for nutrition. They noted that the means for various nutrients leading to protection against cognitive decline is by affecting genetic functioning by causing epigenetic modifications. Indeed, appropriate nutrition toughens.

Chapter 20

# After thoughts

If a new edition of this book were produced just five or ten years from now, other nutrients would undoubtedly need to be included—nutrients such as selenium and NAD+ that may ultimately prove to be wonderful for brain and cognition. Today we do not know everything, and surely we will not in another 10 years either. But even with the things we know with confidence today about various individual nutrients, wise nutritionists and many successful randomized-control trials suggest that benefits to brain and mind are maximized in complex diets that feature combinations of nutrients—diets such as the Med and the MIND (e.g., Panza et al., 2018).

**Research issues (again).** The randomized-control trials that assess individual nutrients have often been less consistent than the correlational ones. In fact, even after successful cross-sectional and longitudinal studies of individual nutrients, and even after physiological studies that showed how the studied nutrient benefits neurochemistry and/or brain structure, we have seen numerous instances of well-constructed randomized-control studies with people that failed to support those results. At least some of those disappointing results may be due to the randomized-control trials studying single nutrients, often as supplements, rather than studying them as components of food in complete diets.

But of course, some of those weak or null results may have resulted from the studies just being too short. For example, recall that the studies of ginkgo reviewed in Chapter 12 were successful only when treatments lasted at least 22 weeks; most of the shorter studies failed. One of the take-away lessons is that when we begin any new dietary regime, perhaps we should not expect new foods or supplements (or the new rhythm of our meals) to be wildly beneficial until we have been using the new regimes for months, or even years. As with toughening activities, both long-term practice and patience may be required.

Before I offer my conclusions about nutrients that maintain toughness, brain health, cognitive capacities, and resilience, consider that by this point, you too have seen the conclusions from the more than 300 research papers and reviews that have provided this book's sustenance. Thus your own well-informed conclusions and perhaps even those of your physician may better fit your own unique circumstances. In these concluding thoughts, I avoid repeating the citations that are sequestered in the relevant chapters.

## Major dietary approaches

**Fats and phytonutrients.** Foremost, mimic the Med and the MIND diets as much as possible. Recall that some nutritionists believe that olive oil is the most important single ingredient in the Med, and recall too the research showing that the Med seemed most effective for boosting cognition when supplemented with extra olive oil. But use olive oil or other unsaturated oils in place of less-admirable fats (not in addition to them), especially replacing butter, and other saturated fats. Forget transfats completely.

To further honor the Med, emphasize veggies and fruits. Especially, as emphasized in the MIND, seek out the highly colored fruits, like most berries, for the phytonutrients known as polyphenols. And to gain the brain benefits from the other major branch of the phytonutrients—the carotenoids—munch yellow and red veggies too. The green leafies are a requirement. Thus the veg and fruit salad with the olive oil dressing is a winner. All those veggies and fruits contribute to the various types of phytonutrients that have been shown to be major contributors to neurochemistry and cognition. Many have proven effective as antioxidants and anti-inflammatories, and in the bargain, they often support great neurotropins such as BDNF, and assure supplies of our favorite neurotransmitters, including serotonin, dopamine, and especially acetylcholine.

Given that there are literally thousands of different phytonutrients, it follows that relatively few have been identified as especially effective and have been singled out for intensive study. Many of the phytonutrients that have been studied intensively include the flavonoids (specifically the flavonols) of cacao, the polyphenol resveratrols from grapes and red wine, and the carotenoid β carotene for its impacts on eyes, the immune system, and (thought the research is scanty) the brain. As hinted above, almost everything good about the Med and MIND diets depends upon adequate consumption of phytonutrients.

Med and MIND diets also ask us that whenever possible, we avoid processed foods. Take to heart the huge international meta-analysis that damned processed meats for causing cardiovascular and mortality problems. And avoid foods with added sugar, especially avoiding those with a high glycemic index. Apparently (and painfully), my chocolate croissant has been ruled out, but dark chocolate, with its generous dollop of cacao, seems to be one of the few foods where some added sugar is worth the exchange for its flavonoid benefits. The cacao-derived flavonoids benefit brain neurochemistry (e.g., BDNF), brain structure, brain circulation, and cognition. (Consider, as I do, whether cacao benefits could be evidence of beneficent celestial intervention.)

**Carbohydrates, glucose and ketones.** Surges of blood glucose are certainly not good for brain, and become more problematic for our health as we edge towards old, elderly, or (hopefully) even ancient. But surges are not the only issue. When diets such as the Western have us systematically consuming sugar by the handfuls, both the high base-rate levels of blood glucose and the high insulin levels that result are horrible for brain and cognition. Perhaps we should solve these issues with ketones.

Besides adhering to the keto or other carbohydrate restricting diets, other means of controlling blood glucose and substituting brain-benefiting ketones were described in Chapter 17. Of the various approaches, restricting the window for eating each day seemed the most humane, with even daily 14-hour fasts encouraging the ketone production that substitutes for glucose, with attendant benefits for mitochondria and brains. I strongly suspect that adding some glucose-consuming exercise during that fasting window would enhance the effectiveness of that approach by further depleting our stores of carbohydrates, and thus stimulating ketone production.

**Protein.** As urged by Med-like diets, aspire to get most of your protein from plants, but as long as you and the environment can afford it, at a minimum consume a serving of fish per week, or even better, two. To maximize omega 3s, fatty ocean fish are best. And even though the randomized-control trials with omega 3s do not conclusively demonstrate great impacts on human brains and cognition, the correlational studies and other forms of research do. Thus nutritionists generally agree that omega 3s, either from fish or fish oil supplements, will buttress our neural-cell membranes and keep our brains operating smoothly. The omega 3s seem especially effective for people already experiencing some cognitive decline.

However, if resisting protein (perhaps in the form of a 16-ounce Nebraska T-bone) creates anguish, remember the evidence that meat from grass-fed animals seems to be much better for brain, and for healthspan. Forget "well marbled;" marble is for your sarcophagus, and "well marbled" may lead to it. Besides the grass-eaters eulogized here, consider chicken. It is even encouraged in some of the Med variations.

## Other nutrients

**Caffeine, coffee, and tea.** Caffeine certainly offers us energy. And depending on our genes and other factors, those short-term benefits may become long-term benefits for some of us, but the research is not consistent. Coffee is different. Coffee definitely provides polyphenols that benefit the brain and cognition. If those nutrients were the sole reason for the benefits derived from coffee, then decaf should be equally great, but some studies showed only modest (or no) benefits from decaf. In both short-term and long-term studies, caffeinated coffee benefited brain and cognition with two *major caveats*. First, (especially long-term) coffee benefits accrue only if it is *filtered* through paper filters; studies that do not account for filtration methods may account for some of the conflicting results in that research literature. Second, like almost everything that we consume, coffee can be overdone. More than six cups per day will apparently dull even well-sharpened cognitive processes. Benefits from coffee (and possibly from caffeine) are also likely to be affected by our genes and the composition of our individual microbiomes. Remember that variations between us in our biomes are much greater than our genetic variations.

Like coffee, tea with its EGCG is great for both lifespan and healthspan, including the (I'll use it only once) "smartspan" we all crave. Drink any kind of tea—green, black, or maté, and don't worry about filters. Obviously, neither the tea nor the coffee is worth it if the caffeine causes problems, but the tea has half the caffeine of the coffee and the decaf coffee is probably an appropriate alternative. (Unfortunately, there are so many kinds of herbal and decaffeinated teas that there is no substantial body of research on their impacts on brain or cognition.)

**Alcohol and red wine.** As said in the Chapter 14 summary, moderate drinking may protect the brain and cognition in some people, depending on genetics, age, one's physical condition, the rhythm of drinking, and the beverage chosen. However, the evidence for any brain/cognitive benefits from any amount of alcohol is very inconsistent. Red wine is clearly an exception. The wine supplies resveratrol, quercetin, and other beneficial polyphenols; other beneficial nutrients from the wine are manufactured by our gut bacteria. Remember, however, that adequate resveratrol levels can be achieved by regularly eating grapes. A combination barely mentioned in the relevant literature is that combining melatonin with resveratrol boosts its powerful impacts, and there is some similar evidence that vitamin D also potentiates resveratrol's positive impacts on the brain.

But even for red wine, some caveats apply: First, benefits accrue if a moderate amount of wine is consumed in a manner that slows its passage through the gut. That means drinking it with food, as recommended in the Med diet. The second caveat begins the next section.

**Vitamins.** For people who regularly consume any type or amount of alcohol, vitamin B levels must be adequate, whether those Bs are derived from food or from supplements. Remember that the Bs are absorbed poorly in the presence of alcohol.

That is not a trivial issue, because several of the Bs are absolutely essential for brain health and for sensible cognition. In fact, as discussed below, when thorough reviewers address the broad question of nutrients that delay or prevent age-related cognitive decline and depression, their conclusions sometimes emphasize the impact of the B vitamins above all other nutrients (Moore et al., 2018; Fenech, 2017).

Whether you drink alcohol or not, seek out those vitamin B supplements especially if your nation does not mandate fortifying flour with B-vitamins. Recall too from Chapter 8 that cognitive benefits from caffeinated coffee were greatest for people taking vitamin B supplements.

Beside those B-vitamins, other vitamins and metals are strongly implicated in brain health, often by nurturing our mitochondria that decline with aging and are overworked during stressful episodes. Vitamin C is important for many brain functions, and it defends the mitochondria through its antioxidant activities and by sustaining adequate levels of glutathione, the master endogenous antioxidant.

Vitamin D is special, not merely because it is actually a hormone, but also by virtue of its effectiveness for reducing depression in (especially) depressed older people who are deficient in vitamin D. Having said that, remember that many nutritionists believe that most of us actually are deficient in vitamin D, and that as we age such deficiencies increase. It is not easy to overdose on D, so consider specific D supplements even beyond the multivitamin.

Another consideration for aging and multis is that if you are over 50 years old, make sure your multi is crafted for older people. The multi's for younger people usually include iron, and we people over 50 should *usually* avoid extra iron.

**Mitochondria.** Nothing is more important for the health of brain (and body) and the wellbeing of cognition and resilience than well-functioning mitochondria. Besides the nutrients mentioned above, other ingredients that maintain mitochondria include zinc and magnesium, urolithin-A (pomegranates), and CoQ10. Of that list, the evidence is high for the importance of adequate zinc to compensate for the frequently noted deficiencies in our diets. Beyond that, although deficiencies in urolithin-A are not a frequent topic in the nutrition literature, it may turn out to be a wonder food; remember, pomegranate juice is cheaper than wine, and undoubtedly better for you. Other nutrients to keep in mind for happy mitochondria include mushrooms and avocados; both keep glutathione levels high, but with mushrooms, we enhance ergothioneine and spermidine too. (Other nutrition that future research may establish to be especially helpful for mitochondria and for brains are MitoQ and NAD+.)

**Spices.** A really brief review of the spices with either proven or promising impact would highlight vast semi-proven potential for ginger. One study (but only one) found spectacular cognitive impacts in women. In animals, it increases both our beloved neurotropins and neurotransmitters, and results in various other identified physiological benefits.

Although the randomized-control trials with people for benefits from curcumin from turmeric and sodium benzoate from cinnamon are not yet convincing, their standing is boosted by animal research that shows that they both cause reductions in the nasty and twisted Alzheimer's proteins (i.e., β-amyloid and tau). Besides, cooking with turmeric and adding a dash of cinnamon to various things (like tea or coffee) cannot be a hardship.

Because saffron is not as frequently touted in nutrition media outlets, its very positive impacts on brain and cognition were (to me) surprising. Saffron also seems to be a powerful antidepressant rivaling the impacts of established antidepressants. But it can be expensive, and nothing in the research suggests it should be substituted for established therapeutics for depression.

**Major reviews of the "best" nutrients.** Although omitted from the lists of some reviewers (who are undoubtedly more sophisticated than me), choline is near the top of my list. Because it is a vital component of acetylcholine (one of the favorite neurotransmitters of the hippocampi), choline is essential for brain function, especially memory. Some nutritionists assert that most of us get insufficient amounts in our food. Unless taking some form of anticholinergic medication, an egg a day (or so) will boost your levels. But also consider taking some form of choline supplement. Multivitamins do not supply it—at least mine doesn't.

But now, I turn to conclusions from real nutritionists. In their review in *Pharmacological Research*, titled "Botanicals and phytochemicals active on cognitive decline ..." Cicero et al. 2018) identified seven nutrients that research has shown to effectively resist cognitive decline. All seven are in my list too, although in this final chapter, I have not summarized any information about ginkgo or bacopa. Their list: cacao, EGCG (tea), ginkgo, bacopa, curcumin (turmeric), saffron, and resveratrol (grapes and red wine).

Fenech (2017) emphasized mainly vitamins. He presented his thorough review titled "Vitamins associated with brain aging, mild cognitive impairment, and Alzheimer disease..." in *Advances in Nutrition*. His list began with the B vitamins, already celebrated above, plus vitamin A (and β-carotene), and vitamin C, vitamin D, and vitamin E. Beyond the vitamins, he listed the Mediterranean diet, flavonoids, omega 3s, and unsaturated fats.

Moore et al. (2018) provided a similar review in the *Proceedings of the Nutrition Society* titled "Diet, nutrition and the ageing brain: Current evidence and new directions." Their list of the most potent nutrients for maintaining cognition and reducing depression began with the Med diet. They described as emerging evidence the current research support for omega 3s, the polyphenols, and vitamin D. However, they noted that:

*the totality of evidence is strongest in support of a role for folate [B-9] and the metabolically related B-vitamins (vitamin B-12, vitamin B-6 and riboflavin [B-2]) in slowing the progression of cognitive decline and possibly reducing the risk of depression in ageing.*

**Contented microbes.** The statement that opened this chapter about the likelihood of new material quickly overtaking our current knowledge about nutrition applies especially to the microbiome. The things we know with certainty are limited, and not very specific. Our gut bacteria regulate and actually produce some neurotransmitters, especially producing the vast majority of our serotonin, some GABA, and even the great neurotropin BDNF. Through such causal paths plus the two-way traffic from gut to brain and back along the vagus nerve, the microbiome has major impacts on moods, especially depression.

Variety in our lives and travel encourages microbial diversity in our gut, and greater diversity of gut bacteria leads to more positive impacts on brain and body. Thus we must be cautious around treatments with antibiotics that can reduce numbers in our microbiome and disrupt the (hopefully balanced) mix of bacteria. Probiotics containing bacteria of the genus *Lactobacillus* and some strains of *Bifidobacteria* seem good for brain, cognition, and moods, and both probiotics and prebiotics are especially recommended after a course of antibiotics (or other factors) have killed or eliminated our bacterial friends. For contented bacteria, consume foods with lots of fiber, and perhaps the occasional avocado. Consider some guacamole with your whole-grain chips and red wine.

**Sources and amounts.** Keep in mind that even after showing effectiveness in well-constructed randomized-control trials, adding certain supplements could be unnecessary, or occasionally even harmful to some individuals. And as you contemplate the animal studies sprinkled throughout the chapters, remember that not all of the pharmaceuticals or nutrients that have proven to boost cognition in critters (or slow their dementias) have proven to be effective for people.

The same cautions apply to quantities; even though small or moderate amounts of some nutrient may have proven to be beneficial, larger doses may be harmful. For example, Chapter 7 provided examples of that curvilinear relationship indicating cognitive benefits from moderate levels of both tea and caffeinated coffee but problems from too much of either. Similarly, in Chapter 14 I noted that low or moderate levels of red wine seem to benefit brain and cognition, but that large amounts of ethanol from any source will eventually remove the shine from our cognitive brilliance.

## Saving the world thru food selection

The dietary possibilities discussed throughout the book are assessed only for their potential impacts on our brain, cognition, and resilience, not for whether they lead to more sustainable agriculture, or climate stability, or other aspects of global stability and wellbeing. Yet it is essential to remain aware that our world population will add three billion people, to top out at around 10 billion by mid-century. Those additional billions will require 40% more food, and that production will affect climate and other aspects of our environment.

If followed, some of the dietary advice that has been available for decades, such as consuming less red meat, would certainly enhance food security and confer environmental benefits. Obviously, obtaining protein from mammals leads to inefficiencies in land use, excessive energy consumption, methane production, and other economic costs. Some estimates are that over 80% of the earth's current agricultural land is devoted to production of dairy products and meat. That land use ignores the gains that could be achieved for food security and climate control by instead converting some of that land to farming veggies, grains (for people, not animals), and fruit, and allowing forests to grow in the rest (Hayek et al., 2020). Remember too that the long-lived people who inhabit the "blue zones" derive most of their protein from beans, whole grains, and other plant sources rather than from mammals (e.g., Buettner, 2008). Our own longevity awaits similar transitions.

While most of the recommendations from Med-style diets are likely to benefit climate and environment, some do not. Consider, for example, the recommendation made for one to two servings of omega 3-rich fish per week. Only some subset of us can follow that recommendation—a subset that is sufficiently wealthy and with the availability of diverse foods sourced from near and far. It is too easy to forget the realities for the third of humanity living on less than US $2.00 per person per day. (For more on these issues, see "The healthiness and sustainability of national and global food based dietary guidelines" by Springmann et al., 2020.)

## Becoming tough, smart, and resilient

**A new drug?** After decades with no new drugs available for treating Alzheimer's dementia, a new one was hurriedly approved in the US in June, 2021—at anticipated costs for patients of tens of thousands of dollars per year. Controversy about the approval process then erupted in July, 2021, but never mind that. Initial research suggested the new drug might *slow* cognitive decline by 22%. That small and not-well-established impact for a "cure" appears to be far less than achieved for prevention from many of the nutrients described throughout the previous chapters. The effect sizes and risk ratios for preventing or slowing cognitive decline and dementias from even single nutrients were often as large or larger than the 22% to be *possibly* gained from that new and astronomically-expensive drug.

**Nutrition and toughening.** Besides great nutrition, I have emphasized other vital ingredients to lifespan, healthspan, brain health, and robust cognition and resilience. Those other avenues most certainly include some assortment of cognitively challenging activities, very regular doses of at least moderate physical exercise, and although not elaborated here, social and nurturing activities, and activities that require self-control (such as meditation and tai chi).

Of all those activities, current research indicates that the most substantial impacts for cognitive capacities and resilience are derived from regular exercise—at least, that is the case for those of us living in technically advanced circumstances where many of us do almost anything to avoid exercise. Adequate sleep, although not detailed in the text, is also an essential ingredient. Note that sleep, like exercise and various veggies, increases levels of the master antioxidant glutathione; and sleep is when our glycemic system is finally allowed to clean waste from the brain. Certainly, those aspects of healthy lifestyles also have better prospects for avoiding cognitive decline and dementia (to say nothing of depression, and stress intolerance) than the new Alzheimer's drug.

**Purpose.** But there are psychological factors that also play important roles in sustaining our cognitive capacities and resilience as we age. Having goals and purpose in life is essential to well-being, including cognitive preservation and resilience. In short, as we age and possibly either retire or scale back some activities, we should have reasons to get up in the morning—things to do that seem to be important and that we want to do. Other benefits to the health of body and brain include cultivating optimism, reducing stress as much as possible, and having positive relationships with family and/or friends, and perhaps pets. All of those ingredients contribute to lifespan, healthspan, cognitive preservation and resilience as well. Your brain-healthy diet may be as important as some of those factors, but it certainly will not be an adequate substitute for them.

# Glossary

**Acetylation.** This is an epigenetic process that quiets the future sensitivity of the affected gene, making that gene less responsive to transcription (activation). It happens when an acetyl-group molecule affects the histone protein complex that forms the "spool" around which the DNA is "wrapped."

**Acetylcholine.** Within the brain's prefrontal cortex and hippocampi the neurotransmitter acetylcholine is vital for long-term memory formation and consolidation. Low acetylcholine levels are implicated in the memory problems of Alzheimer's disease, but low acetylcholine does *not* actually cause Alzheimer's.

**Adenosine and adenosine receptors.** Adenosine is a neuromodulator that attenuates responses of neurons to neurotransmitters, thereby slowing neural activity. Thus the presence of adenosine enhances sleep and alertness. Caffeine occupies adenosine receptors and therefore prevents adenosine from slowing us down and decreasing alertness.

**Alcohol unit.** It is 10cc or eight grams of alcohol. A typical bottle (a "fifth") of table wine at 13% alcohol would contain about 10 units, so splitting that bottle between you and your dinner partner would give you five units each. A 12-oz can of decent craft beer at 6% would have two units. An ounce of 86 proof liquor would have 1.4 alcohol units.

**Alcoholic drink.** This is approximately 12 grams of alcohol, or 150% of an "alcohol unit." It is usually thought of as a large glass of beer or typical glass of wine.

**ALS.** Amyotrophic lateral sclerosis, or more commonly, Lou Gehrig's disease results from the deterioration of the neurons that activate muscles, so that muscular control is lost. One of its most famous victims was Stephen Hawking.

**Alzheimer's dementia.** Nothing is good here. Hippocampal functions decline such as the ability to form new episodic memories and to retrieve memories. Prefrontal cortical functions such as reasoning decline. The brain itself shrinks dramatically as twisted proteins of β-amyloid build plaques between neurons and distorted tau proteins cause tangles within neurons. Destructive inflammation accompanies those processes. Efficiency of all brain processes suffers until the brain cannot maintain vital physical processes and death ultimately ensues.

**Amygdala.** Our two amygdala get lots of bad press. On each side of the brain, they are located near the outside ends of the hippocampi. Various nuclei (centers) within the amygdala are involved with the detection, generation, and expression of survival-relevant emotions such as fear and anger. Thus factors that reduce their functioning are generally thought to be positive. During stress responses the emotions they stimulate keep us focused on the stressors and motivate coping.

**Astrocytes.** They are a vital type of the brain's glia. They contribute to the glymphatic system—the system that flushes waste products from the brain, and they seem to protect and regulate synaptic functions. In addition, the astrocytes absorb excess expended neurotransmitters, regulate glucose, and play some role in regulating the brain's electrical rhythms. They may be the most numerous of all brain cells. See glymphatic system.

*APOE* **gene.** The apolipoprotein E gene comes to us in several variants (alleles) that affect our likelihood of being afflicted by Alzheimer's dementia. The *APOE-4* (sometimes written APOE ε4) is the allele that disposes us to develop Alzheimer's. Lots of us have one copy of it, which is not too bad, although probabilities for Alzheimer's are increased with the one, but having two copies is awful and often leads to early-onset Alzheimer's.

*APP* **gene.** This gene makes amyloid precursor protein. That protein is (obviously) the precursor to the β amyloid protein described below in the β amyloid section.

**BDNF (brain-derived neurotropic factor).** BDNF is an essential neurotropin that is responsible for the maintenance of neuronal health and growth. BDNF increases in and around neurons when those neurons are highly active. When made in the body in response to activities like exercise it crosses the blood-brain barrier to the benefit of brain. The receptors for BDNF called TrkB (reflecting an obvious shortage of vowels) usually are increased too by the same activities (such as exercise) that increase BDNF itself. Seek out activities and/or nutrition that benefit BDNF.

**β-amyloid.** "Beta-amyloid" is sometimes written "amyloid-β" or more simply AB or Aβ. It is an essential brain protein that becomes distorted in shape as Alzheimer's dementia develops. It is derived from the amyloid precursor protein and can consist of from 36 to 43 amino acids. The plaques formed as Alzheimer's develops are mostly composed of the variant with 42 amino acids, even though the most prevalent variant in the brain is the 40 variant. Although the Glymphatic system attempts to remove excess accumulations of that distorted protein, when the molecules accumulate they form tangles outside of the neurons. Those tangles inhibit neural efficiency and degrade synaptic connections between neurons. Those β-amyloid tangles may facilitate tau protein distortion and accumulations within neurons—another of the components of Alzheimer's.

**Blood-brain barrier.** When working correctly, the blood-brain barrier prevents unwanted (usually large) molecules from passing through the brain's capillary walls into the cerebro-spinal fluid that surrounds the neurons. The blood-brain barrier is effective in-so-far as the endothelial cells lining the capillaries remain closely linked together and in-so-far as some glial cells (oligodendrocytes) help to close those gaps. Those processes become less efficient as we age.

**BMI.** BMI or body-mass index is an indicator of how round we are (i.e., ratio of waist circumference to height) and is an approximate indicator of the belly fat we carry (i.e., the fat behind the abdominal muscles).

**C-reactive protein.** This evil protein is created in the liver in response to inflammation anywhere in the body. Thus it is an indicator of potential inflammation damage, and high levels are decidedly unwelcome.

**Cohen's d.** That measure of effect size is described in the "effect size" entry.

**Corpus callosum.** The two hemispheres of our brain are connected by this tract of 200 million myelin-coated axons. Despite often-exaggerated differences in function between the two hemispheres, the hemispheres activities are closely coordinated through the corpus callosum.

**Cortex.** This is the thin (4mm to 6mm) outer layer of gray matter consisting of neural cell bodies and dendrites that reside on the brain's surface and in the folds of the cerebrum. Some structures that are clearly deep inside the brain, such as the cingulate and the hippocampus, are actually cortical material folded deeply into the cerebrum. Thus even though the cortex is considerably less than a centimeter thick, it is still more than a half of the brain's total volume. The cortex is where our mental activities occur.

**Cortisol.** It is a hormone released by the adrenal cortex in the very early morning in a diurnal (24-hour) rhythm. But it is also released in large doses in response to stressors, and then it increases blood glucose in several ways and contributes to brain arousal. Long-term cortisol elevations associated with intense and/or chronic stress damage brain and body, contributing to insulin insensitivity and diabetes, cardiovascular problems, muscle atrophy, the buildup of abdominal fat, and even the deterioration of hippocampal and prefrontal structures. Cortisol's half life in humans is about 90 minutes, so once generated it hangs around.

**CREB.** This protein is properly named cAMP response element-binding protein. It acts as a transcription factor for lots of the brain's genetic activities.

**CRH.** Corticosteroid releasing hormone is a hypothalamic hormone that during stress asks the pituitary to generate ACTH to eventually stimulate the adrenal glands to release cortisol. CHR that is released in the brain during stress (some from amygdala) elicits and maintains negative moods.

**Crystallized intelligence.** Not problem solving (fluid intelligence), but rather the things we know, such as vocabulary, and whether we should consume leafy greens.

**Cytokines.** These are signaling molecules of the immune system that elicit various bodily responses. Some important ones such as interleukin-1, -2, and -6 and tumor necrosis factor alpha cause inflammation. Others function like the anti-inflammatory nutrients discussed throughout the text, opposing inflammation in the body and brain.

**Dendrites.** Dendrites are the projections from the bodies of neurons. They receive impulses from sending neurons. A typical cortical neuron may have 10,000 synapses. When enough synapses on enough dendrites are activated almost simultaneously, the neuron becomes a sending neuron, firing off its own impulse to other neurons.

**Dentate gyrus.** This is an area of the hippocampus involved in memory formation that receives input from the entorhinal cortex. New neurons are created in even adult human brains from neural stem cells in the dentate gyrus.

**DNA.** Deoxyribonucleic acid is the double helix. Sections of a long strand of DNA comprise the genes.

**Dopamine.** Dopamine is one of the neurotransmitters that decline with aging. After release by the ventral tegmental area it motivates us to seek rewards and avoid losses. Dopamine availability and the densities and efficiencies of dopamine receptors regulate motivation generally, and specifically stimulation seeking, reward-seeking, and addictions. Dopamine is deficient in some brain areas in Parkinson's, and overly present in other structures in schizophrenia. Its decline with aging may contribute to cognitive decline and the shrinkage of the prefrontal cortex.

**Dorsal attention network (DAN).** This network of several brain structures is activated when one undertakes consciously direct attention. Because the active focusing of attention is the essence of most meditation, it is not surprising that fMRI scans show increased connectivity between DAN structures in meditators, even in a resting state.

**Double-blind research.** This term means that until all the research data is processed neither the participants nor the researchers interacting with them are aware of the research condition of any study participant (e.g., receiving a nutrient versus placebo), ideally.

**EEG.** Electroencephalogram measures are of the electrical activity of the brain, commonly called "brain waves." That electrical activity is sampled through electrodes attached to the scalp. Different electrical wave forms occur with different levels of rest, attention, arousal, etc. The P-300 wave referred to in the text arises in response to an unusual or unexpected signal.

**EGCG.** Epigallocatechin Gallate is found in all kinds of tea, but (some say) in green tea especially. EGCG is the most abundant catechin in tea and is widely studied as the nutrient that is good for brain. It is.

**Effect size.** This measure tells us how much impact the experimental procedure had on the typical person experiencing that procedure—whether it changed them a little or a lot compared to themselves at an earlier point, or compared to the typical person in the control group. Of course, the "little or lot" judgment is up to us to interpret, and when the dependent measure is a really-important one, such as executive functions or hippocampal size, we should be impressed by even modest effect sizes.

Two effect-size measures seen frequently in the nutrition literature are Cohen's d, and somewhat less frequently, Hedges g. Both d and g are calculated as the difference between the means of the two conditions divided by the (sort of) average of the standard deviations of the two distributions. To actually calculate d or g, don't; instead, Google "effect size calculator" and plug in your numbers for automatic calculation. Effect sizes do not depend upon the number of participants in the research, although when studies have few participants, effect sizes become less reliable.

An easy (and approximate) way to interpret effect sizes for cognitive measures is to think of them as IQ measures. For example, an effect size of Cohen's d of d = .50 (or Hedges g of g = .50) on a composite cognitive measure would be roughly equivalent to a difference of 7.5 IQ points. Remember that the population mean for IQ is usually considered to be 100, and the standard deviation is 15, indicating that about 2/3 of all people have IQs between 85 and 115. Generally, I consider an effect size of around d = .50 for a cognitive measure to be very substantial and meaningful—a really big deal.

Three of the other effect size measures used in the text are risk ratio (RR in text) or the odds ratio (OR), or the hazard ratio (HR). A simple correlation can also be interpreted as showing effect size. See other Glossary entries for those measures.

**Endocannabinoid system.** The endocannabinoid system consists of neurochemicals and receptors that impact physical functioning throughout the brain and body. They are newly studied, but they can influence mood, cognition, and immune functions. The endocannabinoids are lipid-based molecules that activate receptors that are also sensitive to molecules from marijuana (i.e., both THC and CBD). New research shows that physical exercise increases endocannabinoid levels and that those increased levels may account for the "runner's high."

**Entorhinal cortex.** This area in the temporal lobe feeds information from other cortical areas to the hippocampus. Thus it plays a role in the formation of spatial and episodic memories. (Possibly check out the hippocampi glossary entry.)

**Episodic memories.** These are memories of the episodes of our lives. Those life stories gradually leave us with dementia.

**Epigenetics.** The term describes the science of the changes in the sensitivity of our genes to transcribing or activating factors. Acetylation describes an acetyl-group molecule affecting the histone that forms the spool around which the gene winds. Acetylation makes the gene more responsive to future transcription. Methylation occurs when a methyl-group molecule attaches to the gene, making it less sensitive to transcription. Those epigenetic modifications can last days, years, or a lifetime.

**Ergothioneine.** It is an important antioxidant found especially in mushrooms. Whether it is vital is not known for certain, but probably helps to account for positive impacts of mushrooms on cognition.

**Executive functions.** These are usually conscious and sometimes effortful mental activities employed in non-routine situations. They formulate goals and construct plans to accomplish those goals by consciously organizing the required subgoals and operating procedures. They attempt to control emotions, impulses, and the focus of attention. Working memory is an overlapping concept. The executive functions (and working memory) process cognitive activities sequentially, rather than as simultaneous parallel processes.

**Fluid intelligence.** The term means our ability to solve usually-novel problems. It requires developed executive functions, including especially a robust working memory. It is contrasted with crystallized intelligence.

**fMRI.** Functional magnetic resonance imaging of the brain is a scan that shows what parts of the brain are activated by the mental processes occurring during the scan. (See MRI for more.)

**Free radicals.** Also known as reactive oxygen species, they are oxygen molecules that have an extra electron, making them more reactive than may be good for us. They are created in the mitochondria as those organelles produce energy from glucose or fatty acids. If left to accumulate by insufficient anti-oxidants, they cause mutations and damage to cells and mitochondria.

**GABA.** Gamma aminobutyric acid is a central nervous system neurotransmitter that serves more as an inhibitor of neural activation than an activator. Low levels of GABA then allow high levels of activation that may manifest as anxiety and, if excessive, result in neural damage.

**Glia.** There are several types of these the tiny brain cells that do many important services for the neurons and the brain. Some types of glial cells mop up excess glutamate from around the neurons and some create the myelin sheaths that allow efficient neural transmission down long axons. Others make some neurotransmitters; some participate in establishing the blood-brain barrier, and some store glycogen for later use by neighboring neurons. Acting much like proud grandmothers, neuroscientists continue to discover and celebrate new glial accomplishments.

**Glutamate.** Glutamate is the most ubiquitous excitatory neurotransmitter in the brain, playing a key role in many mental processes including memory and learning. However, it can be a neurotoxin if not cleared out of brain structures that have sustained high levels of recent activation.

**Glutathione.** It is a powerful antioxidant manufactured in all of our cells. We could probably not survive without it (i.e., lab animals who cannot produce it do not live). Other antioxidants like vitamin C influence its concentration by relieving some of its burden through their own antioxidant activities. Mushrooms are good dietary sources that supplement our endogenous levels.

**Glycemic index.** When carbohydrate-based foods that are high in glycemic index are digested, they dispense glucose quickly into our blood and thus may tax the ability of our insulin to lower blood glucose to acceptable levels. Added sugars and simple starches such as those from highly refined wheat flower have high glycemic indices. Some fruits are high but still may be a net benefit for health due to their various phytonutrients. (Thus the fruits themselves are far more recommended than fruit juices.)

**Glymphatic system.** Only discovered and described within the last decade or so, at first in mice, this is a brain cleaning system. During sleep, the cells of the brain shrink, leaving more space for the interstitial fluid to circulate through the brain. That circulating fluid picks up and flushes out stray bits of unneeded or deformed proteins (such as excessive β-amyloid and deformed tau) and other crap. Another waste removal system depends on **lysosomes**. Enzymes within lysosomes break down waste products into smaller component parts for later reuse within the cells. When lysosomes become dysfunctional within aging neurons, waste products accumulate and block circulation into and down neural axons.

**Grey matter.** This is the neural tissue of the thin cortex. It consists mostly of neural cell bodies and dendrites. In contrast, white matter, consisting of axons covered by fatty myelin sheaths, connects different grey-matter structures.

**Hazard ratio.** HRs are one index of effect size. See the "effect size" entry if this seems insufficient. HRs are ratios that compare the number of people who developed the condition in the "experimental" group with the number who developed it in the "control" group *within a certain time span.* It can be interpreted as a percent. For example, in the study by Sanchez-Villages et al. (2016; described in Chapter 20) the hazard ratio for the impact of the Med diet on depression was HR = .84. Using their method of dividing participants into thirds (high, medium and low adherence to the Med), for every 100 people developing depression in the low-adherence third, there were only 84 (or 84%) depressed folks in the high-adherence third *within the time of the study.* See risk ratio if this excites you.

**Hedges' g.** See "Effect Size."

**HGH.** Human growth hormone is dispensed by the pituitary gland. It declines remarkably with age and is a general workhorse by positively affecting the health of most tissue types in our bodies. It serves as a neurotropin for neural tissue.

**Hippocampi.** These are the two brain structures responsible for assembling the components of episodic memories but they are not the location where those memories are stored. The hippocampi also play a role in re-assembling memories during recall. Hippocampal damage leaves one without any new episodic memories, and lousy (if any) access to old ones. The singular is hippocampus.

**Homocysteine.** This amino acid results from protein breakdown. It increases with stress. High levels damage the cardiovascular system and cause brain atrophy, increasing Alzheimer's risk. The text offers much more.

**Hormones.** These are molecules released by endocrine glands that circulate via the cardiovascular system, and then affecting organs that have receptors for them. Even very low concentrations can have big impacts.

**Hypothalamus**. This brain structure is directly responsible for all kinds of homeostasis and basic services. It has many nuclei that play roles in hunger, satiation, and sexuality. It releases the hormone CRH to signal the pituitary to begin the steps needed for pituitary-adrenals-cortical (PAC) system arousal and it activates and deactivates sympathetic nervous system arousal. Thus indirectly it controls both adrenaline and cortisol. The hypothalamus is responsive to inputs from cortical structures and from limbic structures such as the nearby amygdala and the distant locus coeruleus.

**Insulin.** This is a hormone that is released by the pancreas when blood glucose levels need to be reduced. It allows blood glucose to be taken into and then used or stored within cells. Insensitivity to insulin or too-little insulin results in high blood glucose (hyperglycemia) and perhaps eventually to diabetes. Too much insulin can lead to hypoglycemia and a lack of energy in body and brain.

**International unit (IU).** This term is a strange shifting one because it is calculated differently for different vitamins. I usually avoid using it in favor of simply using mgs and mcgs along with RDA.

*In vitro.* The term means literally "within the glass" and describes research done with tissue (etc.) that is outside of the body it was taken from. Most of the *in vitro* studies described in the text were done with neurons extracted from rodent brains.

*In vivo.* The complement to the previous term, it implies research done on the whole organism or at least within the living organism.

**Leukocytes.** They are white blood cells with immune-system responsibilities. They are of concern to us mostly because when research assesses impacts from nutrition on genes, whereas it is difficult to induce people to give up brain tissue, leukocytes are easy to harvest from even nervous people.

**Limbic system.** This is a changing and imprecise term that connotes the mostly-lower brain areas that generate and process emotions, basic instincts, and impulses. Its functions are usually contrasted with functions of the cortex.

**Mcg's or micrograms.** A 1/1,000,000 of a gram or a 1/1,000 of a milligram.

**Metabolomics and the metabolome.** The metabalome consists of the small molecules that are produced by the metabolism of food and nutrients by the organisms of our microbiome. As we learn more about those transformations of foods and nutrients the science of metabolomics emerges.

**Meta analysis.** That is a sophisticated statistical technique for combining related studies to determine just how much impact some independent variable (like consuming coffee) has on some dependent variable (such as cognitive ability or hippocampal expansion). That measure of impact is termed the "effect size" (see that entry, above).

**Methionine.** It is an essential amino acid that is a component of the antioxidant glutathione. It is important in angiogenesis (blood vessel growth), and plays a role in the epigenetic process of methylaton.

**Methylation.** When a methyl molecular group is attached to the promoter region of a gene, the gene then becomes resistant to future activation by a transcription molecule that would otherwise activate it. Methylation can last a lifetime, so the protein normally produced by the target gene may never be produced at all. Acetylation has the opposite impact by enhancing genetic transcription.

**Methylglyoxal.** This is a byproduct of carbohydrate conversion to energy by the mitochondria. In excessive quantities, it is highly toxic to the brain and body, causing the array of health issues mentioned in Chapter 17. High levels are considered an indicator of cancer. By substituting ketones for glucose, especially in the brain, the keto diet (or other methods of encouraging ketones) may protect against methylglyoxal toxicity.

**Mgs or milligrams.** A 1/1000 of a gram. Recall that there are 1000 grams of water in a liter (just over a quart).

**Microbiome.** It consists of the microscopic flora and fauna (i.e., bacteria, fungi, protozoa and viruses) that live in our body—mostly in our gut. They may be helpful or harmful, but they are largely symbiotic and many are absolutely essential. They play a major role in converting some of the nutrients we consume, sometimes creating wonderful products (metabolites) and sometimes not so much. We replenish them (whether needed or not) when we consume probiotics, and we feed them with prebiotics and the normal foods we consume, especially food high in fiber.

**Microglia.** These are tiny brain cells that act as the brain's immune system, and they play a role in removing the β-amyloid plaques that build up as Alzheimer's develops. Unfortunately, the microglia can sometimes cause damaging brain inflammation by over-reacting to problems such as excessive β-amyloid and tau proteins.

**MicroRNAs.** These are RNA molecules that regulate the expression of genes.

**Mitochondria.** Bless those organelles found in quantity in each mammalian cell that convert nutrients (especially glucose but also ketons) into energy. They have their own genes, independent of those carried by our 23 pairs of chromosomes, and they are inherited only from our mothers, with around a million in each egg.

**MRI (magnetic resonance imaging).** This scanning method can accurately assess the structure of the brain or body, including the amount of material in various parts of the brain. (See fMRI for more.)

**Myelin.** Myelin is the fatty material that coats the axons of many neurons. The myelin acts metaphorically like the insulator on an electric wire, allowing impulses to proceed down the axon quickly and free from interference. Neurons of the brain have their myelin provided by oligodendrocytes—a type of glial cell. The process of developing myelin coats is called myelination.

**NAD+ or nicotinamide adenine dinucleotide.** It is a coenzyme that is found in all living cells and that plays a major role in activating the sirtuins, proteins that play major roles in cell metabolism and homeostasis (and described in the sirtuin entry below). NAD+ is responsive to levels of flavonoids, and thought to extend longevity.

**NGF or neural growth factor.** NGF is one of the important neurotropins that are enhanced by toughening activities and some nutrients (e.g., ginger). NGF builds and preserves neurons in brain and body.

**Neurochemicals.** They are both the chemicals that are produced by neurons and those that affect neurons. As used throughout the book, this generic term includes the neuromodulators neurotransmitters, and neurotropins.

**Neurons.** Neurons are cells that transmit electrical messages. With the glial cells and the brain's portion of the cardiovascular system, they constitute most of the brain.

**Neurotransmitters.** These are the molecules that are released by a sending neuron into a synapse. When enough of them are detected by receptors on the receiving neuron, they cause an impulse to travel toward the cell body of the neuron, combining with other such impulses to increase the probability that the receiving neuron will discharge or "fire."

**Neurotropins.** They are the neural growth factors that facilitate neural growth, preservation, and repair. (See BDNF.)

**Noradrenaline.** It doubles as a neurotransmitter and a hormone. In the brain, it arouses various structures after it is released from the axon ends of neurons that originate in the locus coeruleus. Too much is associated with anxiety, but deficiencies are associated with depression and neural insufficiency. In fact, deficient noradrenaline levels mimic many of the cognitive changes that result from aging, such as compromised executive processing. It is the neurotransmitter of the Sympathetic NS. In response to Sympathetic NS stimulation, the adrenal medulla also releases even more noradrenaline to act as a hormone that increases blood pressure and energizes the body.

**Oddball paradigm.** This strange term describes an attention task that can be auditory or visual. During a sequence of similar visual images or sounds an "odd" (visual or auditory, respectively) stimulus occurs at unexpected intervals. The P-300 EEG wave occurs at 300 milliseconds after that "odd" stimulus if the participant is attending to the task, with the amplitude of the P-300 wave being higher when attention to the task is better. If the P-300 is delayed past 300 milliseconds, the detection of "oddness" is taking longer. The wave's amplitude is considered a measure of the capacity of working memory. According to Saenghong et al. (2012) the regions of the brain that are apparently responsible for the generation of the P-300 are the temporal and parietal lobes, and the hippocampi.

**Odds ratio (OR).** When some treatment (like consuming the Med diet) enhances some outcome measure (say executive processes) the OR will be greater than one (OR > 1). If the treatment (say vitamin B-12) decreases the outcome (say dementia), then OR < 1. Consider an example from Chapter 13: Moderate Drinkers had an odds ratio of OR = .65 for being mentally "slow." That means that within the crowd of only the Moderate Drinkers, for every 65 who developed dementia, there were 100 who developed dementia in the group of non-drinkers. In short, moderate drinking was cognitively protective. Another way of looking at the numbers is that moderate drinking reduced the chances of slipping into "slow" by 35%.

**Pituitary-adrenal-cortcal (PAC) arousal.** In humans, both stressors and extraordinary energy demands elicit PAC arousal. Unlike the arousal of the Sympathetic NS, PAC arousal develops slowly. It begins when the hypothalamus sends hormones (CRH) to the pituitary. The pituitary in turn releases hormones into general circulation (ACTH) that cause the cortex of the adrenal glands to release the hormone cortisol. Cortisol increases blood glucose levels and arouses neural activity in various brain structures. In the short term, those physiological responses tend to be adaptive, but sustained PAC arousal is dangerous to the brain. See Dienstbier (2015) for much more—perhaps too much more.

$p = .05$ **or** $p < .05$**, etc.** See statistical significance.

**RDA.** Recommended daily allowance of a food or nutrient is determined by the US Food and Nutrition Board of the Institute of Medicine. It is the minimum amount needed to prevent a deficiency disease for 97.5% of people in the specified population.

**Risk ratio (RR).** The RR is very similar to hazard ratio (see that entry) and to odds ratio, except not restricted to any particular time interval. E.g., What is the *risk ratio* of developing Alzheimer's across one's lifetime if in the upper half of the population in pomegranate consumption, compared to being in the lower half in consumption. In contrast, compared to controls on a normal diet what was the *hazard ratio* of rats developing Alzheimer's during three months of vitamin B-12 deficiency?

**RNA.** Ribonucleic acid is a molecule produced from DNA when the relevant gene is transcribed. RNA travels out of the nucleus of the cell into a ribosome where it guides the production of the relevant protein. See also microRNA.

**Serotonin.** It is a neurotransmitter. Serotonin molecules are projected into vast areas of the brain via axons that originate in the several raphe nuclei that are located in the brain stem. Serotonin seems important for just about all mental processing. Deficiencies are associated with depression, and with aggression and impulse-control deficits. Most of our serotonin is actually made by the microbiome. Drugs such as MAOIs and SSRIs also up-regulate serotonin and thus serve as anti-depressants.

**Sirtuins.** The seven sirtuins constitute a family of proteins that are involved in literally hundreds of functions from cell metabolic processes to homeostasis and even protecting against damage from reactive oxygen species and repair of damaged DNA. For more see the NAD+ entry, above and the material of Chapter 15.

**Statistical significance.** Statistical significance tells us whether we should believe that an experimental procedure really made a difference, or whether that observed difference could be due to chance alone. In the text, I do not usually mention experimental results unless they were statistically significant—that is, unless the differences between an experimental and control condition (usually with random assignment of participants into conditions) had at least a 95 per cent probability of being due to the experimental procedures. The "$p$" stands for probability. So $p = .05$ or $p < .05$ means that there is at most a 5% probability that a difference that large could be due to chance alone. Thus there is a 95% (or greater) likelihood that the impact of the target diet or supplement, etc. really did cause the differences observed.

Statistical significance depends, in part, on the numbers of people in the research, so that a very small difference between the performance of Experimental- and the Control-condition participants may still be statistically significant if there were (say) 1000 participants in the study, whereas a very large difference between the two groups may not be statistically significant if there were (say) only ten participants per condition.

Contrast that explanation with "effect size."

**Sympathetic NS.** This branch of the autonomic nervous system is responsible for many aspects of arousal in the body. It originates in the brain stem and follows the spinal column, exiting at regular intervals to affect the gut, the cardiovascular system, bladder, genitals and most anything else that is worthwhile in the body. Its arousal is balanced by the parasympathetic nervous system's relaxation of that arousal.

**Synapses.** These are the places where neurons stimulate each other. Neurotransmitter molecules are released when a neural impulse reaches the axon terminals of an impulse-sending neuron. When enough neurotransmitter molecules are detected by receptors across the synaptic gap on the receiving neuron, an impulse may start in the receiving neuron. A typical cortical neuron has 10,000 synapses. That's lots.

**Tau.** This important brain protein becomes misshapen as Alzheimer's dementia develops. Those misshapen tau molecules clump together inside neurons, interfering with efficient neural function and thus contributing to the neural deterioration and cognitive decline that develops. As Alzheimer's develops, distorted tau protein molecules are passed from neuron to neuron in a manner that resembles a spreading infection.

**Telomeres.** These are complexes of protein and DNA that cap the ends of chromosomes, protecting them from picking up stray and unhelpful bits of DNA, and from acquiring the errors in our genes that would result. The telomeres also allow the chromosomes to replicate themselves completely, as they must when cells divide. Telomeres shrink as we age, so their length is thought to be an indicator of how long we have to live.

**Trail-marking test.** It is a measure of visual attention and processing speed (in Part I) and decision-making (or executive processes, in Part II). A continuous line is drawn from number to number to connect somewhat scrambled numbers in order in Part I, but in sequence from numbers to alternating letters in Part II.

**Transcription factors.** These are molecules that activate the promoter region of genes, ultimately (after a couple more steps) causing the gene to produce its protein. Transcription factors are often formed when neurochemicals combine with receptors. That often happens on cell membranes but in other cases can happen inside cells.

**Transgenic animals.** These star-crossed beasts are usually mice or rats that have been given genes—often human genes—that (usually) dispose them to develop abnormal dispositions. Those most often cited in the text usually dispose the animals to develop Alzheimer's dementia at a fairly young age. The animals are used in studies of nutrients or therapies that may delay or even reverse the progression of Alzheimer's.

**Translation.** It is not for language majors. After a gene is transcribed, the code carried by the RNA to the ribosome becomes "translated" by the ribosome so that ultimately the proper protein is produced.

**Virome.** Like the biome for bacteria, virome describes the collection of viruses living in the gut. According to the unique Ohio State lab, almost 98% of those viruses are phages—viruses that invade bacteria.

**White matter.** It consists of axons covered with myelin. Those axons provide the communication channels that connect diverse structures in the brain and that connect the brain to the body, and vice versa.

**Working memory.** This concept overlaps with "executive functions." Working memory is akin to the popular notion of consciousness. It is where we do our conscious thinking. Within working memory our current goal-relevant observations and thoughts are brought together with relevant memories while goal-irrelevant mental elements are screened out to conserve our limited sequential-processing resources. When working memory is assessed, it is usually by seeing how many elements can be held. (E.g., how long a sequence of newly-presented numbers can be remembered in tests of immediate recall.)

# References

Alam, A. B., Lutsey, P. L., Gottesman, R. F., Tin, A., & Alonso, A. (2020). Low serum magnesium is associated with incident dementia in the ARIC-NCS Cohort. *Nutrients, 12*(10), 70-79. https://doi.org/10.3390/nu12103074

Al-Amin, M., Bradford, D. K., Sullivan, R. K. P., Kurniawan, N. D., Moon, Y., Han, S-H., Zalesky, A., & Burne, T. H. J. (2019). Vitamin D deficiency is associated with reduced hippocampal volume and disrupted structural connectivity in patients with mild cognitive impairment. *Human Brain Mapping, 40*(2), 394-406. https://doi.org/10.1002/hbm.24380

Alavi, N. M., Khademalhoseini, S., Vakili, Z., & Assarian, F. (2019). Effect of vitamin D supplementation on depression in elderly patients: A randomized clinical trial. *Clinical Nutrition, 38*(5), 2065-2070. http://eprints.kaums.ac.ir/4022/1/1-s2.0-S026156141832449X-main.pdf

Ali, Y. O., Bradley, G., & Lu, H-C. (2017). Screening with an NMNAT2-MSD platform identifies small molecules that modulate NMNAT2 levels in cortical neurons. *Scientific Reports, 7*, 43846. https://doi.org/10.1038/srep43846

Alisi, L., Cao, R., DeAngelis, C., Cafolla, A., Caramia, F., Cartocci, G., Librando, A., & Fiorelli, M. (2019). The relationships between vitamin K and cognition: A review of current evidence. *Frontiers of Neurology, 10*, 239. https://doi.org/10.3389/fneur.2019.00239

Amen, D. J., Harris, W. S., Kidd, P. M., Meysami, S., & Raji, C. A. (2017). Quantitative erythrocyte Omega-3 EPA plus DHA levels are related to higher regional cerebral blood flow on brain SPECT. *Journal of Alzheimer's Disease, 58*(4), 1189-1199. https://doi.org/10.3233/JAD-17028

Anderson, R. A., Qin, B., Canini, F., Poulet, L., & Roussel, A. M. (2013). Cinnamon counteracts the negative effects of a high fat/high fructose diet on behavior, brain insulin signaling and Alzheimer-associated changes. *PLoS One, 8*(12), e83243. https://doi.org/10.1371/journal.pone.0083243

Andreux, P. A., Blanco-Bose, W., Ryu, D., Burdet, F., Ibberson, M., Aebischer, P., Auwerx, J., Singh, A., & Rinsch, C. (2019). The mitophagy activator urolithin A is safe and induces a molecular signature of improved mitochondrial and cellular health in humans. *Nature Metabolism, 1*(6), 595-603. https://doi.org/10.1038/s42255-019-0073-4

Anjum, I., Jaffery, S. S., Fayyaz, M., Samoo, Z., & Anjum, S. (2018). The role of vitamin D in brain health: A mini literature review. *Cureus, 10*(7), e2960. https://doi.org/10.7759/cureur.2960

Appleton, K. M., Sallis, H. M., Perry, R., Ness, A. R., & Churchill, R. (2015). Omega-3 fatty acids for depression in adults. *Cochrane Database Systematic Reviews, 2015*(11), *Article* CD004692. https://doi.org/10.1002/14651858.CD004692.pub4

Appleton, K. M, Voyias, P. D, Sallis, H. M., Dawson, S., Ness, A. R., Churchill, R., & Perry, R. (2021). Omega-3 fatty acids for depression in adults. *Cochrane Database of Systematic Reviews, 2021*(11).

Avallone, R., Vitale G., & Bartolotti, M. (2019). Omega-3 fatty acids and neurodegenerative diseases: New evidence in clinical trials. *International Journal of Molecular Science, 20,* 4256. https://doi.org/10.3390/ijms2017 4256

Avgerinos, K. I., Vrysis, C., Chaitidis, N., Kolotsiou, K., Myserlis, P. G., & Kapogiannis, D. (2020). Effects of saffron (*Crocus sativus* L.) on cognitive function. A systematic review of RCTs. *Neurological Sciences, 41*(10), 2747–2754. https://doi.org/10.1007/s10072-020-04427-0

Ayati, Z., Yang, G., Ayati, M. H., Emami, S. A., & Chang, D. (2020). Saffron for mild cognitive impairment and dementia: A systematic review and meta-analysis of randomised clinical trials. *BMC Complementary Medicine and Therapies, 20*(1), 333. https://doi.org/10.1186/s12906-020-03102-3

Bae, J. H., & Kim, G. (2018). Systematic review and meta-analysis of omega-3-fatty acids in elderly patients with depression. *Nutrition Research. 50,* 1-9. https://doi.org/10.1016/j.nutres.2017.10.013.

Ballarini, T., Van Lent, D. M., Brunner, J., Schröder, A., Wolfsgruber, S., Altenstein, S., Brosseron, F., Buerger, K., Dechent, P., Dobisch, L., Duzel, E., Ertl-Wagner, B., Fliessbach, K., Freiesleben, S. D., Frommann, I., Glanz, W., Hauser, D., Haynes, J. D., Heneka, M. T., … Delcode Study Group. (2021). Mediterranean diet, Alzheimer disease biomarkers and brain atrophy in old age. *Neurology, 96*(24), e2920–e2932. Advance online publication. https://doi.org/10.1212/WNL.0000000000012067

Basak, C., Boot, W. R., Voss, M. W., & Kramer, A. F. (2008). Can training in a real-time strategy videogame attenuate cognitive decline in older adults? *Psychology and Aging, 23*(4), 767–777. https://doi.org/10.1037/a0013494

Basambombo, L. L., Carmichael, P.-H., Côté, S., & Laurin, D. (2017). Use of vitamin E and C supplements for the prevention of cognitive decline. *Annals of Pharmacotherapy, 51*(2), 118-124. https://doi.org/10.1177/106002801667 3072

Baynham, R., van Zanten, J. J. C. S. V., Johns, P. W., Pham, Q. S., & Rendeiro, C. (2021). Cocoa flavanols improve vascular responses to acute mental stress in young healthy adults. *Nutrients, 13*(4), 1103. https://doi.org/10.3390/nu1 3041103

Berman, M. E., McCloskey, M. S., Fanning, J. R., Schumacher, J. A., & Coccaro, E. F. (2009). Serotonin augmentation reduces response to attack in aggressive individuals. *Psychological Science, 20*(6), 714-720. https://doi.org/10.1111/ j.1467-9280.2009.02355.x

Beydoun, M. A., Gamaldo, A. A., Beydoun, H. A., Tanaka, T., Tucker, K. A., Talegawkar, S. A., Ferrucci, L., & Zonderman, A. B. (2014). Caffeine and alcohol intakes and overall nutrient adequacy are associated with longitudinal cognitive performance among U.S. adults. *The Journal of Nutrition: Nutritional Epidemiology, 144*(6), 890-901. https://doi.org/10.394 5/jn.113.189027

Bhattacharyya, R., Black, S. E., Lotlikar, M. S., Fenn, R. H., Jorfi, M., Kovacs, D. M., & Tanzil, R. E. (2021). Axonal generation of amyloid-β from palmitoylated APP in mitochondria-associated endoplasmic reticulum membranes. *Cell Reports, 35*(7), 109134. https://doi.org/10.1016/j.celrep.2021.109134

Blake-Mortimer, J., Winefield, A. H., & Chalmers, A. H. (1998). Evidence for free radical-mediated reduction of lymphocytic 5'-ectonucleotidase during stress. *International Journal of Stress Management, 5*(1), 57-75.

Block, G., Jensen, C. D., Dalvi, T. B., Norkus, E. P., Hudes, M., Crawford, P. B., Holland, N., Fung, E. B., Schumacher, L., & Harmatz, P. (2008). Vitamin C treatment reduces elevated C-reactive protein. *Free Radical Biology and Medicine, 46*(1) 70-77.

Boehme, M., Guzzetta, K. E., Bastiaanssen, T. F. S., van de Wouw, M., Moloney, G. M., Gual-Grau, A. Spichak, S., Olavarría-Ramírez, L., Fitzgerald, P., Morillas, E., Ritz, N. L., Jaggar, M., Cowan, C. S. M., Crispie, F., Donoso, F., Halitzki, E., Neto, M. C., Sichetti, Golubeva, A. V. ... Cryan, J. F. (2021). Microbiota from young mice counteracts selective age-associated behavioral deficits. *Nature Aging, 1*(8), 660-676. https://doi.org/10.1038/s43587-021-00093-9

Borota, D., Murray, E., Keceli, G., Chang, A., Watabe, J. M., Ly, M., Tosscno, J. P., & Yassa, M. A. (2014). Post-study caffeine administration enhances memory consolidation in humans. *Nature Neuroscience, 17*(2), 201–203. https://doi.org/10.1038/nn.3623

Bowman, G. L., Silbert, L. C., Howieson, D., Dodge, H. H., Traber, M. G., Frei, B., Kaye, J. A., Shannon, J., & Quinn, J. F. (2012). Nutrient biomarker patterns, cognitive function, and MRI measures of brain aging. *Neurology, 78*(4), 241-249. https://doi.org/10.1212/WNL.0b013e3182436598

Braakhuis, A. J., Nagulan, R., & Somerville, V. (2018). The effect of MitoQ on aging-related biomarkers: A systematic review and meta-analysis. *Oxidative Medicine and Cellular Longevity, 2018*, 8575263. https://doi.org/10.1155/2018/8575263

Braidy, N., & Liu, Y. (2020). NAD+ therapy in age-related degenerative disorders: A benefit/risk analysis. *Experimental Gerontology, 132*, 110831. https://doi.org/10.1016/j.exger.2020.110831

Brainard, J. S., Jimoh, O. F., Deane, K. H. O., Biswas, P., Donaldson, D., Maas, K., Abdelhamid, A. S, Hooper, L. & PUFAH group. (2020). Omega-3, omega-6, and polyunsaturated fat for cognition: Systematic review and meta-analysis of randomized trials. *Journal of the American Medical Directors Association, 2020*(10), 1439-1450.e21. https://doi.org/10.1016/j.jamda.2020.02.022. Epub 2020 Apr 15. PMID: 32305302

Bravo, J. A., Forsythe, P., Chew, M. V., Escaravage, E., Savignac, H. M., Dinan, T. G., Bienenstock, J. & Cryan, J. F. (2011). Ingestion of *Lactobacillus* strain regulates emotional behavior and central GABA receptor expression in a mouse via the vagus nerve. *Proceedings of the National Academy of Sciences of the United States of America, 108*(38), 16050-16055. https://doi.org/10.1073/pnas.1102999108

Bredesen, D. E., Amos, E. C., Canick, J., Ackerley, M., Raji, C., Fiala, M., & Ahdidan, J. (2016). Reversal of cognitive decline in Alzheimer's disease. *Aging, 8*(6), 1250–1258. https://doi.org/10.18632/aging.100981

Brown, B. S., Payne, T., Kim, C., Moore, G., Krebs, P., & Martin, W. (1979). Chronic response of rat brain norepinephrine and serotonin levels to endurance training. *Journal of Applied Physiology, 46*(1), 19–23. https://doi.org/10.1152/jappl.1979.46.1.19

Buettner, D. (2008). *The blue zones: Lessons for living longer from the people who've lived the longest.* National Geographic Society.

Buffington, S. A., Dooling, S. W., Sgritta, M., Noecker, C., Murillo, O. D., Felice, D. F., Turnbaugh, P. J., & Costa-Mattioli, M. (2021). Dissecting the contribution of host genetics and the microbiome in complex behaviors. *Cell, 184*(7), 1740-1756. https://doi.org/10.1016/j.cell.2021.02009

Burdette, J. H., Laurienti, P. J., Espeland M. A., Morgan, A., Telesford, Q., Vechlekar, C. D., Hayasaka, S., Jennings, J. M., Katula, J. A., Kraft, R. A., & Rejeski, J. (2010). Using network science to evaluate exercise-associated brain changes in older adults. *Frontiers in Aging Neuroscience, 2*, 23, https://doi.org/10.3389/fnagi.2010.0023

Burton, C., Campbell, P., Jordan, K., Strauss, V., & Mallen, C. (2013). The association of anxiety and depression with future dementia diagnosis: A case-control study in primary care. *Family Practice, 30*(1), 25-30.

Calabrese, C., Gregory, W. L., Leo, M., Kraemer, D., Bone, K., & Oken, B. (2008). Effects of a standardized *Bacopa monnieri* extract on cognitive performance, anxiety, and depression in the elderly: a randomized, double-blind, placebo-controlled trial. *Journal of Alternative and Complementary Medicine, 14*(6), 707–713. https://doi.org/10.1089/acm.2008.0018

Calderone, J. (2018, February 5). Do memory supplements really work? *Consumer Reports.* https://www.consumerreports.org/dietary-supplements /do-memory-supplements-really-work-a1023445146/

Campbell, N. L., Boustani, M. A., Lane, K. L., Gao, S., Hendrie, H., Khan, B. C., Murrell, J. R., Unverzagt, F. W., Hake, A., Smith-Gamble, V., & Hall, K. (2010). Use of anticholinergics and the risk of cognitive impairment in an African American population. *Neurology, 75*(2), 152-159. https://doi.org/10.1212/ WNL.0b013e3181e7f2ab

Canfield, C.-A., & Bradshaw, P. C. (2019). Amino acids in the regulation of aging and age-related diseases. *Translational Medicine of Aging, 3*, 70-89. https://doi.org/10.1016/j.tma.2019.09.001

Cawthon, R. M., Meeks, H. D, Sasani, T. A., Smith, K. R., Kerber, R. A., O'Brien, E., Baird, L., Dixon, M. M., Peiffer, A. P., Leppert, M. F., Quinlan, A. R., & Jorde, L. B. (2020). Germline mutation rates in young adults predict longevity and reproductive lifespan. *Scientific Reports, 10*(1), 10001. https://doi.org/10.10 38/s41598-020-66867-0

Champagne, F. A. (2010). Early adversity and developmental outcomes: Interaction between genetics, epigenetics, and social experiences across the life span. *Perspectives on Psychological Science, 5*(5), 564-574. https://doi. org/10.1177/1745691610383494

Chapman, T. R., Barrientos, R. M., Ahrendsen, J. T., Maier, S. F., & Patterson, S. L. (2010). Synaptic correlates of increased cognitive vulnerability with aging: Peripheral immune challenge and aging interact to disrupt theta-burst late-phase long-term potentiation in hippocampal area CA1. *Journal of Neuroscience, 30*(22), 7598-7603. https://doi.org/10.1523/JNEUROSCI.5172-09.2010

Chaudhari, K. S., Tiwari, N. R., Tiwari, R. R., & Sharma, R. S. (2017). Neurocognitive effect of nootropic drug *Brahmi* (*Bacopa monnieri*) in

Alzheimer's disease. *Annals of Neurosciences, 24*(2), 111-122. https://doi.org/10.1159/000475900

Chevalier, G., Siopi, E., Guenin-Macé, L., Pascal, M., Laval, T., Rifflet, A., Boneca, I. G., Demangel, C., Colsch, B., Pruvost, A., Chu-Van, E., Messager, A., Leulier, F., Lepousez, G., Eberl, G., & Lledo, P.-M. (2020). Effect of gut microbiota on depressive-like behaviors in mice is mediated by the endocannabinoid system. *Nature Communications, 11*(1), 6363. https://doi.org/10.1038/s41467-020-19931-2

Chida, Y., & Hamer, M. (2008). Chronic psychosocial factors and acute physiological responses to laboratory-induced stress in healthy populations: A quantitative review of 30 years of investigations. *Psychological Bulletin, 134*(6), 829-885. https://doi.org/10.1037/a0013342

Cicero, A. F. G., Fogacci, F., & Banach, M. (2018). Botanicals and phytochemicals active on cognitive decline: The clinical evidence. *Pharmacological Research, 130,* 204-212. https://doi.org/10.1016/j.phrs.2017.12.029

Colcombe, S. J., Ericksen, K. I., Scalf, P. E., Kim, J. S., Prakash, R., McAuley, E., Elavsky, S., Marquez, D. X., Hu, L., & Kramer, A. F. (2006). Aerobic exercise training increases brain volume in aging humans. *The Journals of Gerontology Series A: Biological Sciences and Medical Sciences, 61*(11), 1166–1170. https://doi.org/10.1093/gerona/61.11.1166

Colcombe, S. J., & Kramer, A. F. (2003). Fitness effects on the cognitive function of older adults: A meta-analytic study. *Psychological Science, 14*(2), 125–130. https://doi.org/10.1111/1467-9280.t01-1-01430

Colcombe, S. J., Kramer, A. F., Ericksen, K. I., Scalf, P., McAuley, E., Cohen, N. J., Webb, A., Jerome, G. J., Marquez, D. X, & Elavsky, S. (2004). Cardiovascular fitness, cortical plasticity, and aging. *Proceedings of the National Academy of Sciences of the United States of America, 101*(9), 3316–3332. https//:doi.org/10.1073/pans0400266101

Colucci, L., Bosco, M., Rosario Ziello, A., Rea, R., Amenta, F., & Fasanaro, A. M. (2012). Effectiveness of nootropic drugs with cholinergic activity in treatment of cognitive deficit: a review. *Journal of Experimental Pharmacology, 4,* 163–172. https://doi.org/10.2147/JEP.S35326

Cotman, C. W., Berchtold, N. C., & Christie, L. A. (2007). Exercise builds brain health: Key roles of growth factor cascades and inflammation. *Trends in Neurosciences, 30*(9), 464–472. https://doi.org/10.1016/j.tins.2007.06.011

Coupland, C. A. C., Hill, T., Dening, T., Morriss, R., Moore, M., & Hippisley-Cox, J. (2019). Anticholinergic drug exposure and the risk of dementia: A nested case-control study. *Journal of the American Medical Association: Internal Medicine, 179*(8), 1084-1093. https://doi.org/10.1001/jamainternmed.2019.0677

Craik, F. I. M., Bialystok, E., & Freeman, M. (2010). Delaying the onset of Alzheimer disease: Bilingualism is a form of cognitive reserve. *Neurology, 75*(19), 1726–1729. https://doi.org/10.1212/WNL.0b013e3181fc2a1c

Crane, P. K., Walker, R., Hubbard, R. A., Li, G., Nathan, D. M., Zheng, H., Heneuse, S., Craft, S., Montine, T. J., Kahn, S. E., McCormick, W., McCurry, S. M., Bowen, J. D., & Larson, E. B. (2013). Glucose levels and risk of dementia. *New England Journal of Medicine, 369*(6), 540–548. https://doi.org/10.1056/NEJMoa1215740

Cunnane, S. C., Courchesne-Loyer, A., St-Pierre, V., Vandenberghe, C., Pierotti, T., Fortier, M., Croteau, E., & Castellano, C. A. (2016). Can ketones compensate for deteriorating brain glucose uptake during aging? Implications for the risk and treatment of Alzheimer's disease. *Annals of the New York Academy of Science, 1367*(1), 12–20. https://doi.org/10.1111/nyas.12999

D'Amelio, P., & Quacquarelli, L. (2020). Hypovitaminosis D and aging: Is there a role in muscle and brain health? *Nutrients, 12*(3), 628. https://doi.org/10.3390/nu12030628

Danker, J. F., & Anderson, J. R. (2010). The ghosts of brain states past: Remembering reactivates the brain regions engaged during encoding. *Psychological Bulletin, 136*(1), 87–102. https://doi.org/10.1037/a0017937

Daviet, R., Aydogan, G., Jagannathan, K., Spilka, N., Koellinger, P. D., Kranzler, H. R., Nave, G., & Wetherill, R. R. (2022). Associations between alcohol consumption and gray and white matter volumes in the UK Biobank. *Nature communications, 13*(1), 1175. https://doi.org/10.1038/s41467-022-28735-5

Dcruz, M. M., Mamidipalli, S. S., Thakurdesai, A., & Andrade, C. (2018). Curcumin for neuroprotection: Taking a second look at results. *American Journal of Geriatric Psychiatry, 26*(6), 715. https://doi.org/10.1016/j.jagp.2018.03.015

de Cabo, R., & Mattson, M. P. (2020). Effects of intermittent fasting on health, aging, and disease. *New England Journal of Medicine, 381*(26), 2541–2551. https://doi.org/10.1056/NEJMra1905136

de Jager, C. A., Oulhaj, A., Jacoby, R., Refsum, H., & Smith, A. D. (2012). Cognitive and clinical outcomes of homocysteine-lowering B-vitamin treatment in mild cognitive impairment: a randomized controlled trial, *International Journal of Geriatric Psychiatry, 27*(6), 592-600. https://doi.org/10.1002/gps.2758

de J.R. De-Paula, V., Forlenza, A. S., & Forlenza, O. V. (2018). Relevance of gutmicrobiota in cognition, behaviour and Alzheimer's disease. *Pharmacological Research, 136*, 29-34. https://doi.org/10.1016/j.phrs.2018.07.007

de Lucia, C., Murphy, T., Steves, C. J., Dobson, R. J. B., Proitsi, P., & Thuret, S. (2020). Lifestyle mediates the role of nutrient-sensing pathways in cognitive aging: cellular and epidemiological evidence. *Communications Biology, 3*(1), 157. https://doi.org/10.1038/s42003-020-0844-1

Deng, J., Zhou, D. H. D., Li, J., Wang, Y. J., Gao, C., & Chen, M. (2006). A 2-year follow-up study of alcohol consumption and risk of dementia. *Clinical Neurology and Neurosurgery 108*(4), 378–383. https://doi.org/10.1016/j.clineuro.2005.06.005

Derbyshire, E. (2019). Could we be overlooking a potential choline crisis in the United Kingdom. *British Medical Journal: Nutrition, Prevention & Health, 2*(2), 86-89. https://doi.org/10.1136bjnph-2019-000037

Dhana, K., James, B. D., Agarwal, P., Aggarwal, N. T., Cherian, L. J., Leurgans, S. E., Barnes, L. L., Bennett, D. A., & Schneider, J. A. (2021). MIND Diet, common brain pathologies, and cognition in community-dwelling older adults. *Journal of Alzheimer's Disease, 83*(2): 683. https://doi.org/10.3233/JAD-210107

Dhir, A. (2018). Red wine retards abeta deposition and neuroinflammation in Alzheimer's disease. In Farooqui, T., & Farooqui, A. (Eds.) *Role of the*

*Mediterranean diet in the brain and neurodegenerative diseases*, (pp. 285-299). Academic Press.

Di Castelnuovo, A., Costanzo, S., Bonaccio, M., Rago, L., De Curtis, A., Persichillo, M., Bracone, F., Olivieri, M., Cerletti, C., Donati, M. B., de Gaetano, G., Iacoviello, L., & Moli-sani Investigators (2017). Moderate alcohol consumption is associated with lower risk for heart failure but not atrial fibrillation. *Journals of the American College of Cardiology. Heart Failure. 5*(11), 837–844. https://doi.org/10.1016/j.jchf.2017.08.017

Dickerson, S. S., & Kemeny, M. E. (2004). Acute stressors and cortisol responses: A theoretical integration and synthesis of laboratory research, *Psychological Bulletin, 130*(3), 355–391. https://doi.org/10.1037/0033-2909.130.3.355

Dienstbier, R. A., & PytlikZillig, L. M. (2021). Building emotional stability and mental capacity: The toughness model. In Snyder, C. R, Lopez, S. J., Edwards, L. M., & Marques, S. C. (Eds.) *Oxford handbook of positive psychology* (3rd ed., pp. 687-702). Oxford University Press.

Dienstbier, R. A. (2015). *Building resistance to stress and aging: The toughness model.* Palgrave Macmillan.

Douaud, G., Refsum, H., de Jager, C. A., Jacoby, R., Nichols, T. E., Smith, S. M., & Smith, A. D. (2013). Preventing Alzheimer's disease-related gray matter atrophy by B-vitamin treatment. *Proceedings of the National Academy of Sciences of the United States of America, 110*(23), 9523-9528. https://doi:10.1073/ pnas.1301816110

Draganski, B., Gaser, C., Kempermann, G., Kuhn, H. G., Winkler, G., Buchel, C., & Arne, M. (2006). Temporal and spatial dynamics of brain structural changes during extensive learning. *The Journal of Neuroscience, 26*(23), 6314–6317. https://doi.org/10.1523/JNEUROSCI.4628-05.2006

Driscoll, I., Shumaker, S. A., Snively, B. M., Margolis, K. L., Manson, J. E., Vitolins, M. Z., Rossom, R. C., & Espeland, M. A. (2016). Relationships between caffeine intake and risk for probable dementia or global cognitive impairment: The Women's Health Initiative Memory Study. *The Journals of Gerontology: Series A, 71*(12), 1596-1602. https://doi.org/10.1093/gerona/ glw078

Droste, S. K., Chandramohan, Y., Hill, L. E., Linthorst, A. C. E., & Reul, J. M. (2007). Voluntary exercise impacts on the rat hypothalamic-pituitary-adrenocortical axis mainly at the adrenal level. *Neuroendocrinology, 86*(1), 26–37. https://doi.org/10.1159/000104770, 26–37.

Du, L., Zhao, Z., Cui, A., Zhu, Y., Zhang, L., Liu, J., Shi, S., Fu, C., Han, X., Gao, W., Song, T., Xie, L., Wang, L., Sun, S., Guo, R., & Ma, G. (2018). Increased iron deposition on brain quantitative susceptibility mapping correlates with decreased cognitive function in Alzheimer's disease. *ACS Chemical Neuroscience, 9*(7), 1849–1857. https://doi.org/10.1021/acschemneuro.8b00194

Epel, E. S. (2009). Telomeres in a life-span perspective: A new "psychobiomarker"? *Current Directions in Psychological Science, 18*(1), 6-10. https://doi.org/10.1111/ j.1467-8721.2009.01596.x

Erickson, K. I., Banducci, S. E., Weinstein, A. M., MacDonald, A. W. III, Ferrell, R. E., Halder, I., Flory, J. D., & Manuck, S. B. (2013). The brain-derived neurotropic factor Val66Met polymorphism moderates an effect of physical activity on working memory performance. *Psychological Science, 24*(9), 1770–1779. https://doi.org/10.1177/0956797613480367

Erickson, K. I., Prakash, R. S., Voss, M. W., Chaddock, L., Heo, S., McLaren, M., Pence, B. D., Martin, S. A., Vieira, V. J., Woods, J. A., McAuley, E., & Kramer, A. F. (2010). Brain-derived neurotropic factor is associated with age-related decline in hippocampal volume. *The Journal of Neuroscience, 30*(15), 5368-5375. https://doi.org/10.1523/JNEUROSCI.6251-09.2010

Erickson, K. I., Voss, M. W., Prakash, R. S., Basak, C., Szabo, A., Chaddock, L., Kim, J. S., Heo, S., Alves, H., White, S. M., Wojcicki, T. R., Mailey, E., Vieira, V. J., Martin, S. A., Pence, B. D., Woods, J. A., McAuley, E., & Kramer, A. F. (2011). Exercise training increases size of hippocampus and improves memory. *Proceedings of the National Academy of Sciences of the United States of America, 108*(7), 3017–3022. https://doi.org/10.1073/pnas.1015950108

Esteban-Fernández, A., Rendeiro, C., Spencer, J. P. E., Gigorro del Coso, D., González de Llano, M. D., Bartolomé, B., & Moreno-Arribas, M. V. (2017). Phenolic metabolites and aroma compounds from wine in human SH-SY5Y neuroblastoma cells and their putative mechanisms of action. *Frontiers in Nutrition, 4*(3). https://doi.org/10.3389/fnut.2017.00003

Fadnes, L. T., Økland, J.-M., Haaland, Ø. A., & Johansson, K. A. (2022) Estimating impact of food choices on life expectancy: A modeling study. *PLoS Medicine 19*(2), e1003889. https://doi.org/10.1371/journal.pmed.1003889

Farooqui, T., & Farooqui, A. (2017). *Role of the Mediterranean diet in the brain and neurodegenerative diseases.* Academic Press.

Farzaei, M. H., Rahimi, R., Nikfar, S., & Abdollahi, M. (2018). Effects of resveratrol on cognitive and memory performance and mood: A meta-analysis of 225 patients. *Pharmacological Research, 128*, 338-344. https://doi.org/10.1016/j.phrs.2017.08.009

Feeney, J., O'Leary, N., Moran, R., O'Halloran, A. M., Nolan, J. M., Beatty, S., Young, I. S., & Kenny, R. A. (2017). Plasma lutein and zeaxanthin are associated with better cognitive function across multiple domains in a large population-based sample of older adults: Findings from the Irish Longitudinal Study on Aging. *The Journals of Gerontology: Series A, 72*(10), 1431–1436. https://doi.org/10.1093/gerona/glw330

Fenech, M. (2017). Vitamins associated with brain aging, mild cognitive impairment, and Alzheimer disease: Biomarkers, epidemiological and experimental evidence, plausible mechanisms, and knowledge gaps. *Advances in Nutrition, 8*(6), 958-970. https://doi.org/10.3945/an.117.015610

Firth, J., Marx, W., Dash, S., Carney, R., Teasdale, S. B., Solmi, M., Studds, B., Schuch, F. B., Carvalho, A. F., Jacka, F., & Sarris, J. (2019). The effects of dietary improvements on symptoms of depression and anxiety: A meta-analysis of randomized controlled trials. *Psychosomatic Medicine, 81*(3), 265-280. https://doi.org/10.1097/PSY.0000000000000673

Fitzgerald, K. N., Hodges, R., Hanes, D., Stack, E., Cheishvili, D., Szyf, M., Henkel, J., Twedt, M. W., Giannopoulou, D., Herdell, J., Logan, S., & Bradley, R. (2021). Potential reversal of epigenetic age using a diet and lifestyle intervention: a pilot randomized clinical trial. *Aging, 13*(7), 9419–9432. https://doi.org/10.18632/aging.202913

Fliton, M., Macdonald, I. A., & Knight, H. M. (2019). Vitamin intake is associated with improved visuospatial and verbal semantic memory in middle-aged individuals. *Nutritional Neuroscience, 22*(6), 401-408.

Forsythe, P., Bienenstock, J., & Kunze, W. A. (2014). Vagal pathways for microbiome-brain-gut axis communication. In Lyte, M., & Cryan, J. F. (Eds.) *Microbial endocrinology: The microbiota gut-brain access in health and disease*, (pp. 115-133). Springer.

Fraga, M. F., Ballestar, E., Paz, M. F., Ropero, S., Setien, F., Ballestar, M. L., Heine-Suner, D., Cigudosa, J. C., Urioste, M., Benitez, J., Boix-Chornet, M., Sanchez-Aguilera, A., Ling, C., Carlsson, E., Poulsen, P., Vaag, A., Stephan, Z., Spector, T. D., Wu, Y.-Z., Plass, C., & Esteller, M. (2005). Epigenetic differences arise during the lifetime of monozygotic twins. *Proceedings of the National Academy of Sciences of the United States of America, 102(30)*, 10604-10609. https://doi.org/10.1073/pnas.0500398102

Frasure-Smith, N., & Lesperance, F. (2005). Reflections on depression as a cardiac risk factor. *Psychosomatic Medicine, 67*, Suppl 1, S19-S25. https://doi.org/10.1097/01.psy.0000162253.07959.db

Freedman, R., Hunter, S. K., Law, A. J., D'Alessandro, A., Noonan, K., Wyrwa, A., & Hoffman, M. C. (2020). Maternal choline and respiratory coronavirus effects on fetal brain development. *Journal of Psychiatric Research, 128*, 1-4. https://doi.org/10.1016/j.jpsychires.2020.05.019

Fulton, J. L., Dinas, P. C., Carrillo, A. E., Edsall, J. R., Ryan, Emily J., & Ryan, Edward J. (2018). Impact of genetic variability on physiological responses to caffeine in humans: A systematic review. *Nutrients, 10*(10), 1373. https://doi.org/10.3390/nu10101373

Ganesan, K. & Xu, B. (2017). Polyphenol-rich lentils and their health promoting effects. *International Journal of Molecular Sciences, 18*(11), 2390. https://doi.org/10.3390/ijms18112390

Gardener, S. L., Rainey-Smith, S. R., Villemagne, V. L., Fripp, J., Doré, V., Bourgeat, P., Taddei, K., Fowler, C., Masters, C. L., Maruff, P., Rowe, C. C., Ames, D., & Martins, R. N. (2021). Higher coffee consumption is associated with slower cognitive decline and less cerebral Aβ-amyloid accumulation over 126 months: Data from the Australian Imaging, Biomarkers, and Lifestyle Study. *Frontiers in Aging Neuroscience, 13*, 744872. https://doi.org/10.3389/fnagi.2021.744872

Geary, D. C. (2019). The spark of life and the unification of intelligence, health, and aging, *Current Directions in Psychological Science, 28*(3), 223-228. https://doi.org/10.1177/0963721419829719

Gong, Z., Huang, J., Xu, B., Ou, Z., Zhang, L., Lin, X., Ye, X., Kong, X., Long, D., Sun, X., Xu, L., Li, Q., & Xuan, A. (2019). Urolithin A attenuates memory impairment and neuroinflammation in APP/PS1 mice. *Journal of Neuroinflammation, 16*(1), 62. https://doi.org/10.1186/s12974-019-1450-3

González-Domínguez, R., Castellano-Escuder, P., Carmona, F., Lefèvre-Arbogast, S., Low, D. Y., Du Preez, A., Ruigrok, S. R., Manach, C., Urpi-Sarda, M., Korosi, A., Lucassen, P. J., Aigner, L., Pallàs, M., Thuret, S., Samieri, C., Sánchez-Pla, A., & Andres-Lacueva, C. (2021). Food and microbiota metabolites associate with cognitive decline in older subjects: A 12-year prospective study. *Molecular*

*Nutrition & Food Research, 65*(23), e2100606. https://doi.org/10.1002/mnfr. 202100606

Goodwill A. M., & Szoeke C. A. (2017). Systematic review and meta-analysis of the effect of low vitamin D on cognition. *Journal of the American Geriatric Society, 65*, 2161–2168. https://doi.org/10.1111/jgs.15012

Grabowska, W., Sikora, E., & Bielak-Zmijewska, A. (2017). Sirtuins, a promising target in slowing down the aging process. *Biogerontology, 18*(4), 447–476. https://doi.org/10.1007/s10522-017-9685-9

Grammatikopoulou, M. G., Goulis, D. G., Gkiouras, K., Theodoridis, X., Gkouskou, K. K., Evangeliou, A., Dardiotis, E., & Bogdanos, D. P. (2020). To keto or not to keto? A systematic review of randomized controlled trials assessing the effects of ketogenic thereapy on Alzheimer disease. *Advances in Nutrition, 11*(6), 1583–1602. https://doi.org/10.1093/advances/nmaa073

Gratton, G., Weaver, S. R., Burley, C. V., Low, K. A., Maclin, E. L., Johns, P. W., Pham, Q. S., Lucas, S. J. E., Fabiani, M., & Rendeiro, C. (2020). Dietary flavanols improve cerebral cortical oxygenation and cognition in healthy adults. *Scientific Reports, 10*(1), 1-13. https://doi.org/10.1038/s41598-020-76160-9

Greenwood, B. N., Foley, T. E., Burhans, D., Maier, S. F., & Fleshner, M. (2005). The consequences of uncontrollable stress are sensitive to duration of prior wheel running. *Brain Research, 1033*(2), 164–178. https://doi.org/10.1016/j.brainres.2004.11.037

Gregory, A. C., Zablocki, O., Zayed, A. A., Howell, A., Bolduc, B., & Sullivan, M. B. (2020). The gut virome database reveals age-dependent patterns of virome diversity in the human gut. *Cell Host and Microbe, 28*(5), 724-740. https://doi.org/10.1016/j.chom.2020.08.003

Grodstein, F., Lemos, B., Yu, L., Iatrou, A., De Jager, P. L., & Bennett, D. A. (2020). Characteristics of epigenetic clocks across blood and brain tissue in older women and men. *Frontiers of Neuroscience, 14*, 555307. https://doi.org/10.3389/fnins.2020.555307

Grossmann, I., Karasawa, M., Izumi, S., Na, J., Varnum, M. E. W., Kitayama, S., & Nisbett, R. E. (2012). Aging and wisdom: Culture matters. *Psychological Science, 23*(10), 1059-1066. https/doi.org/10.1177/0956797612446025

Gunter, M. J., Murphy, N., Cross, A. J., Dossus, L., Dartois, L., Fagherazzi, G., Kaaks, R. et al. (2017). Coffee drinking and mortality in 10 European countries: A multinational cohort study. *Annals of Internal Medicine, 167*(4), 236–247. https://doi.org/10.7326/M16-2945

Hanna-Pladdy, B., & Gajewski, B. (2012). Recent and past musical activity predicts cognitive aging variability: Direct comparison with general lifestyle activities. *Frontiers in Human Neuroscience, 6*, 198. https://doi.org/10.3389/fnhum.2012.00198. eCollection 2012

Harrington, K. D., Aschenbrenner, A. J., Maruff, P., Masters, C. L., Fagan, A. M., Benzinger, T. L. S., Gordon, B. A., Cruchaga, C., Morris, J. C., & Hassenstab, J. (2021). Undetected neurodegenerative disease biases estimates of cognitive change in older adults. *Psychological Science, 32*(6), 849-860. https://doi.org/10.1177/0956797620985518

Harvanek, Z. M., Fogelman, N., Xu, K., & Sinha, R. (2021). Psychological and biological resilience modulates the effects of stress on epigenetic aging.

*Translational Psychiatry, 11*(1). Article 601 (2021). https://doi.org/10.1038/s41398-021-01735-7

Haussler, M. R., Whitfield, G. K., Haussler, C. A., Sabir, M. S., Khan, Z., Sandoval, R., & Jurutka, P. W. (2016). 1,25-Dihydroxyvitamin D and klotho: A tale of two renal hormones coming of age. *Vitamins and Hormones, 100*, 165-230. https://doi.org/10.1016/bs.vh.2015.11.005

Hawkins, M. A. W., Keirns, N. G., & Helms, Z. (2018). Carbohydrates and cognitive function. *Current Opinion in Clinical Nutrition and Metabolic Care, 21*(4), 302–307. https://doi.org/10.1097/MCO.0000000000000471

Hayek, M. N., Harwatt, H., Ripple, W. J., & Mueller, N. D. (2020). The carbon opportunity cost of animal-sourced food production on land. *Nature Sustainability, 4*, 21-24. https://doi.org/10.1038/s41893-020-00603-4

Hennebelle, M., Champeil-Potokar, G., Lavialle, M., Vancassel, S., & Denis, I. (2014). Omega-3 polyunsaturated fatty acids and chronic stress-induced modulations of glutamatergic neurotransmission in the hippocampus. *Nutrition Reviews, 72*(2), 99–112. https://doi.org/10.1111/nure.12088

Hertzog, C., Kramer, A. F., Wilson, R. S., & Lindenberger, U. (2008). Enrichment effects on adult cognitive development: Can the functional capacity of older adults be preserved and enhanced. *Psychological Science in the Public Interest, 9*(1), 1–65. https://doi.org/10.1111/j.1539-6053.2009.01034.x

Hess, T. M. (2005). Memory and aging in context. *Psychological Bulletin, 131*(3), 383–406. https://doi.org/10.1037/0033-2909.131.3.383

Heyn, P., Abreu, B. C., & Ottenbacher, K. J. (2004). The effects of exercise training on elderly persons with cognitive impairment and dementia: A meta-analysis. *Archives of Physical Medicine and Rehabilitation, 85*(10), 1694–1704. https://doi.org/10.1016/j.apmr.2004.03.019

Ho L., Chen L. H., Wang, J., Zhao, W., Talcott, S. T., Ono, K., Teplow, D., Humala, N., Cheng, A., Percival, S. S., Ferruzzi, M., Janle, E., Dickstein, D. L., & Pasinetti, G. M. (2009). Heterogeneity in red wine polyphenolic contents differentially influences Alzheimer's disease-type neuropathology and cognitive deterioration. *Journal of Alzheimers Disease, 16*(1), 59–72. https://doi.org/10.3233/JAD-2009-0916

Hole, K. L. & Williams, R. J. (2021). Flavonoids as an intervention for Alzheimer's disease: Progress and hurdles toward defining a mechanism of action. *Brain Plasticity, 6*(2), 167-192. https://doi.org/10.3233/BPL-200098

Holland, T. M., Agarwal, P., Wang, Y., Leurgans, S. E., Bennett, D. A., Booth, S. L., & Morris, M. C. (2020). Dietary flavonols and risk of Alzheimer dementia. *Neurology, 94*(16), e1749–e1756. https://doi.org/10.1212/WNL.0000000000008981

Horn, J. L., & Masunaga, H. (2000). New directions for research into aging and intelligence: the development of expertise. In Perfect, T. J., & Maylor, E. A. (Eds.) *Models of cognitive aging,* (pp. 125-159). Oxford University Press.

Huang, Y., Huang, X., Zhang, L., Han, F., Pang, K. L., Li, X., & Shen, J. Y. (2018). Magnesium boosts the memory restorative effect of environmental enrichment in Alzheimer's disease mice. *CNS Neuroscience & Therapeurics, 24*(1):70-79. https://doi.org/10.1111/cns.12775

Icahn School of Medicine at Mount Sinai (2022). Best to get your vitamins from your food. *Focus on Healthy Aging, 25*(2), 1-6.

Iqbal, R., Dehghan, M., Mente, A., Rangarajan, S., Wielgosz, A., Avezum, A., Seron, P., AlHabib, K. F., Lopez-Jaramillo, P., Swaminathan, S., Mohammadifard, N., Zatońska, K., Bo, H., Varma, R. P., Rahman, O., Yusufali, AH., Lu, Y., Ismail, N., Rosengren, A., ... Yusuf, S., on behalf of the PURE study. (2021). Associations of unprocessed and processed meat intake with mortality and cardiovascular disease in 21 countries [Prospective Urban Rural Epidemiology (PURE) Study]: a prospective cohort study, *The American Journal of Clinical Nutrition, 114*(24), 1049-1058. https://doi.org/10.1093/ajcn/nqaa448

Jacka, F. N., Cherbuin, N., Anstey, K. J., Schdev, P., & Butterworth, P. (2015). Western diet is associated with a smaller hippocampus: A longitudinal investigation. *BMC Medicine, 13*, 215. https://doi.org/10.1186/s12916-015-0461-x

Jacobs, T. L., Epel, E. S., Lin, J., Blackburn, E. H., Wolkowitz, O. M., Bridwell, D. A., Zanesco, A. P., Aiche, S. R., Sahdra, D. K., MacLean, K. A., King, B. G., Shaver, P. R., Rosenberg, E. L., Ferrer, E., Wallace, B. A., & Saron, C. D. (2010). Intensive meditation training, immune cell telomerase activity, and psychological mediators. *Psychoneuroendocrinology, 36*(5), 664-681. https://doi.org/10.1016/j.psyneuen.2010.09.010

Jefferson, A. L., Himali, J. J., Beiser, A. S., Au, R., Massaro, J. M., Seshadri, S., Gona, P., Salton, C. J., DeCarli, C., O'Donnel, C. J., Benjamin, E. J., Wolf, P. A., & Manning, W. J. (2010). Cardiac index is associated with brain aging: The Framingham Heart Study. *Circulation, 122*(7), 690–697. https://doi.org/10.1161/CIRCULATIONAHA.109.905091

Jernerén, F., Cederholm, T., Refsum, H., Smith, A. D., Turner, C., Palmblad, J., Eriksdotter, M., Hjorth, E., Faxen-Irving, G., Wahlund, L.-O., Schultzberg, M., Basun, H., & Freund-Levi, Y. (2019). Homocysteine status modifies the treatment effect of Omega-3 fatty acids on cognition in a randomized clinical trial in mild to moderate Alzheimer's disease: The OmegAD Study. *Journal of Alzheimer's Disease, 69*(1), 189-197. https://doi.org/10.3233/JAD-181148

Kalaras, M. D., Richie, J. P., Calcagnotto, A., & Beelman, R. B. (2017). Mushrooms: A rich source of the antioxidants ergothioneine and glutathione. *Food Chemistry, 233.* https://doi.org/101016j.foodchem.2017.04.109

Kamkaew, N., Scholfield, C. N., Ingkaninan, K., Taepavarapruk, N., & Chootip, K. (2013). *Bacopa monnieri* increases cerebral blood flow in rat independent of blood pressure. *Phytotherapy Research, 27*(1), 135–138. https://doi.org/10.1002/ptr.4685

Kaplan, B. J., Rucklidge, J. J., Romijn, A., & McLeod, K. (2015). The emerging field of nutritional mental health: Inflammation, the microbiome, oxidative stress, and mitochondrial function. *Clinical Psychological Science, 3*(6), 964-980. https://doi.org/10.1177/2167702614555413

Karlamangla, A. S., Singer, B. H., Chodosh, J., McEwen, B. S., & Seeman, T. S. (2005). Urinary cortisol excretion as a predictor of incident cognitive impairment. *Neurobiology of Aging, 26*, Suppl 1, 80-84. https://doi.org/10.1016/j.neurobiolaging.2005.09.037

Kazdin, A. E. (2016). Editor's introduction: Special series on nutrition and mental health. *Clinical Psychological Science, 4*(6), 1080-1081. https://doi.org/10.1177/2167702616651051

Kiechl, S., Pechlaner, R., Willeit, P., Notdurfter, M., Paulweber, B., Willeit, K., Werner, P., Ruckenstuhl, C., Iglseder, B., Weger, S., Mairhofer, B., Gartner, M., Kedenko, L., Chmelikova, M., Stekovic, S., Stuppner, H., Oberhollenzer, F., Kroemer, G., Mayr, M., ... Willeit, J. (2018). Higher spermidine intake is linked to lower mortality: A prospective population-based study. *American Journal of Clinical Nutrition, 108*(2), 371-380. https://doi.org/10.1093/ajcn/nqy102

Kiely, A., Ferland, G., Ouliass, B., O'Toole, P. W., Purtill, H., & O'Connor, E. M. (2020). Vitamin K status and inflammation are associated with cognition in older Irish adults, *Nutritional Neuroscience, 23*(8), 591-599. https://doi.org/10.1080/1028415X.2018.1536411

Kirkland, A. E., Sarlo, G. L., & Holton, K. (2018). The role of magnesium in neurological disorders. *Nutrients, 10*(6), 730. https://doi.org/10.3390/nu10060730

Klinedinst, B. S., Le, S. T., Larsen, B., Pappas, C., Hoth, N. J., Pollpeter, A., Wang, Q., Wang, Y., Yu, S., Wang, L., Allenspach, K., Mochel, J. P., Bennett, D. A., & Willette, A. A. (2020). Genetic factors of Alzheimer's disease modulate how diet is associated with long-term cognitive trajectories: A UK Biobank study. *Journal of Alzheimer's Disease, 78*(3), 1245-1257. https://doi.org/10.3233/JAD-201058

Kongkeaw, C., Dilokthornsakul, P., Thanarangsarit, P., Limpeanchob, N., & Scholfield, N. (2014). Meta-analysis of randomized controlled trials on cognitive effects of *Bacopa Monnieri* extract. *Journal of Ethnopharmacology, 151*(1), 528-535. https://doi.org/10.1016/j.jep.2013.11.008

Konttinen, H., Cabral-da-Silva, M., Ohtonen, S., Wojciechowski, S., Shakirzyanova, A., Caligola, S., Giugno, R., Ishchenko, Y., Hernandez, D., Fazaludeen, M. F., Eamen, S., Budia, M. G., Fagerlund, I., Scoyni, F., Korhonen, P., Huber, N., Haapasalo, A., Hewitt, A. W., Vickers, J., ... Malm, T. (2019). PSEN1∆E9, APPswe, and APOE4 confer disparate phenotypes in human iPSC-derived microglia. *Stem Cell Reports, 13*(4), 669-683. https://doi.org/10.1016/j.stemcr.2019.08.004

Krikorian, R., Shidler, M. D., Dangelo, K., Couch, S. C., Benoit, S., C., & Clegg, D. J. (2012). Dietary ketosis enhances memory in mild cognitive impairment. *Neurobiology of Aging, 33*(2), 425.e19–425.e27. https://doi.org/10.1016/j.neurobiolaging.2010.10.006

Kumar, N., Abichandani, L. G., Thawani, V., Gharpure, K. J., Naidu, M. U. R., & Ramana, G. V. (2016). Efficacy of standardized extract of Bacopa monnieri (Bacognize®) on cognitive functions of medical students: a six-week, randomized placebo-controlled trial. *Evidence Based Complementary and Alternative Medicine, eCAM, 2016*, 4103423. https://doi.org/10.1155/2016/4103423

Kumar, P., Liu, C., Hsu, J. W., Chacko, S., Minard, C., Jahoor, F., & Sekhar, R. V. (2021). Glycine and N-acetylcysteine (GlyNAC) supplementation in older adults improves glutathione deficiency, oxidative stress, mitochondrial dysfunction, inflammation, insulin resistance, endothelial dysfunction, genotoxicity, muscle strength, and cognition: Results of a pilot clinical trial. *Clinical and Translational Medicine, 11*(3), e372. https://doi.org/10.1002/ctm2.372

Laird, E., O'Halloran, A., Molloy, A., Healy, M., Hernandez, B., O'Connor, D., Kenny R. A. & Briggs, R. (2021). Low vitamin B12 but not folate is associated with incident depressive symptoms in community-dwelling older adults: A 4-year longitudinal study. *British Journal of Nutrition*, 1-22. Advance online publication. https://doi.org/10.1017/S0007114521004748

Lam, A. B., Kervin, K., & Tanis, J. E. (2021). Vitamin B12 impacts amyloid beta-induced proteotoxicity by regulating the methionine/S-adenosylmethionine cycle. *Cell Reports*. *36*(13), 109753. https://doi.org/10.1016/j.celrep.2021.10 9753

Lam, V., Takechi, R., Hackett, M. J., Francis, R., Bynevelt, M., Celliers, L. M., Nesbit, M., Mamsa, S., Arfuso, F., Das, S., Koentgen, F., Hagan, M., Codd, L., Richardson, K., O'Mara, B., Scharli, R. K., Morandeau, L., Gauntlett, J., Leatherday, C., Boucek, J., & Mamo, J. C. L. (2021). Synthesis of human amyloid restricted to liver results in an Alzheimer disease–like neurodegenerative phenotype. *PLoS Biology 19*(9): e3001358. https://doi.org/10.1371/journal.pbio.3001358

Lassale, C., Batty, G. D., Baghdadli, A., Jacka, F., Sánchez-Villegas, A., Kivimäki, M., & Akbaraly, T. (2019). Healthy dietary indices and risk of depressive outcomes: a systematic review and meta-analysis of observational studies. *Molecular Psychiatry 24*, 965–986. https://doi.org/10.1038/s41380-018-0237-8

Lauretti, E., Iuliano, L., & Pratic D. (2017). Extra-virgin oive oil ameliorates cognition and neuropathology of the 3xTg mice: Role of autophagy. *Annals of Clinical and Translational Neurology 4*(8), 564–574. https://doi.org/10.1002/acn3.431

Leclerc, E., Trevizol, A. P., Grigolon, R. B., Subramaniapillai M., McIntyre, R. S., Brietzke, E., & Mansur, R. G. (2020). The effect of caloric restriction on working memory in healthy non-obese adults. *CNS Spectrum*, *25*(1), 2–8. https://doi.org/10.1017/S1092852918001566, 2-8.

LeDoux, J. (2002). *Synaptic self: How our brains become who we are*. Penguin Books.

Lee, H., & Birks, J. S. (2018). Ginkgo biloba for cognitive improvement in healthy individuals. *Cochrane Database Systematic Reviews*, *2018*(8), CD004671. https://doi.org/10.1002/14651858.CD004671

Li, J., Romero-Garcia, R., Suckling, J., & Feng, L. (2019). Habitual tea drinking modulates brain efficiency: Evidence from brain connectivity evaluation. *Aging, 11*, 3876. https://doi.org/10.18632/aging.102023

Li, Z., Li, B., Song, X., & Zhang, D. (2017). Dietary zinc and iron intake and risk of depression: A meta-analysis. *Psychiatry Research, 251*, 41-47. https://doi.org/10.1016/j.psychres.2017.02.006

Listabarth, S., König, D., Vyssoki, B., & Hametner, S. (2020). Does thiamin protect the brain from iron overload and alcohol-related dementia? *Alzheimer's & Dementia, 16*(11), 1591-1595. https://doi.org/10.1002/alz.12 146

Liu, H., Ye, M., & Guo, H. (2019). An updated review of randomized clinical trials testing the improvement of cognitive function of *Ginkgo biloba* extract in healthy people and Alzheimer's patients. *Frontiers of Pharmacology, 10*, 1668. https://doi.org/10.3389/fphar.2019.01688

Liu, Q. P., Wu, Y. F., Cheng, H. Y., Xia, T., Ding, H., Wang, H., Wang, Z. M., & Xu, Y. (2016). Habitual coffee consumption and risk of cognitive decline/

dementia: A systematic review and meta-analysis of prospective cohort studies. *Nutrition, 32*(6), 628-636. https://doi.org/10.1016/j.nut.2015.11.015

Loma Linda University Adventist Health Sciences Center (2018, April 24). Dark chocolate consumption reduces stress and inflammation: Data represent first human trials examining the impact of dark chocolate consumption on cognition and other brain functions. *ScienceDaily*. Retrieved March 27, 2022 from www.sciencedaily.com/releases/2018/04/180424133628.htm

Lundgaard, I., Wang, W., Eberhardt, A., Vinitsky, H. S., Reeves, B. C., Peng, S., Lou, N., Hussain, R., & Nedergaard, M. (2018). Beneficial effects of low alcohol exposure, but adverse effects of high alcohol intake on glymphatic function. *Scientific Reports, 8*(1), 2246. https://doi.org/10.1038/s41598-018-20424-y

Lupien, S. J., DeLeon, M. J., DeSanti, S., Convit, A., Tarshish, C., Nair, N. P. V., Thakur, M., McEwen, B. S., Hauger, R. L., & Meaney, M. J. (1998). Cortisol levels during human aging predict hippocampal atrophy and memory deficits. *Nature Neuroscience, 1*(1), 69-73. https://doi.org/10.1038/271

McIntosh, C., & Chick, J. (2004). Alcohol and the nervous system. *Journal of Neurology, Neurosurgery & Psychiatry, 75*(Issue Supplement 3). http://dx.doi.org/10.1136/jnnp.2004.045708

Madeo, F., Hofer, S. J., Pendl, T., Bauer, M. A., Eisenberg, T., Carmona-Gutierrez, D., & Kroemer, G. (2020). Nutritional aspects of spermidine. *Annual Review of Nutrition, 40*, 135-159. https://doi.org/10.1146/annurev-nutr-120419-015419

Manap, A. S. A., Madhavan, P., Chia, Y. Y., Arya, A., Wong, E. H., Rizwan, F., Bindal, U., & Koshy, S. (2019). *Bacopa monnieri*, a neuroprotective lead in Alzheimer disease: A review on its properties, mechanisms of action, and preclinical and clinical studies. *Drug Target Insights, 13*, 1-13. https://doi.org/10.1177/1177392819866412

Martensson, J., Eriksson, J., Bodammer, N. C., Lindgren, M., Johansson, M., Nyberg, L., & Lovden, M. (2012). Growth of language-related brain areas after foreign language learning. *Neuroimage, 63*(1), 240–244. https://doi.org/10.1016/j.neuroimage.2012.06.043

Martikainen, J., Jalkanen, K., Heiskanen, J., Lavikainen, P., Peltonen, M., Laatikainen, T., & Lindström, J. (2021). Type-2 diabetes-related health economic impact associated with increased whole grains consumption among adults in Finland. *Nutrients, 13*, 3583. https://doi.org/10.3390/nu13103583

Martinez-Lapiscina, E. H., Clavero, P., Toledo, E., Estruch, R., Salas-Salvado, J., San Julian, B., Sanchez-Tainta, A., Ros, E., Valls-Pedret, C., & Martinez-Gonzalez, M.A. (2013). Mediterranean diet improves cognition: the PREDIMED-NAVARRA randomised trial. *Journal of Neurology, Neurosurgery, and Psychiatry, 84*(12), 1318–1325. https://doi.org/10.1136/jnnp-2012-304792

Marx, W., Lane, M., Rocks, T., Ruusunen, A., Loughman, A., Lopresti, A., Marshall, S., Berk, M., Jacka, F., & Dean, O. M. (2019). Effect of saffron supplementation on symptoms of depression and anxiety: A systematic review and meta-analysis. *Nutrition Reviews, 77*(8), 557-571. [nuz023]. https://doi.org/10.1093/nutrit/nuz

Maserejian, N. N., Hall, S. A., & McKinlay, J. B. (2012). Low dietary or supplemental zinc is associated with depression symptoms among women, but not men, in a population-based epidemiological survey. *Journal of Affective Disorders, 136*(3), 781-788. https://doi.org/10.1016/j.jad.2011-09-039

Mather, M., & Lighthall, N. R. (2012). Both risk and reward are processed differently in decisions made under stress. *Current Directions in Psychological Science, 21*(2), 36–41. https://doi.org/10.1177/0963721411429452

Matsui, T., Ishikawa, T., Hitoshi, I., Okamoto, M., Inoue, K., Min-chul, L., Fujikawa, T., Ichitani, Y., Kawanaka, K., & Soya, H. (2012). Brain glycogen supercompensation following exhaustive exercise. *Journal of Physiology, 590*(3), 607–616. https://doi.org/10.1113/jphysiol.2011.217919

Mayne, P. E. & Burne, T. H. J. (2019). Vitamin D in synaptic plasticity, cognitive function, and neuropsychiatric illness. *Trends in Neurosciences, 42*(4), 293-306. https://doi.org/10.1016/j.tins.2019.01.003

Mayneris-Perxachs, J., Castells-Nobau, A., Arnoriaga-Rodríguez, M., Garre-Olmo, J., Puig, J., Ramos, R., Martínez-Hernández, F., Burokas, A., Coll, C., Moreno-Navarrete, J. M., Zapata-Tona, C., Pedraza, S., Pérez-Brocal, V., Ramió-Torrentà, L., Ricart, W., Moya, A., Martínez-García, M., Maldonado, R., & Fernández-Real, J-M. (2022). Caudovirales bacteriophages are associated with improved executive function and memory in flies, mice, and humans. *Cell Host & Microbe, 30*(3), 340-356.e8. https://doi.org/10.1016/j.chom.2022.01.013

Mazidi, M., Kengne, A. P., & Banach, M. (2017). Mineral and vitamin consumption and telomere length among adults in the United States. *Polish Archives of Internal Medicine, 127*, 87-90. https://doi.org/10.20452/pamw.3927

McBurney, M. I., Tintle, N. L., Vasan, R. S., Sala-Vila, A., & Harris, W. S. (2021). Using an erythrocyte fatty acid fingerprint to predict risk of all-cause mortality: the Framingham Offspring Cohort. *The American Journal of Clinical Nutrition, 114*(6) https://doi.org/10.1093/ajcn/nqab195

McCleery, J., Abraham, R. P., Denton, D. A., Rutjes, A. W., Chong, L-Y., Al-Assaf, A. S., Griffith, D. J., Rafeeq, S., Yaman, H., Malik, M. A., Di Nisio, M., Martinez, G., Vernooij, R. W., & Tabet, N. (2018). Vitamin and mineral supplementation for preventing dementia or delaying cognitive decline in people with mild cognitive impairment. *The Cochrane Database of Systematic Reviews, 11*(11), CD011905. *https://doi.org/10.1002/14651858.CD011905.pub2*

Meaney, M. J., Aitken, D. H., Bhatnagar, S., & Sapolsky, R. M. (1990). Postnatal handling attenuates neuroendocrine, anatomical, and cognitive dysfunctions associated with aging in female rats. *Neurobiology of Aging, 12*(1), 31–38. https://doi.org/10.1016/0197-4580(91)90036-j

Metcalfe-Roach A., Yu, A. C., Golz, E., Cirstea, M., Sundvick, K., Kliger, D., Foulger, L. H., Mackenzie, M., Finlay, B. B., & Appel-Cresswell, S. (2021). MIND and Mediterranean diets associated with later onset of Parkinson's disease. *Movement Disorders, 36*(4), 977-984. https://doi.org/10.1002/mds.28464.

Mielech, A., Puścion-Jakubik, A., Markiewicz-Żukowska, R., & Socha, K. (2020). Vitamins in Alzheimer's disease: Review of the latest reports. *Nutrients, 12*(11), 3458. https://doi.org/10.3390/nu12113458

Miller, G. E., & Blackwell, E. (2006). Turning up the heat: Inflammation as a mechanism linking chronic stress, depression, and heart disease. *Current Directions in Psychological Science, 15*(6), 269–272. https://doi.org/10.1111/j.1467-8721.2006.00450.x

Mitra, S., Rauf, A., Tareq, A. M., Jahan, S., Emran, T. B., Shahriar, T. G., Dhama, K., Alhumaydhi, F. A., Aljohani, A. S. M., Rebezov, M., Uddin, M. S., Jeandet, P., Shah, Z. A., Shariati, M. A., & Rengasamy, K. R. R. (2021). Potential health benefits of carotenoid lutein: An updated review. *Food and Chemical Toxicology, 154*, 112328. https://doi.org/10.1016/j.fct.2021.112328

Mock, J. T., Chaudhari, K., Sidhu, A., & Sumien, N. (2017). The influence of vitamins E and C and exercise on brain aging. *Experimental Gerontology, 94*, 69-72. https://doi.org/10.1016/j.exger.2016.12.008

Modi, K. K., Rangasamy, S. B., Dasarathi, S., Roy, A., & Pahan, K. (2016). Cinnamon converts poor learning mice to good learners: Implications for memory improvement. *Journal of Neuroimmune Pharmacology, 11*(4), 693-707. https://doi.org/10.1007/s11481-016-9693-6

Modi, K. K., Roy, A., Brahmachari, S., Rangasamy, S. B., & Pahan, K. (2015). Cinnamon and its metabolite sodium benzoate attenuate the activation of p21rac and protect memory and learning in an animal model of Alzheimer's disease. *PLoS One_10*(6), e0130398. https://doi.org/10.1371/journal.pone.0130398.eCollection 2015 10:e0130398

Momtaz, S., Hassani, S., Khan, F., Ziaee, M., & Abdollahi, M. (2018). Cinnamon, a promising prospect towards Alzheimer's disease. *Pharmacological Research, 130*, 241-258. https://doi.org/10.1016/j.phrs.2017.12.011

Moore, K., Hughes, C. F., Ward, M., Hoey, L. & McNulty, H. (2018). Diet, nutrition and the ageing brain: Current evidence and new directions. *Proceedings of the Nutrition Society, 77*(2), 152–163. https://doi.org/10.1017/S0029665117004177

Moore, L., Le, T., & Fan, G. (2013). DNA methylation and its basic function. *Neuropsychopharmacology, 38*, 23–38. https://doi.org/10.1038/npp.2012.112

Morley, J. E. (2004). The top 10 hot topics in aging. *The Journals of Gerontology: Series A, 59*(1), M24–M33. https://doi.org/10.1093/gerona/59.1.M24

Morris, M. C., Tangney, C. C., Wang Y., Sacks, F. M., Bennett, D. A., & Aggarwal, N. T. (2015). MIND diet associated with reduced incidence of Alzheimer's disease. *Alzheimer's and Dementia, 11*(9), 1007–1014. https://doi.org/10.1016/j.jalz.2014.11.009

Naoi, M., Shamoto-Nagai, M., & Maruyama, W. (2019). Neuroprotection of multifunctional phytochemicals as novel therapeutic strategy for neurodegenerative disorders: antiapoptotic and antiamyloidogenic activities by modulation of cellular signal pathways. *Nature Neurology, 14*(1), FLN9. https://doi.org/10.2217/fnl-2018-0028

Napoletano, F., Schifano, F., Corkey, J. M., Guirguis, A., Arillotta, D., Zangani, C., & Vento, A. (2020). The psychonauts' world of cognitive enhancers. *Frontiers in Psychiatry, 11*, 546796. https://doi.org/10.3389/fpsyt.2020.546796

Nemetchek, M. D., Stierle, A. A., Stierle, D. B., & Lurie, D. I. (2017). The Ayurvedic plant *Bacopa monnieri* inhibits inflammatory pathways in the brain. *Journal of Ethnopharmacology, 197*, 92-100. https://doi.org/10.1016/j.jep.2016.07.073

Neshatdoust, S., Saunders, C., Castle, S. M., Vauzour, D., Williams, C., Butler, L., Lovegrove, J. A., & Spencer, J. P. E. (2017). High-flavonoid intake induces cognitive improvements linked to changes in serum brain-derived neurotrophic factor: Two randomised, controlled trials. *Nutrition and Healthy Aging, 4*(1), 81-93. https://doi.org/10.3233/NHA-1615

Ng, Q. X., Venkatanarayanan, N., & Ho, C. Y. (2017). Clinical use of *Hypericum perforatum* (St John's wort) in depression: A meta-analysis. *Journal of Affective Disorders, 210*, 211–221. https://doi.org/10.1016/j.jad.2016.12.048

Nishida, K., Sawada, D., Kuwano, Y., Tanaka, H., Sugawara, T., Aoki, Y., Fujiwara, S., & Rokutan, K. (2017). Daily administration of paraprobiotic *Lactobacillus gasseri* CP2305 ameliorates chronic stress-associated symptoms in Japanese medical students. *Journal of Functional Foods, 36*, 112-121. https://doi.org/10.1016/j.jff.2017.06.031

Niu, Y., Na, L., Feng, R., Gong, L., Zhao, Y., Li, Q., Li, Y., & Sun, C. (2013). The phytochemical, EGCG, extends lifespan by reducing liver and kidney function damage and improving age-associated inflammation and oxidative stress in healthy rats. *Aging Cell, 12*(6), 1041-1049. https://doi.org/10.11 11/acel.2013.12.issue-6/issuetoc

Noonan, S., Zaveri, M., Macaninch, E., & Martyn, K. (2020). Food & mood: a review of supplementary prebiotic and probiotic interventions in the treatment of anxiety and depression in adults. *BMJ Nutrition, Prevention & Health, 2020*. bmjnph-2019-000053. https://doi.org/10.1136/bmjnph-2019-000053

Nooyens, A. C. J., Bueno-de-Mesquita1, H. G., van Gelder, B. M., van Boxtel, M. P. J., & Verschuren, W. M. M. (2014). Consumption of alcoholic beverages and cognitive decline at middle age: the Doetinchem Cohort Study. *British Journal of Nutrition, 111*(4), 715–723. https://doi.org/10.1017/S00071145130 02845

Nouchi, R., Suiko, T., Kimura, E., Takenaka, H., Murakoshi, M., Uchiyama, A., Aono, M., & Kawashima, R. (2020). Effects of lutein and astaxanthin intake on the improvement of cognitive functions among healthy adults: A systematic review of randomized controlled trials. *Nutrients, 12*(3), 617. https://doi.org/10.3390/nu12030617

Ntranos, A., Park, H.-J., Wentling, M., Tolstikov, V., Amatruda, M., Inbar, B., Kim-Schulze, S., Frazier, C., Button, J., Kiebish, M. A., Lublin, F., Edwards, K., & Casaccia, P. (2021). Bacterial neurotoxic metabolites in multiple sclerosis cerebrospinal fluid and plasma. *Brain*, awab320. https://doi.org/10.1093/brain/awab320

Nurk, E., Refsum, H., Drevon, C. A., Tell, G. S., Nygaard, H. A., Engedal, K., & Smith, A. D. (2009). Intake of flavonoid-rich wine, tea, and chocolate by elderly men and women is associated with better cognitive test performance. *Journal of Nutrition, 139*(1), 120–127. https://doi.org/10.3945/jn.108.095182

Nurk, E., Refsum, H., Drevon, C. A., Tell, G. S., Nygaard, H. A., Engedal, K., & Smith, A. D. (2010). Cognitive performance among the elderly in relation to the intake of plant foods. The Hordaland Health Study. *British Journal of Nutrition, 104*(8), 1190-1201. https://doi.org/10.1017/S0007114510001807

Okereke, O. I., Vyas, C. M., Mischoulon, D., Chang, G., Cook, N. R., Weinberg, A., Bubes, V., Copeland, T., Friedenberg, G., Lee, I-M., Buring, J. E., Reynolds

III, C. F., & Manson, J. E. (2021). Effect of long-term supplementation with marine Omega-3 fatty acids vs placebo on risk on depression or clinically-relevant depressive symptoms and on change in mood scores: A randomized clinical trial. *Journal of the American Medical Association, 326*(23), 2385-2394. https://doi.org/10.1001/jama.2021.21187

Oliver, A., Chase, A. B., Weihe, C., Orchanian, S. B., Riedel, S. F., Hendrickson, C. L., Lay, M., Sewall, J. M., Martiny, J. B. H., & Whiteson, K. (2021). High-fiber, whole-food dietary intervention alters the human gut microbiome but not fecal short-chain fatty acids. *mSystems, 6*(2): e00115-21. https://doi.org/10.1128/mSystems.00115-21

O'Rourke, M. F. (2008). Brain microbleeds, amyloid plaques, intellectual deterioration, and arterial stiffness. *Hypertension, 51,* e20. https://doi.org/10.1161/HYPERTENSIONAHA.107.109199

Oulhaj, A., Jernerén, F., Refsum, H., Smith, A. D., & de Jager, C. A. (2016). Omega-3 fatty acid status enhances the prevention of cognitive decline by B vitamins in Mild Cognitive Impairment. *Journal of Alzheimer's Disease, 50*(2), 547-557. https://doi.org/10.3233/JAD-150777

Ozawa, M., Shipley, M., Kivimaki, M., Singh-Manoux, S., & Brunner, E. J. (2017). Dietary pattern, inflammation and cognitive decline: The Whitehall II prospective cohort study. *Clinical Nutrition, 36*(2), 506-512. https://doi.org/10.1016/j.clnu.2016.01.013

Pagano, G., Pallardó, F. V., Lyakhovich, A., Tiano, L., Fittipaldi, M. R., Toscanesi, M., & Trifuoggi, M. (2020). Aging-related disorders and mitochondrial dysfunction: A critical review for prospect mitoprotective strategies based on mitochondrial nutrient mixtures. *International Journal of Molecular Sciences, 21*(19), 7060. https://doi.org/10.3390/ijms21197060

Pak, H. H., Haws, S. A., Green, C. L., Koller, M., Lavarias, M. T., Richardson, N. E., Yang, S. E., Dumas, S. N., Sonsalla, M., Bray, L., Johnson, M., Barnes, S., Darley-Usmar, V., Zhang, J., Yen, C-L. E., Denu, J. M., & Lamming, D. W. (2021). Fasting drives the metabolic, molecular and geroprotective effects of a calorie-restricted diet in mice. *Nature Metabolism, 3*(10), 1327-1341. https://doi.org/10.1038/s42255-021-00466-9

Panza, F., Lozupone, M., Solfrizzi, V., Custodero, C., Valiani, V., D'Introno, A., Stella, E., Stallone, R., Piccininni, M., Bellomo, A., Seripa, D., Daniele, A., Greco, A., & Logroscino, G., (2018). Contribution of Mediterranean diet in the prevention of Alzheimer's disease. In Farooqui, T., & Farooqui, A. (Eds.) *Role of the mediterranean diet in the brain and neurodegenerative diseases,* (pp. 139-155). Academic Press.

Park, D. C., Lodi-Smith, J., Drew, L., Haber, S., Hebrank, A., Bischof, G. N., & Aamodt, W. (2014). The impact of sustained engagement on cognitive function in older adults: The synapse project. *Psychological Science, 25*(1), 103–112. https://doi.org/10.1177/0956797613499592

Park, S-Y., Freedman, N. D., Haiman, C. A., LeMarchand, L., Wilkens, L. R., & Setiawan, W. (2017). Association of coffee consumption with total and cause-specific mortality among nonwhite populations. *Annals of Internal Medicine, 167*(4), 228–235. https://doi.org/10.7326/M16-2472

Parkin, A. J. & Rosalind, I. J. (2000). Determinants of age-related memory loss. In Perfect, T. J., & Maylor, E. A. (Eds.) *Models of cognitive aging*, (pp. 188-203). Oxford University Press.

Pase, M. P., Kean, J., Sarris, J., Neale, C., Scholey, A. B., & Stough, C. (2012). The cognitive-enhancing effects of *Bacopa monnieri:* A systematic review of randomized, controlled human clinical trials. *Journal of Alternative and Complementary Medicine, 18*(7), 647-652. https://doi.org/10.1089/acm.2011.0367

Patel, P. & Shah, J. (2017). Role of vitamin D in amyloid clearance via LRP-1 upregulation in Alzheimer's disease: A potential therapeutic target? *Journal of Chemical Neuroanatomy, 85*, 36-42. https://doi.org/10.1016/j.jchemneu.2017.06.007

Pavlopoulos, E., Jones, S., Kosmidis, S., Close, M., Kim, C., Kovalerchik, O., Small, S. A., & Kandel, E. R. (2013). Molecular mechanism for age-related memory loss: The histone-binding protein RbAp48. *Science Translational Medicine, 5*, 200ra115. https://doi.org/10.1126/scitranslmed.3006373

Peeri, N. C., Egan, K. M., Chai, W., & Tao, M-H. (2020). Association of magnesium intake and vitamin D status with cognitive function in older adults: an analysis of US National Health and Nutrition Examination Survey (NHANES) 2011 to 2014. *European Journal of Nutrition, 60*(1), 465–474. https://doi.org/10.1007/s00394-020-02267-4

Pekar, T., Wendzel, A., Flak, W., Kremer, A., Pauschenwein-Frantsich, S., Gschaider, A., Wantke, F., & Jarisch, R. (2020). Spermidine in dementia: Relation to age and memory performance. *Wien Klin Wochenschr 132*(1-2), 42–46. https://doi.org/10.1007/s00508-019-01588-7

Peth-Nui, T., Wattanathorn, J., Muchimapura, S., Tong-Un, T., Piyavhatkul, N., Rangseekajee, P., Ingkaninan, K., & Vittaya-areekul, S. (2012). Effects of 12-week *Bacopa monnieri* consumption on attention, cognitive processing, working memory, and functions of both cholinergic and monoaminergic systems in healthy elderly volunteers. *Evidence-Based Complementary and Alternative Medicine: eCAM 2012*, 606424. https://doi.org/10.1155/2012/606424

Pham, K., Mulugeta, A., Zhou, A., O'Brien, J. T., Llewellyn, D. J., & Hyppönen, E. (2021). High coffee consumption, brain volume and risk of dementia and stroke. *Nutritional Neuroscience*, 1-12, Advance online publication. https://doi.org/10.1080/1028415X.2021.1945858

Piao, M., Cong, X., Lu, Y., Feng, C., & Ge, P. (2017). The role of zinc in mood disorders. *Neuropsychiatry, 7*(4), 378-386. https://doi.org/10.1097/MCO.0b013e32833df61a

Picard, M., McManus, M. J., Gray, J. D., Nasca, C., Moffat, C., Kopinskia, P. K., Seifert, E. L., McEwen, B. S., & Wallace, D. C. (2015). Mitochondrial functions modulate neuroendocrine, metabolic, inflammatory, and transcriptional responses to acute psychological stress. *Proceedings of the National Academy of Sciences of the United States of America, 112*(48), E6614-E6623. https://doi.org/10.1073/pnas.1515733112

Pivina, L., Semenova, Y., Doşa, M. D., Dauletyarova, M., & Bjorklund, G. (2019). Iron deficiency, cognitive functions, and neurobehavioral disorders in children. *Journal of Molecular Neuroscience, 68*(1), 1–10. https://doi.org/10.1007/s12031-019-01276-1

Prinelli, F., Fratiglioni, L., Kalpouzos, G., Musicco, M., Adorni, F., Johansson, I., Marseglia, A., & Xu W. (2019). Specific nutrient patterns are associated with higher structural brain integrity in dementia-free older adults. *Neuroimage, 199*, 281-288. doi:10.1016/j.neuroimage.2019.05.066

Qin, X.-Y., Cao, C., Cawley, N. X., Liu, T.-T., Yuan, J., Loh, Y. P., & Cheng, Y. (2017). Decreased peripheral brain-derived neurotrophic factor levels in Alzheimer's disease: A meta-analysis study (N=7277). *Molecular Psychiatry, 22*(2), 312-320. https//doi.org/10.1038/mp.2016.62.

Quach, A., Levine, M. E., Tanaka, T., Lu, A. T., Chen, B. H., Ferrucci, L., Ritz, B., Bandinelli, S., Neuhouser, M. L., Beasley, J. M., Snetselaar, L., Wallace, R. B., Tsao, P. S., Absher, D., Assimes, T. L., Stewart, J. D., Li, Y., Hou, L., Baccarelli, A. A., Whitsel, E. A., ... Horvath, S. (2017). Epigenetic clock analysis of diet, exercise, education, and lifestyle factors. *Aging, 9*(2), 419–446. https://doi.org/10.18632/aging.101168

Rainey-Smith, S., Brown, B., Sohrabi, H., Shah, T., Goozee, K., Gupta, V., & Martins, R. (2016). Curcumin and cognition: A randomised, placebo-controlled, double-blind study of community-dwelling older adults. *British Journal of Nutrition, 115*(12), 2106-2113. https://doi.org/10.1017/S0007114516001203

Rangel-Huerta, O. D. & Gil, A. (2018). Effect of omega-3 fatty acids on cognition: an updated systematic review of randomized clinical trials. *Nutrition Reviews, 76*, 1–20. https://doi.org/10.1093/nutrit/nux064

Razazan, A., Karunakar, P., Mishra, S. P., Sharma, S., Miller, B., Jain, S., & Yadav, H. (2021). Activation of microbiota sensing – free fatty acid receptor 2 signaling ameliorates amyloid-β induced neurotoxicity by modulating proteolysis-senescence axis. *Frontiers in Aging Neuroscience, 13*, 735933. https://doi.org/10.3389/fnagi.2021.735933

Redford, K. E., Rognant, S., Jepps, T. A., & Abbott, G. W. (2021). KCNQ5 potassium channel activation underlies vasodilation by tea. *Cellular Physiology and Biochemistry, 55*(S3), 46–64. https://doi.org/10.33594/000000337

Redman, L. M., Smith, S. R., Burton, J. H., Martin, C. K., Il'yasova, D., & Ravussin, E. (2018). Metabolic slowing and reduced oxidative damage with sustained caloric restriction support the rate of living and oxidative damage theories of aging. *Cell Metabolism, 27*(4), 805-815. https://doi.org/10.1016/j.cmet.2018.02.019

Rezai-Zadeh, K., Arendash, G. W., Hou, H., Fernandez, F., Jensen, M., Runfeldt, M., Shytle, R. D., & Tan, J. (2008). Green tea epigallocatechin-3-gallate (EGCG) reduces β-amyloid mediated cognitive impairment and modulates tau pathology in Alzheimer transgenic mice. *Brain Research, 1214*, 177-187. https://doi.org/10.1016/j.brainres.2008.02.107

Richard, E. L., Kritz-Silverstein, D., Laughlin, G. A., Fung, T. T., Barrett-Connor, E., & McEvoy, L. K. (2017). Alcohol intake and cognitively healthy longevity in community-dwelling adults: the Rancho Bernardo study. *Journal of Alzheimer's Disease, 59*(3), 803-814. https://doi.org/10.1093/geroni/igx004.1686

Rivas, A. (2013, August 4). More people than ever chose wine over beer: Did wine's health benefits win over drinkers? *Medical Daily.*

Rodrigues, R. R., Gurung, M., Li, Z., García-Jaramillo, M., Greer, R., Gaulke, C., Bauchinger, F., You, H., Pederson, J. W., Vasquez-Perez, S., White, K. D., Frink, B., Philmus, B., Jump, D. B., Trinchieri, G., Berry, D., Sharpton, T. J., Dzutsev, A., Morgun, A., & Shulzhenko, N. (2021). Transkingdom interactions between *Lactobacilli* and hepatic mitochondria attenuate western diet-induced diabetes. *Nature Communications, 12*(1), 101. https://doi.org/10.1038/s414 67-020-20313-x

Roodenrys, S., Booth, D., Bulzomi S., Phipps, A., Micallef, C., & Smoker, J. (2002). Chronic effects of Brahmi (*Bacopa monnieri*) on human memory. *Neuropsychopharmacology, 27*(2), 279–281. https://doi.org/10.1016/S0893-133X(01)00419-5

Rossman, M. J., Santos-Parker, J. R., Steward, C. A. C., Bispham, N. Z., Cuevas, L. M., Rosenberg, H. L., Woodward, K. A., Chonchol, M., Gioscia-Ryan, R. A., Murphy, M. P., & Seals, D. R. (2018). Chronic supplementation with a mitochondrial antioxidant (MitoQ) improves vascular function in healthy older adults. *Hypertension. 71*(6), 1056–1063. https://doi.org/10.1161/hypertensionaha.117.10787

Roth, T. L., Lubin, F. D., Funk, A. J., & Sweatt, J. D. (2009). Lasting epigenetic influence of early-life adversity on the BDNF gene. *Biological Psychiatry, 65*(9), 760–769. https://doi.org/10.1016/j.biopsych.2008.11.028

Ruan, Q., Ruan, J., Zhang, W., Qian, F., & Yu, Z. (2018). Targeting NAD+ degradation: The therapeutic potential of flavonoids for Alzheimer's disease and cognitive frailty. *Pharmacological Research, 128*, 345-358. https://doi.org/10.1016/j.phrs.2017.08.010

Ryu, D., Mouchiroud, L., Andreux, P. A., Katsyuba, E., Moullan, N., Nicolet-dit-Félix, A. A., Williams, E. G., Jha, P., Sasso, G. L., Huzard, D., Aebischer, P., Sandi, C., Rinsch, C., & Auwerx J. (2016). Urolithin A induces mitophagy and prolongs lifespan in *C. elegans* and increases muscle function in rodents. *Nature Medicine, 22*(8), 879–888. https://doi.org/10.1038/nm.4132

Saenghong, N., Wattanathorn, J., Muchimapura, S., Tongun, T., Piyavhatkul, N., Banchonglikitkul, C., & Kajsongkram, T. (2012). *Zingiber officinale* improves cognitive function of the middle-aged healthy women. *Evidence-Based Complementary and Alternative Medicine, 2012*(9), Article ID 383062. https://doi.org/10.1155/2012/383062

Sahardi, N. F. N. M., & Makpol, S. (2019). Ginger (*Zingiber officinale* Roscoe) in the pevention of ageing and degenerative diseases: Review of current evidence. *Evidence-Based Complementary and Alternative Medicine: eCAM, 2019*, 5054395. https://doi.org/10.1155/2019/5054395

Sakurai, K., Shen, C., Shiraishi, I., Inamura, N., & Hisatsune, T. (2021). Consumption of oleic acid on the preservation of cognitive functions in Japanese elderly individuals. *Nutrients, 13*(2), 284. https://doi.org/10.3390/nu13020284

Salomón, T., Sibbersen, C., Hansen, J., Britz, D., Svart, M. V., Voss, T. S., Møller, N., Gregersen, N., Jørgensen, K. A., Palmfeldt, J., Poulsen, T. B., & Johannsen, M. (2017). Ketone body acetoacetate buffers methylglyoxal via a nonenzymatic conversion during diabetic and dietary ketosis. *Cell Chemical Biology, 24*(8), 935–943.e7. https://doi.org/10.1016/j.chembiol.20 17.07.012

Sánchez-Villegas, A., Ruíz-Canela, M., Geak A., Lahortiga, L., & Martínez-Gonz, M. A. (2016). The association between the Mediterranean lifestyle and depression. *Clinical Psychological Science, 4*(6), 1085-1093. https://doi.org/10.1177%2F2167702616638651

Sarker, M. R., & Franks, S. F. (2018). Efficacy of curcumin for age-associated cognitive decline: a narrative review of preclinical and clinical studies. *GeroScience, 40*(2), 73–95. https://doi.org/10.1007/s11357-018-0017-z

Savage, K., Firth, J., Stough, C., & Sarris, J. (2018). GABA-modulating phytomedicines for anxiety: A systematic review of preclinical and clinical evidence. *Phytotherapy Research, 32*(1) 3-18. https://doi.org/10.1002/ptr.59 40

Sawada, D., Kawai, T., Nishida, K., Kuwano, Y., Fujiwara, S., & Rokutan, K. (2017). Daily intake of *Lactobacillus gasseri* CP2305 improves mental, physical and sleep quality among Japanese medical students enrolled in a cadaver dissection course. *Journal of Functional Foods, 31*, 188–197. https://doi.org/10.1016/j.jff.2017.01.042.

Schulkin, J., Gold, P. W., & McEwen, B. S. (1998). Induction of corticotropin-releasing hormone gene expression by glucocorticoids: Implications for understanding the states of fear and anxiety and allostatic load. *Psychoneuroendocrinology, 23*(3), 219–243. https://doi.org/10.1016/s0306-4530(97)00099-1

Schumacher, B., Pothof, J., Vijg, J. & Hoeijmakers (2021). The central role of DNA damage in the ageing process. *Nature, 592*(7856), 695–703. https://doi.org/10.1038/s41586-021-03307-7

Schwarz, C., Horn, N., Benson, G., Calzado, I. W., Wurdack, K., Pechlaner, R., Grittner, U., Wirth, M., & Flöel, A. (2020). Spermidine intake is associated with cortical thickness and hippocampal volume in older adults. *Neuroimage, 221*, 117132. https://doi.org/10.1016/j.neuroimage.2020.117132

Shafie, A., Rahimi, A. M., Ahmadi, I., Nabavizadeh, F., Ranjbaran, M., & Ashabi, G. (2020). High-protein and low-calorie diets improved the anti-aging Klotho protein in the rats' brain: the toxic role of high-fat diet. *Nutrition & Metabolism, 17*, Article 86. https://doi.org/10.1186/s12986-020-00508-1

Shalev, I., Entringer, S., Wadhwa, P. D., Wolkowitz, O. M., Puterman, E., Lin, J., & Epel, E. S. (2013). Stress and telomere biology: A life span perspective. *Psychoneuroendocrinology, 38* (9), 1835–1842. https://doi.org/10.1016/j.psy neuen.2013.03.010

Sherwin, B. B. & Henry, J. F. (2008). Brain aging modulates the neuroprotective effects of estrogen on selective aspects of cognition in women: A critical review. *Frontiers of Neuroendocrinology, 29* (1), 88–113. https://doi.org/10.1016/j.yfrne.2007.08.002

Shi, L., Brunius, C., Johansson, I., Bergdahl, I. A., Rolandsson, O., Guelpen, B., Winkvist, A., Hanhineva, K., & Landberg R. (2019). Plasma metabolite biomarkers of boiled and filtered coffee intake and their association with type 2 diabetes risk. *Journal of Internal Medicine, 287*(4), 405–421. https://doi.org/10.1111/joim.13009

Shi, Z., Li, M., Wang, Y., Liu J., & El-Obeid, T. (2019). High iron intake is associated with poor cognition among Chinese old adults and varied by weight status—a 15-y longitudinal study in 4852 adults. *The American Journal of Clinical Nutrition, 109*(1), 109–116. https://doi.org/10.1093/ajcn/nqy254

Shishtar, E., Rogers, G. T., Blumberg, J. B., Au, R., & Jacques, P. F. (2020). Long-term dietary flavonoid intake and risk of Alzheimer disease and related dementias in the Framingham Offspring Cohort. *The American Journal of Clinical Nutrition, 112*(2), 343–353. https://doi.org/10.1093/ajcn/nqaa079

Shively, C. A., Appta, S. E., Chenb, H., Dayc, S. M., Fryea, B. M., Shaltoutd, H. A., Silverstein-Metzlera, M. G., Snyder-Macklere, N., Ubersedera, B., Vitolinsf, M. Z., & Registera, R. C. (2020). Mediterranean diet, stress resilience, and aging in nonhuman primates. *Neurobiology of Stress, 13,* 100254. https://doi.org/10.1016/j.ynstr.2020.100254

Singh, B., Parsaik, A. K., Mielke, M. M., Erwin, P. J., Knopman, D. S., Petersen, R. C., & Roberts, R. O. (2014). Association of Mediterranean diet with mild cognitive impairment and Alzheimer's disease: A systematic review and meta-analysis. *Journal of Alzheimer's Disease, 39*(2): 271-282. https://doi.org/10.3233/JAD-130830

Skvarc, D. R., Dean, O. M., Byrne, L. K., Gray, L., Lane, S., Lewis, M., Fernandes, B. S., Berk, M., & Marriott, A. (2017). The effect of N-acetylcysteine (NAC) on human cognition – A systematic review. *Neuroscience and Biobehavioral Reviews, 78,* 44-56. https://doi.org/10.1016/j.neubiorev.2017.04.013

Slutsky, I., Abumaria, N., Wu, L.-J., Huang, C., Zhang, L., Li, B., Zhao, X., Govindarajan, A., Zhao, M-G., Zhuo, M., Tonegawa, S., & Liu, G. (2010). Enhancement of learning and memory by elevating brain magnesium. *Neuron, 65*(2), 165–177. https://doi.org/10.1016/j.neuron.2009.12.026

Small, G. W., Siddarth, P., Li, Z., Miller, K. J., Ercoli, L., Emerson, N. D., Martinez, J., Wong, K. P., Liu, J., Merrill, D. A., Chen, S. T., Henning, S. M., Satyamurthy, N., Huang, S. C., Heber, D., & Barrio, J. R. (2017). Memory and brain amyloid and tau effects of a bioavailable form of curcumin in non-demented adults: A double-blind, placebo-controlled 18-month trial. *American Journal of Geriatric Psychiatry. 26*(3), 266-277. https://doi.org/10.1016/j.jagp.2017.10.010

Smith, A. D., Smith, S. M., de Jager, C. A., Whitbread, P., Johnston, C., Agacinski, G., Oulhaj, A., Bradley, K. M., Jacoby, R., & Refsum, H. (2010). Homocysteine-lowering by B vitamins slows the rate of accelerated brain atrophy in mild cognitive impairment: a randomized controlled trial. *PLoS One, 5*(9):e12244. https://doi.org/10.1371/journal.pone.0012244. PMID: 20838622; PMCID: PMC2935890.

Smith, A. D., & Refsum, H. (2021). Homocysteine - from disease biomarker to disease prevention. *Journal of Internal Medicine, 290*(4) 826-854. https://doi.org/:10.1111/joim.13279

Smith, L. K., & Wissel, E. F. (2019). Microbes and the mind: How bacteria shape affect, neurological processes, cognition, social relationships, development, and pathology. *Perspectives on Psychological Science 14*(3), 397–418. https://doi.org/10.1177/1745691618809379

Sobesky, J. L., Barrientos, R. M., De May, H. S., Thompson, B. M., Weber, M. D., Watkins, L. R., & Maier, S. F. (2014). High-fat diet consumption disrupts memory and primes elevations in hippocampal IL-1β, an effect that can be prevented with dietary reversal or IL-1 receptor antagonism. *Brain, behavior, and immunity, 42,* 22–32. https://doi.org/10.1016/j.bbi.2014.06.017

Socci, V., Tempesta, D., Desideri, G., DeGennaro, L., & Ferrara, M., (2017). Enhancing human cognition with cocoa flavonoids. *Frontiers in Nutrition, 4,* 19. https://doi.org/10.3389/fnut2017.00019

Sodhi, K., Pratt, R., Wang, X., Lakhani, H. V., Pillai, S. S., Zehra, M., Wang, J., Grover, L., Henderson, B., Denvir, J., Liu, J., Pierre, S., Nelson, T., & Shapiro, J. I. (2021). Role of adipocyte Na,K-ATPase oxidant amplification loop in cognitive decline and neurodegeneration. *iScience, 24*(11), 103262. https://doi.org/10.1016/j.isci.2021.103262

Solfrizzi, V., Custodero, C., Lozupone, M., Imbimbo, B. P., Valiani, V., Agosti, P., Schilardi, A., D'Introno, A., La Montagna, M., Calvani, M., Guerra, V., Sardone, R., Abbrescia, D. I., Bellomo, A., Greco, A., Daniele, A., Seripa, D., Logroscino, G., Sabbá, C., & Panza, F. (2017). Relationships of dietary patterns, foods, and micro- and macronutrients with Alzheimer's disease and late-life cognitive disorders: A Systematic Review. *Journal of Alzheimer's Disease, 59*(3), 815-849. https://doi.org/10.3233/JAD-170248

Springmann, M., Spajic, L., Clark, M. A., Poore, J., Herforth, A., Webb, P., Rayner, M., & Scarborough, P. (2020). The healthiness and sustainability of national and global food based dietary guidelines: modeling study. *British Medical Journal, (Clinical research ed.), 370,* m2322. https://doi.org/10.1136/bmj.m2322

Squitti, R., Pal, A., Picozza, M., Avan, A., Ventriglia, M., Rongioletti, M. C., & Hoogenraad, T. (2020). Zinc therapy in early Alzheimer's disease: Safety and potential therapeutic efficacy. *Biomolecules, 10*(8), 1164. https://doi.org/10.3390/biom10081164

Steiner, J. L., Murphy, E. A., McClellan, J. L., Carmichael, M D., & Davis J. M. (2011). Exercise training increases mitochondria biogenesis in the brain. *Journal of Applied Physiology, 111*(4), 1066–1071. https://doi.org/10.1152/japplphysiol.00343.2011

Strandwitz, P., Kim, K. H., Terekhova, D., Liu, J. K., Sharma, A., Levering, J., McDonald, D., Dietrich, D., Ramadhar, T. R., Lekbua, A., Mroue, N., Liston, C., Stewart, E. J., Dubin, M. J., Zengler, K., Knight, R., Gilbert, J. A., Clardy, J., & Lewis, K. (2019). GABA-modulating bacteria of the human gut microbiota. *Nature Microbiolism, 4*(3), 396–403. https://doi.org/10.1038/s41564-018-0307-3

Stringham, N. T., Holmes, P. V., & Stringham, J. M. (2016). Lutein supplementation increases serum brain-derived neurotropic factor (BDNF) in humans. *The FASEB Journal, 30*(S1), 689.3-689.3. https://doi.org/10.1096/fasebj.30.1_supplement.689.3

Sun, N., Youle, R. J., & Finkel, T. (2016). The mitochondrial basis of aging. *Molecular Cell, 61*(5), 654-666. https://doi.org/10.1016/j.molcel.2016.01.028

Tadokoro, K., Ohta, Y., Inufusa, H., Loon, A. F. N., & Abe, K. (2020). Prevention of cognitive decline in Alzheimer's disease by novel antioxidative supplements. *International Journal of Molecular Sciences.* *21*(6), 1974. https://doi.org/10.3390/ijms21061974

Tan, S., Yu, C. Y., Sim, Z. W., Low, Z. S., Lee, B., See, F., Min, N., Gautam, A., Chu, J. J. H., Ng, K. W., & Wong, E. (2019). Pomegranate activates TFEB to promote autophagy-lysomal fitness and mitophagy. *Scientific Reports, 9*(1), 727. https://doi.org/10.1038s41598-018-37400-1

Teruya, T., Chen, Y-J., Kondoh, H., Fukuji, Y., & Yanagida, M. (2021). Whole-blood metabolomics of dementia patients reveal classes of disease-linked metabolites. *Proceedings of the National Academy of Sciences, 118*(37) e2022857118. https://doi.org/10.1073/pnas.2022857118

Thompson, S., Bailey, M., Taylor, A., Kaczmarek, J., Mysonhimer, A., Edwards, C., Reeser, G., Burd, N., Khan, N., & Holscher, H. (2021). Avocado consumption alters gastrointestinal bacteria abundance and microbial metabolite concentrations among adults with overweight or obesity: a randomized controlled trial. *The Journal of Nutrition, 151*(4), 753–762. https://doi.org/10.1093/jn/nxaa219

Timmers, P. R. H. J., Wilson, J. F., Joshi, P. K., & Deelen, J. (2020). Multivariate genomic scan implicates novel loci and haem metabolism in human aging. *Nature Communications, 11*(1), 3570. https://doi.org/10.1038/s41467-202-17312-3

Topiwala, A., Allan, C. L., Valkanova, V., Zsoldos, E., Filippini, N., Sexton, C. E., Mahmood, A., Fooks, P., Singh-Manoux, A., Mackay, C. E., Kivimaki, M., & Ebmeier, K. P. (2017). Moderate alcohol consumption as risk factor for adverse brain outcomes and cognitive decline: longitudinal cohort study. *British Medical Journal, 357*, j2353. https://doi.org/10.1136/bmj.j2353

Tranter, L. J. & Koutstaal, W. (2008). Age and flexible thinking: An experimental demonstration of the beneficial effects of increased cognitively stimulating activity on fluid intelligence in healthy older adults. *Aging, Neuropsychology, and Cognition, 15*(2), 184–207. https://doi.org/10.1080/13825580701322163

Tsao, C. W., Aday, A. W., Almarzooq, Z. I., Alonso, A., Beaton, A. Z., Bittencourt, M. S., Boehme, A. K., Buxton, A. E., Carson, A. P., Commodore-Mensah, Y., Elkind, M., Evenson, K. R., Eze-Nliam, C., Ferguson, J. F., Generoso, G., Ho, J. E., Kalani, R., Khan, S. S., Kissela, B. M., Knutson, K. L., ... Martin, S. S. (2022). Heart disease and stroke statistics-2022 update: A report from the American Heart Association. *Circulation, 145*(8), e153–e639. https://doi.org/10.1161/CIR.0000000000001052

Tsolaki, M., Lazarou, E., Kozori, M., Petridou, N., Tabakis, I., Lazarou, I., Karakota, M., Saoulidis, I., Melliou, E., & Magiatis, P. (2020). A randomized clinical trial of Greek high phenolic early harvest extra virgin olive oil in mild cognitive impairment: The MICOIL pilot study. *Journal of Alzheimer's Disease, 78*(2), 801–817. https://doi.org/10.3233/JAD-200405

Tucker, L. A. (2017). Caffeine consumption and telomere length in men and women of the National Health and Nutrition Examination Survey (NHANES). *Nutrition and Metabolism, 14*, Article 10. https://doi.org/10.1186/s12986-017-0162-x

Tverdal, A., Selmer, R., Cohen, J. M., & Thelle, D. S., (2020). Coffee consumption and mortality from cardiovascular diseases and total mortality. Does the brewing method matter? *European Journal of Preventive Cardiology, 27*(18), 1986–1993. https://doi.org/10.1177/2047487320914443

Valenzuela, M., & Sachdev, P. (2009). Can cognitive exercise prevent the onset of dementia? Systematic review of randomized clinical trials with longitudinal follow-up. *American Journal of Geriatric Psychiatry, 17*(3), 179–187. https://doi.org/10.1097/JGP.0b013e3181953b57

Valls-Pedret, C., Sala-Vila, A., Serra-Mir, M., Corella, D., de la Torre, R., Martinez-Gonzalez, M. A., Martinez-Lapiscina, E. H., Fito, M., Perez-Heras, A., Salas-Salvado, J., Estruch, R., & Ros, E. (2015). Mediterranean diet and age-related cognitive decline: A randomized clinical trial. *Journal of the American Medical Association, Internal Medicine, 175*(7), 1094–1103. https://doi.org/10.1001/jamainternmed.2015.1668

Velazquez, R., Ferreira1, E., Knowles, S., Fux, C., Rodin, A., Winslow, W., & Oddo, S. (2019). Lifelong choline supplementation ameliorates Alzheimer's disease pathology and associated cognitive deficits by attenuating microglia activation. *Aging Cell, 18*(6), e13037. https://doi.org/10.1111/acel.13037

Vercambre, M-N., Berr, C., Ritchie, K., & Kang, J. H. (2013). Caffeine and cognitive decline in elderly women at high vascular risk. *Journal of Alzheimer's Disease, 35*(2), 413-421. https://doi.org/10.3233/JAD-122371

Vijay, A., Kouraki, A., Gohir, S., Turnbull, J., Kelly, A., Chapman, V., Barrett, D. A., Bulsiewicz, W. J., & Valdes, A. M. (2021). The anti-inflammatory effect of bacterial short chain fatty acids is partially mediated by endocannabinoids. *Gut Microbes, 13*(1), 1997559. https://doi.org/10.1080/19490976.2021.1997559

Vinciguerra, F., Graziano, M., Hagnäs, M., Frittitta, L., & Tumminia, A. (2020). Influence of the Mediterranean and ketogenic diets on cognitive status and decline: A narrative review. *Nutrients, 12*(4), 1019. https://doi.org/10.3390/nu12041019

Vitiello, M. V., Moe, K. E., Merriam, G. R., Mazzoni, G., Buchner, D. H., & Schwartz, R. S. (2006). Growth hormone releasing hormone improves the cognition of healthy older adults. *Neurobiology of Aging, 27*(2), 318–323. https://doi.org/10.1016/j.neurobiolaging.2005.01.010

von Krause, M., Radev, S. T., & Voss, A. (2022). Mental speed is high until age 60 as revealed by analysis of over a million participants. *Nature human behaviour*, 10.1038/s41562-021-01282-7. Advance online publication. https://doi.org/10.1038/s41562-021-01282-7

Voulgaropoulou, S. D., van Amelsvoort, T. A. M. J., Prickaerts, J., & Vingerhoets, C. (2019). The effect of curcumin on cognition in Alzheimer's disease and healthy aging: A systematic review of pre-clinical and clinical studies. *Brain Research, 1725*, 146476. https://doi.org/10.1016/j.brainres.2019.146476

Wade, A. T., Davis, C. R., Dyer, K. A., Hodgson, J. M., Woodman, R. J., Hannah A. D., Keage, H. A. D., & Murphy, K. J. (2019). A Mediterranean diet with fresh, lean pork improves processing speed and mood: Cognitive findings from the MedPork Randomised Controlled Trial. *Nutrients, 11*(7), 1521. https://doi.org/10.3390/nu11071521

Waldstein, S. R., Rice, S. C., Thayer, J. F., Najjar, S. S., Scuteri, A., & Zonderman, A. B. (2008). Pulse pressure and pulse wave velocity are related to cognitive decline in the Baltimore Longitudinal Study of Aging. *Hypertension, 51*(1), 99–104. https://doi.org/10.1161/HYPERTENSIONAHA. 107.093674

Walker, J. M., Klakotskaia, D., Ajit, D., Weisman, G. A., Wood, W. G., Sun, G. Y., Serfozo, P., Simonyi, A., & Schachtman, T. R. (2015). Beneficial effects of dietary EGCG and voluntary exercise on behavior in an Alzheimer's disease mouse model. *Journal of Alzheimer's Disease, 44*(2), 561–572. https://doi.org/10.3233/JAD-140981

Wallenstein, G. (2003). *Mind, stress, & emotion: The new science of mood.* Commonwealth Press.

Wang, D. D., Li, Y., Chiuve, S. E., Stampfer, M. J., Masnson, J. E., Rimm, E. B., Willett, W. C., & Hu, F. B. (2016). Specific dietary fats in relation to total and cause-specific mortality. *Journal of the American Medical Association, Internal Medicine, 176*(8), 1134–1145. https://doi.org/10.1001/jamaintern med.2016.2417

Wang, J., Ho, L., Zhao, Z., Seror, I., Humala, N., Dickstein, D. L., Thiuyagarajan, M., Percival, S. S., Talcott, S. T., & Pasinetti, G. M. (2006). Moderate consumption of Cabernet Sauvignon attenuates Abeta neuropathology in a mouse model of Alzheimer's disease. *Federation of American Society for Experimental Biology. 20*(13), 2313-2320. https://doi.org/10.1096/fj.06-6281com

Wang, J., Um, P., Dickerman, B. A., & Liu, J. (2018). Zinc, magnesium, selenium and depression: A review of the evidence, potential mechanisms and implications. *Nutrients, 10*(5), 584. https://doi.org/10.3390/nu10050584

Wang, Z., Zhu, W., Xing, Y., Jia, J., & Tang, Y. (2021). B vitamins and prevention of cognitive decline and incident dementia: A systematic review and meta-analysis. *Nutrition Reviews, 80*(4), 931–949. https://doi.org/10.1093/nutrit/nuab057

Ward, M. B., Scheitler, A., Yu, M., Senft, L., Zillmann, A. S., Gorden, J. D., Schwartz, D. D., Ivanović-Burmazović, Y., & Goldsmith, C. R. (2018). Superoxide dismutase activity enabled by a redox-active ligand rather than metal. *Nature Chemistry, 10*(12), 1207-1212. https://doi.org/10.1038/s41557-018-0137-1

Wessels, I., Maywald, M., & Rink, L. (2017). Zinc as a gatekeeper of immune function. *Nutrients, 9*(12), 1286. https://doi.org/10.3390/nu9121286

Wilson, K. A., Chamoli, M., Hilsabeck, T. A., Pandey, M., Bansal, S., Chawla, G., & Kapahi, P. (2021). Evaluating the beneficial effects of dietary restrictions: A framework for precision nutrigeroscience. *Cell Metabolism, 33*(11), 2142-2173. https://doi.org/10.1016/j.cmet.2021.08.018

Wilson, R. S., Boyle, P. A., Yu, L., Barnes, L. I., Schneider, J. A., & Bennett, D. A. (2013). Life-span cognitive activity, neuropathologic burden, and cognitive aging. *Neurology, 81*(4), 314–321. https://doi.org/10.1212/WNL.0b013e3182 9c5e8a

Wirth, M., Benson, G., Schwarz, C., Köbe, T., Grittner, U., Schmitz, D., Sigrist, S. J., Bohlken, J., Stekovic, S., Madeo, F., & Flöel, A. (2018). The effect of spermidine on memory performance in older adults at risk for dementia: A randomized controlled trial. *Cortex, 109*, 181-188. https://doi.org/10.1016/j.cortex.2018.09.014

Witte, A. V., Fobker, M., Gellner, R., Knecht, S., & Flöel, A. (2009). Caloric restriction improves memory in elderly humans. *Proceedings of the National Academy of Sciences of the United States of America, 106*(4), 1255-1260. https://doi.org/10.1073/pnas.0808587106

Wood, A. M., Kaptoge, S., Butterworth, A. S., Willeit, P., Warnakula, S., Bolton, T., Paige, E., Paul, D. S., Sweeting, M., Burgess, S., Bell, S., Astle, W., Stevens, D., Koulman, A., Selmer, R. M., Verschuren, W. M. M., Sato, S., Njølstad, I., Woodward, M., ... Emerging Risk Factors Collaboration/EPIC-CVD/UK Biobank Alcohol Study Group. (2018). Risk thresholds for alcohol consumption: Combined analysis of individual-participant data for 599 912 current drinkers in 83 prospective studies. *The Lancet, 391*(10129), 1513–1523. https://doi.org/10.1016/S0140-6736(18)30134-X

Wu, P-Y, Chen, K. M. & Belcastro, F. (2020). Dietary patterns and depression risk in older adults: Systematic review and meta-analysis. *Nutrition Reviews, 79*(9), 976–987. https://doi.org/10.1093/nutrit/nuaa118

Wu, Y., Zhang, L., Li, S., & Zhang, D. (2022). Associations of dietary vitamin B1, vitamin B2, vitamin B6, and vitamin B12 with the risk of depression: A systematic review and meta-analysis. *Nutrition Reviews, 80*(3), 351–366. https://doi.org/10.1093/nutrit/nuab014

Xie, L., Kang, H., Xu, Q., Chen, M. J., Liao, Y., Thiyagarajan, M., O'Donnell, J., Christensen, D. J., Nicholson, C., Iliff, J. J., Takano, T., Deane, R., & Nedergaard, M. (2013). Sleep drives metabolite clearance from the adult brain. *Science, 342*(6156), 373–377. https://doi.org/10.1126/science.1241224

Yamagishi, K., Maruyama, K., Ikeda, A., Nagao, M., Noda, H., Umesawa, M., Hayama-Terada, M., Muraki, I., Okada, C., Tanaka, M., Kishida, R., Kihara, T., Ohira, T., Imano, H., Brunner, E. J., Sankai, T., Okada, T., Tanigawa, T., Kitamura, A., Kiyama, M., ... Iso, H. (2022). Dietary fiber intake and risk of incident disabling dementia: the Circulatory Risk in Communities Study. *Nutritional Neuroscience*, 1–8. Advance online publication. https://doi.org/10.1080/1028415X.2022.2027592

Ylilauri, M. P. T., Voutilainen, S., Lonnroos, E., Virtanen, H. E. K., Tuomainen, T.-P., Salonen, J. T., & Virtanen, J. K. (2019). Associations of dietary choline intake with risk of incident dementia and with cognitive performance: The Kuopio Ischaemic Heart Disease Risk Factor study. *The American Journal of Clinical Nutrition, 110*(6), *1416-1423*. https://doi.org/10.1093/ajcn/nqz148

Yu, J.-Z., Wang, J., Sheridan, S. D., Perlis, R. H., & Rasenick, M. M. (2020). N-3 polyunsaturated fatty acids promote astrocyte differentiation and neurotrophin production independent of cAMP in patient-derived neural stem cells. *Molecular Psychiatry, 26*(9), 4605–4615. https://doi.org/10.1038/s41380-020-0786-56-5

Yulug, B., Kilic, E., Altunay, S., Ersavas, C., Orhan, C., Dalay, A., Tuzcu, M., Sahin, N., Juturu, V., & Sahin, K. (2018). Cinnamon polyphenol extract exerts neuroprotective activity in traumatic brain injury in male mice. *CNS & Neurological Disorders - Drug Targets (Formerly Current Drug Targets - CNS & Neurological Disorders), 17*(6), 439-447. https://doi.org/10.2174/1871527317666180501110918

Zamroziewicz, M. K., Paul, E. J., Zwilling, C. E., Johnson, E. J., Kuchan, M. J., Cohen, N. J., & Barbey, A. K. (2016). Parahippocampal cortex mediates the relationship between lutein and crystallized intelligence in healthy, older adults. *Frontiers in Aging Neuroscience, 8,* 297. https://doi.org/10.3389/fnagi.2016.00297

Zamroziewicz, M. K., Taludar, M. T., Zwilling, C. E., & Barbey, A. K. (2017). Nutritional status, brain network organization, and general intelligence. *Neuroimage, 161,* 241-250. https://doi.org/10.1016/j.neuroimage.2017.08.043

Zapata, F. J., Rebollo-Hernanz, M., Novakofski, J. E., Nakamura, M. T., & de Mejia, E. G., (2019). Caffeine, but not other phytochemicals in mate tea (Ilex paraguariensis St. Hilaire) attenuates high-fat-high-sucrose-diet-driven lipogenesis and body fat accumulation. *Journal of Functional Foods, 64,* 103646. https://doi.org/10.1016/j.jff.2019.103646

Zhang, B., Wang, H. E., Bai, Y. M., Tsai, S. J., Su, T. P., Chen, T. J., Wang, Y. P., & Chen, M. H. (2021). Inflammatory bowel disease is associated with higher dementia risk: A nationwide longitudinal study. *Gut, 70*(1), 85-91. https://doi.org/10.1136/gutjnl-2020-320789

Zhang, L., Reyes, A., & Wang, X. (2018). The role of mitochondria-targeted antioxidant MitoQ in neurodegenerative disease. *Molecular and Cellular Therapies, 6*(1), 1887-1899. https://doi.org/10.26781/2052-8426-2018-01

Zhang, R., Shen, L., Miles, T., Shen, Y., Cordero, J., Qi, Y., Liang, L., & Li, C. (2020). Association of low to moderate alcohol drinking with cognitive functions from middle to older age among US adults. *Journal of the American Medical Association Network Open 3*(6), e207922. https://doi.org/10.1001/jamanetworkopen.2020.7922

Zhang, Y., Yang, H., Li, S., Li, W.-D., & Wang, Y. (2021). Consumption of coffee and tea and risk of developing stroke, dementia, and post stroke dementia: A cohort study in the UK Biobank. *PLoS Medicine, 18*(11), e1003830. https://doi.org/10.1371/journal.pmed.1003830

Zhao, J., Blayney, A., Liu, X., Gandy, L., Jin, W., Yan, L., Ha. J.-H., Canning, A. J., Connelly, M., Yang, C., Liu, X., Xiao, Y., Cosgrove, M. S., Solmaz, S. R., Zhang, Y., Ban, D., Chen, J., Loh, S. N., & Wang, C. (2021). EGCG binds intrinsically disordered N-terminal domain of p53 and disrupts p53-MDM2 interaction. *Nature Communications, 12,* Article 986. https://doi.org/10.1038/s41467-021-21258-5

Zhou, A., Taylor, A. E., Karhunan, V., Zhan, Y., Rovio, S. P., Lahti, J., Sjögren, P., Byberg, L., Lyall, D. M., Auvinen, J., Lehtimäki, T., Kähönen, M., Hurti-Kähönen, N., Perälä, M. M., Michaëlsson, K., Mahajan, A., Lind, L., Power, C., Eriksson, J. G., ... Hyppönen, E. (2018). Habitual coffee consumption and cognitive function: A Mendelian randomization meta-analysis in up to 415,530 participants. *Scientific Reports, 8*(1), 7526. https://doi.org/10.1038/s41598-018-25919-2

Zhu, L.-N., Mei, X., Zhang, Z.-G., Xie, Y.-P., & Lang, F. (2018). Curcumin intervention for cognitive function in different types of peoples: A systematic review and meta-analysis. *Phytotherapy Research, 33*(3), 524-533. https://doi.org/10.1002/ptr.6257

Ziegler, D. A., Piguet, O., Salat, D. H., Prince, K., Connally, E., & Corkin, S. (2010). Cognition in healthy aging is related to regional white matter integrity, but not cortical thickness. *Neurobiology of Aging, 31*(11), 1912–1926. https://doi.org/10.1016/j.neurobiolaging.2008.10.015

Zoladz, J. A., Pilc, A., Majerczak, J., Grandys, M., Zapart-Bukowska, J., & Duda, K. (2008). Endurance training increases plasma brain-derived neurotrophic factor concentration in young healthy men. *Journal of Physiology and Pharmacology, 59, Suppl 7*, 119–132.

Zwilling, C. E., Strang, A., Anderson, E., Jurcsisn, J., Johnson, E., Das, T., Kuchan, M. J., & Barbey, A. K. (2021). Enhanced physical and cognitive performance in active duty airmen: Evidence from a randomized multimodal physical fitness and nutritional intervention. *Scientific Reports, 11*(1), 3820. https://doi.org/10.1038/s41598-021-81800-9

# Index

Lightning Source UK Ltd.
Milton Keynes UK
UKHW010757051222
413416UK00016B/836